Choosing the Correct Radiologic Test

Susanna I. Lee • James H. Thrall

Choosing the Correct Radiologic Test

Case-Based Teaching Files

Springer

Susanna I. Lee
Department of Radiology
Massachusetts General Hospital
Harvard Medical School Boston
Massachusetts
USA

James H. Thrall
Department of Radiology
Massachusetts General Hospital
Harvard Medical School Boston
Massachusetts
USA

ISBN 978-3-662-51974-5 ISBN 978-3-642-15772-1 (eBook)
DOI 10.1007/978-3-642-15772-1
Springer Heidelberg New York Dordrecht London

Softcover reprint of the hardcover 1st edition 2013

Printed on acid-free paper

Springer is part of Springer Science+Business Media (www.springer.com)

Preface

Few areas in medicine have undergone the dramatic expansion of technical capabilities experienced in diagnostic imaging, or radiology, over the past 30 years. As precision cross-sectional imaging has rendered older technologies obsolete, diagnostic imaging has become one of the fastest expanding and rapidly changing component of healthcare, providing the clinician with powerful and precise tools to diagnose and treat illness. The ultimate beneficiary has been the patient, who enjoys earlier detection of and improved outcomes from disease.

Unfortunately, medical education and training has failed to keep pace with these advances. Residency training and continuing medical education requirements rarely include provisions to insure that physicians retain current knowledge on the risks and benefits of radiologic exams and evaluate their utility. Yet appropriate imaging utilization, when integrated into patient management algorithms, may reduce the need for expensive and more invasive alternative investigations, avoid many futile interventions, and provide sensitive monitors for chronic therapies of less than predictable efficacy.

This textbook is a guide to appropriate image ordering for the general medical practitioner. A hard copy and digital versions of the textbook are available. While all organ systems and patient demographics are discussed, the focus is on the commonly encountered scenarios. These are included in the both the hard copy and digital versions. The latter version also contains additional more specialized content (e.g., oncology, surgical subspecialties). Finally, the digital textbook presents the material in an interactive quiz-based format and provides a search engine by each chapter.

The teaching approach is case based. The practitioner is presented with a patient with a specific complaint or physical exam finding and asked to choose the imaging test most applicable to the situation. Once a choice has been made, the solution grades the usefulness of the imaging exam choices according to the American College of Radiology (ACR) Appropriateness Criteria on a nine-point scale as most, usually, sometimes, or rarely appropriate. On occasion, no ideal imaging exam, an option available with every scenario, may be the correct answer should none of the exam choices score as usually appropriate. Each case is accompanied by an image from the correct radiologic exam choice illustrating a possible diagnosis for the patient presented in the case.

Contents

*Indicates content only in digital version.

Introduction

1

1.1 ACR Appropriateness Criteria

The ACR Appropriateness Criteria represents consensus guidelines for the medical practitioner on how to use of imaging in the evaluation of common clinical problems. For each clinical scenario, possible radiology exam choices are ranked on a scale of 1–9 from least to most appropriate as defined in Table 1.1. They have been devised by a series of expert panels comprised of radiologists and treating physicians, with each panel devoted to a specific medical specialty. When available, recommendations for exam ordering are drawn from evidence in the peer-reviewed literature. However, in the absence of relevant science, recommendations are drawn from the expert opinion on the panel, should the majority agree that this represents general medical practice. The guidelines are freely available on the web and are kept current, with updates every 2–3 years.

While comprehensive, the Appropriateness Criteria is far from exhaustive. On many clinical issues where no literature or consensus is available (e.g., surveillance of cancer patients, chronic pain), the Appropriateness Criteria, as well as this textbook, is silent. Finally, for many scenarios, the underlying assumption is that the referring practitioner has evaluated the patient and determined that a radiologic test is indicated. Only rarely do the guidelines speak to the question, "Should imaging be undertaken at all?" Due to the dearth of literature on the topic, only a minority of cases address this query by defining specific clinical criteria (i.e., patient complaints or physical exam findings) that should be present before imaging is likely to prove useful.

1.2 Imaging Modalities

Radiologic exams are generally classified by the imaging modality. These include X-ray and fluoroscopy, ultrasound, computed tomography, magnetic resonance imaging, nuclear medicine scan, and interventional procedures. As diagnostic tests,

S.I. Lee, J.H. Thrall, *Choosing the Correct Radiologic Test*,
DOI 10.1007/978-3-642-15772-1_1, © Springer-Verlag Berlin Heidelberg 2013

Table 1.1 Exam appropriateness rankings

Appropriateness ranking[a]	Definition
1, 2, 3	Exam is rarely appropriate and is inappropriate for most scenarios
4, 5, 6	Exam is sometimes appropriate but would not be the preferred or first-line choice for most scenarios
7, 8, 9	Exam is usually appropriate. The exam with the highest ranking in this category is the most appropriate choice
No ideal imaging exam	Imaging is not indicated or there is no imaging exam considered usually appropriate NA Exam not appropriate and not ranked

[a]Higher number indicates greater appropriateness

each carries known advantages and disadvantages. The language of radiology, similar to that for all other medical specialties, is replete with acronyms. Those commonly used in this textbook have been defined in Table 1.2.

1.2.1 X-Ray and Fluoroscopy

X-ray plain film is the oldest and most widely available radiologic modality with evaluation of certain body parts (e.g., chest or abdomen) possible at the bedside. Images of reasonable diagnostic quality can be obtained even in patients who cannot cooperate with breath-holding instructions as acquisition times are on the order of seconds. Extremely high resolution allows for optimal evaluation of bone and lung. Exams deliver 0.001–1 mSv of ionizing radiation, well below the average annual radiation dose of 3 mSv from background radiation.

With fluoroscopy, the patient is evaluated in real time with X-ray. Thus, movement such as that of bowel, diaphragm, or joints can be assessed. Oral contrast, either barium (non-water soluble) or iodine based (water soluble), is ingested (e.g., X-ray swallow exam) or administered rectally (e.g., X-ray contrast enema) for visualization of the proximal and distal bowel, respectively. X-ray fluoroscopy confers higher radiation doses that plain film with effective doses of 6–8 mSv for abdominal exams. Because exams entail that the patient be able to follow swallowing, positioning, and breath-holding instructions, it cannot be applied to the critically ill or debilitated patient.

1.2.2 Ultrasound

Ultrasound (US) is a modality that is widely available with exams that can be performed at the bedside for critically ill patients. It also has the distinct advantage that no ionizing radiation is involved. No biologic effects have been documented from

Table 1.2 Abbreviation list

ACR	American College of Radiology
β-HCG	β-Human chorionic gonadotropin
CCR	Canadian C-spine Rules
CT	Computed tomography
CTA	Computed tomography angiogram
DMSA	Dimercaptosuccinic acid
DTPA	Diethylenetriaminepentaacetic acid
DXA	Dual energy X-ray absorptiometry
ERCP	Endoscopic retrograde cholangiopancreatogram
Ga	Gallium
HMPAO	Hexamethylpropylenamine oxide
HU	Hounsfield units
MAA	Macroaggregated albumin
MDP	Methylene diphosphonate
MIBG	Metaiodobenzylguanidine
MRA	Magnetic resonance angiogram
MRCP	Magnetic resonance cholangiopancreatogram
MRI	Magnetic resonance imaging
mSv	Milli-Sievert
NEXUS	National Emergency X-Radiography Utilization Study
PET	Positron emission tomography
QCT	Quantitative computed tomography
QUS	Quantitative ultrasound
SPECT	Single photon emission tomography
Tc	Technetium
US	Ultrasound
V/Q	Ventilation perfusion
Xe	Xenon

diagnostic US exams, even in the fetus, despite widespread use over several decades. With Doppler, the theoretical risks to a fetus from heat and cavitation are a consideration; hence, it is used judiciously, minimizing the exposure time and acoustic output. Intravenous contrast, while available for niche indications, is not administered in the routine diagnostic US exam.

US as an imaging tool is hampered by its inability to penetrate through many tissues (e.g., typically <10 cm in soft tissue, 0 cm through air or bone) limiting its ability to image deep visceral organs or large patients. As a diagnostic test, its performance is extremely operator dependent and therefore unpredictable. In this sense, US can be more correctly viewed as an extension of the physical exam, where the reliability of the results is subject to the experience and the expertise of the sonographer.

1.2.3 Computed Tomography

Computed tomography (CT) is widely available both in outpatient and inpatient settings. Exams are well tolerated, as imaging a given body part typically requires <30 s on most scanners. Thus, even in a patient who is unresponsive or unable to cooperate with breathing instructions, CT has a high likelihood of yielding diagnostic quality images. As the modality involves an X-ray beam capable of penetrating through most tissue types (metallic implants being the notable exception), field of view is not a limitation. Bone, soft tissue, fluid, fat, and air are all imaged with high resolution and reproducibility. Intravenous contrast that is iodine based is administered to evaluate vessels and to improve tissue contrast of the solid and ollow viscera, renal collecting systems, and neoplasms.

Ionizing radiation exposure is the most significant drawback of CT. While effective doses administered by a diagnostic CT exam (1–30 mSv in adult) have not been directly shown to pose a health risk, extrapolation from higher levels estimates, for instance, an added fatal cancer risk of approximately 1:1,000 in an adult undergoing an abdomen CT exam. This seems negligible in the context of the general lifetime risk of 1:5 for fatal cancer. However, this risk is thought to be additive with each exam and is predicted to be higher in the pediatric population and in the fetus.

Intravenous iodinated contrast is associated with a 3 % incidence of allergic reaction, the vast majority of which are mild (e.g., itching, hives) and self-limited. However, 0.004–0.04 % incidence of severe reactions (e.g., laryngeal edema, hypotension) requiring hospitalization has been reported. In patients with underlying renal insufficiency, transient acute renal failure also represents a potential complication of intravenous contrast administration. Common predisposing risk factors include age >70 years, diabetes, dehydration, congestive heart failure, and nephrotoxic medications.

1.2.4 Magnetic Resonance Imaging

Magnetic resonance imaging (MRI) affords the best soft tissue contrast of any of the radiologic modalities and involves no ionizing radiation. Brain and spinal cord, bone marrow, joints, muscles, and abdominopelvic solid organs (e.g., liver, kidneys, uterus, prostate) are all optimally depicted with MRI. The electromagnetic field, which is the basis for scanning, allows for multiplanar imaging with an essentially unrestricted field of view. Intravenous contrast that is gadolinium based is administered to better evaluate the vessels, solid viscera, and neoplasms. However, even in a patient who cannot receive intravenous contrast, specific flow-sensitive pulse sequences can be used to evaluate blood vessels.

Disadvantages of MRI include limited access to the scanner itself or the radiologist expertise to implement and interpret the exams in some practice settings. Most exams entail that the patient lie still in an enclosed scanner for up to 20–40 min, although wider bore or "open" scanners, if available, can be used for some indications. For pediatric patients, sedation is usually necessary. In the critically ill patient, monitoring and supportive-care equipment that are compatible with high-field-strength magnets are required. Even in the conscious patient, concerns such as claustrophobia or inability to cooperate with the scanning procedure can hinder successful image acquisition.

Intravenous gadolinium contrast is associated with a much lower incidence (0.07 %) of allergic reactions than iodinated contrast (3 %). Incidence of severe reactions requiring hospitalization is reported as <0.005 %. However, gadolinium contrast administration in patients with renal failure has been associated with nephrogenic systemic fibrosis, a syndrome resulting in progressive fibrosis of the skin, joints, eyes, and organs, which is uniformly fatal. While the magnitude and the pathophysiology of this risk are poorly understood, gadolinium is considered relatively contraindicated in patients with renal dysfunction.

1.2.5 Nuclear Medicine Scan

Nuclear medicine employs the physiologic and biochemical processes in the body to image specific organs and their function. Radiopharmaceuticals are administered most often intravenously, but for some exams by other means such as inhalation (^{133}Xe into lung) or by catheter (^{99}Tc-pertechnetate into bladder). Their uptake and/or excretion by various tissues are then imaged by computer-aided detectors that can acquire and present the information in planar (e.g., anteroposterior, lateral) or tomographic (e.g., SPECT, PET) formats.

Because a physiologically active radiotracer is used, many nuclear medicine exams have the distinct advantage of being able to provide functional as well as anatomic information. Examples include cardiac myocardial perfusion (^{99}Tc-sestamibi), bone turnover (^{99}Tc-MDP), lung ventilation (^{133}Xe) and perfusion (^{99}Tc-MAA), and glucose metabolism (^{18}FDG). These are each tailored to answer a defined diagnostic question. Effective radiation doses range from 1 to 20 mSv and, hence, are comparable to a CT exam. Because the imaging source is emitted from rather than external to the body, whole body evaluation is possible without added radiation.

The major disadvantage of a nuclear medicine scan is poor image resolution, which for some exams has been mitigated by fusing them with concurrently acquired anatomic images (e.g., PET-CT). Availability of many exam types is often limited because a radiopharmacy and, for specific isotopes, a cyclotron, with the attendant radiopharmacist expertise, must be nearby to deliver isotopes with half-lives on the order of several minutes to days. Finally, image acquisition requires upwards of 30 min and up to several hours rendering many of them unsuitable for the uncooperative or a critically ill patient.

1.2.6 Interventional Procedures

Interventional procedures in diagnostic radiology typically use imaging guidance to introduce a catheter or a needle into a particular anatomic space, such as a blood vessel (angiogram), a joint space (arthrogram), the spinal cord (myelogram), or a hollow viscera (e.g., cystogram, hysterosonogram). Contrast material is then introduced thereby allowing for detailed visualization of the opacified lumen. Biopsies comprise the other general category of diagnostic radiologic interventions. Here an aspiration and/or cutting needle is introduced into the lesion or organ of interest under imaging guidance to obtain tissue samples for histologic evaluation.

Most image-guided interventions are performed as same-day outpatient procedures and involve no intravenous anesthesia. Angiograms and deep tissue biopsies, however, usually require conscious sedation for which the patient will need to fast before and be monitored afterwards. Major complications requiring hospitalization are exceedingly rare. Minor complications include bleeding (usually self-limited), localized infection, and allergic reaction to administered contrast.

2 Breast Imaging

2.1 Palpable Breast Mass

A 54-year-old woman with a palpable breast mass.

a. Mammogram diagnostic
b. MRI breast with contrast
c. PET breast
d. Core biopsy breast
e. No ideal imaging exam

S.I. Lee, J.H. Thrall, *Choosing the Correct Radiologic Test*,
DOI 10.1007/978-3-642-15772-1_2, © Springer-Verlag Berlin Heidelberg 2013

A woman 30 years of age or older, initial evaluation.

a. *Mammogram diagnostic* is the most appropriate. Mammogram should be done first for patients in this age group as it may demonstrate additional findings of concern. Ultrasound should be used right after the mammogram to ensure that the palpable finding corresponds to the mammogram finding (9).
b. MRI breast with contrast is usually not appropriate (1).
c. PET breast is usually not appropriate (1).
d. Core biopsy breast is usually not appropriate (1).

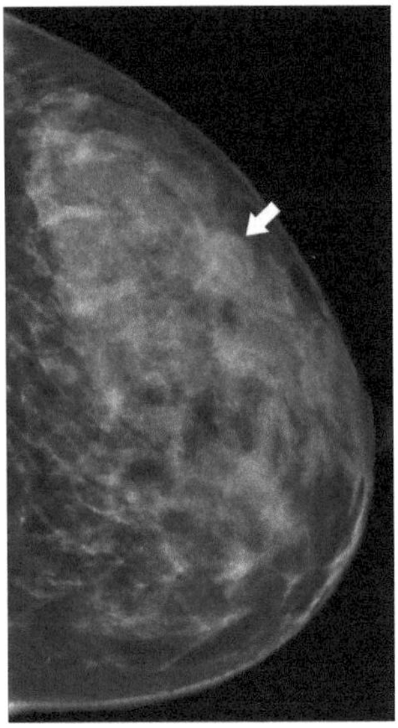

Fig. 2.1 Fibroadenoma. Mammogram lateral view shows a round soft tissue density (*arrow*) corresponding to the palpable mass

An 80-year-old woman with a palpable breast mass. Mammogram shows a finding suspicious for malignancy.

a. US breast
b. MRI breast with contrast
c. PET breast
d. Fine needle aspiration breast
e. No ideal imaging exam

A woman 30 years of age or older, mammogram findings suspicious for malignancy.

a. *US breast* is the most appropriate. Mammogram should be done first for patients in this age group as may demonstrate additional findings of concern. Ultrasound should be used right after the mammogram to ensure that the palpable finding corresponds to the mammogram finding (9).
b. MRI breast with contrast is usually not appropriate (3).
c. PET breast is usually not appropriate (1).
d. Fine needle aspiration breast is usually not appropriate (2).

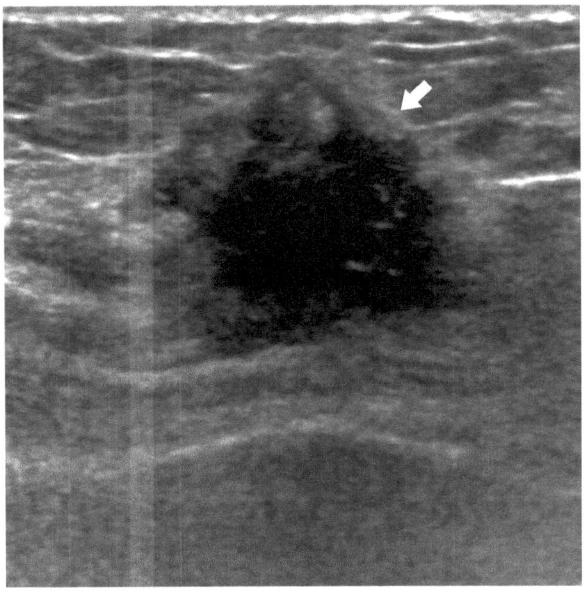

Fig. 2.2 Breast cancer. Breast ultrasound shows a 1-cm irregular hypoechoic solid lesion (*arrow*) corresponding to the palpable mass

A 45-year-old woman with a palpable breast mass. Mammogram shows a probably benign finding.

a. Mammogram short-interval follow-up
b. US breast
c. MRI breast with contrast
d. Core biopsy breast
e. No ideal imaging exam

A woman 30 years of age or older, mammogram findings probably benign.

a. Mammogram short-interval follow-up is usually appropriate, but there is a better choice here. Short-interval follow-up may be appropriate after workup with ultrasound (7).
b. *US breast* is the most appropriate. Ultrasound is important to ensure that the palpable finding corresponds to the mammogram finding (9).
c. MRI breast with contrast is usually not appropriate (2).
d. Core biopsy breast may sometimes be appropriate. The decision to biopsy depends on the suspicion for malignancy based on clinical findings and ultrasound (5).

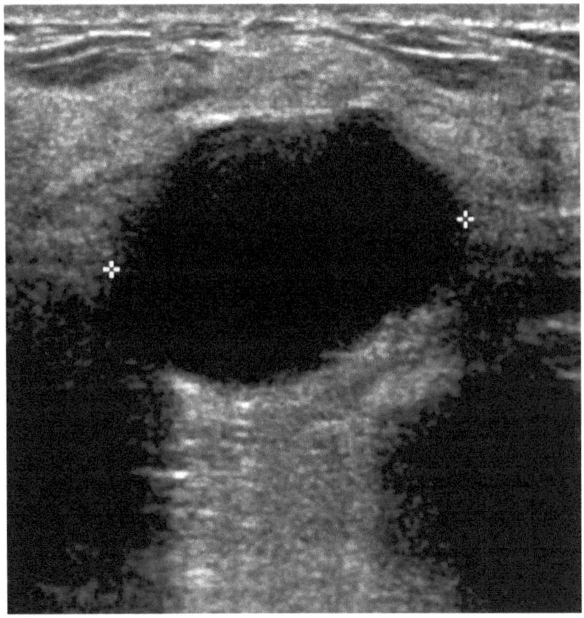

Fig. 2.3 Breast cyst. Breast ultrasound shows a 3-cm anechoic cyst (*calipers*) corresponding to the palpable mass

A 50-year-old woman with a palpable breast mass. Mammogram shows a benign finding.

a. Mammogram short-interval follow-up
b. US breast
c. MRI breast with contrast
d. PET breast
e. No ideal imaging exam

A woman 30 years of age or older, mammogram finding benign.

a. Mammogram short-interval follow-up is usually not appropriate (2).
b. *US breast* is the most appropriate (7).
c. MRI breast with contrast is usually not appropriate (1).
d. PET breast is usually not appropriate (1).

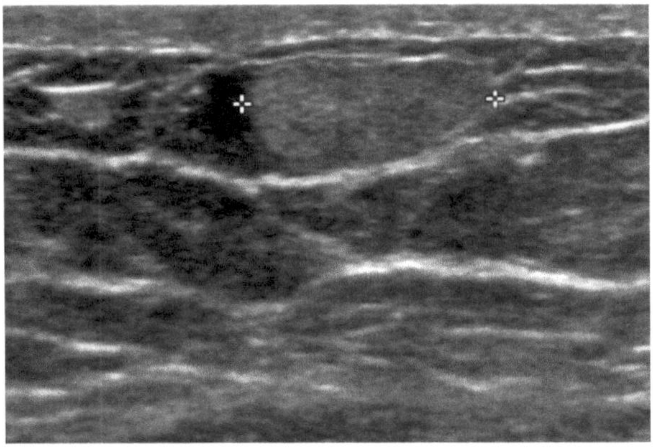

Fig. 2.4 Breast lipoma. Breast ultrasound shows a 1.2-cm echogenic well-circumscribed solid lesion (*calipers*) corresponding to the palpable mass

A 57-year-old woman with a palpable breast mass. Mammogram is negative.

a. Mammogram short-interval follow-up
b. US breast
c. MRI breast with contrast
d. Core biopsy breast
e. No ideal imaging exam

A woman 30 years of age or older, mammogram finding negative.

a. Mammogram short-interval follow-up is usually not appropriate (1).
b. *US breast* is the most appropriate (9).
c. MRI breast with contrast is usually not appropriate (2).
d. Core biopsy breast is usually not appropriate (1).

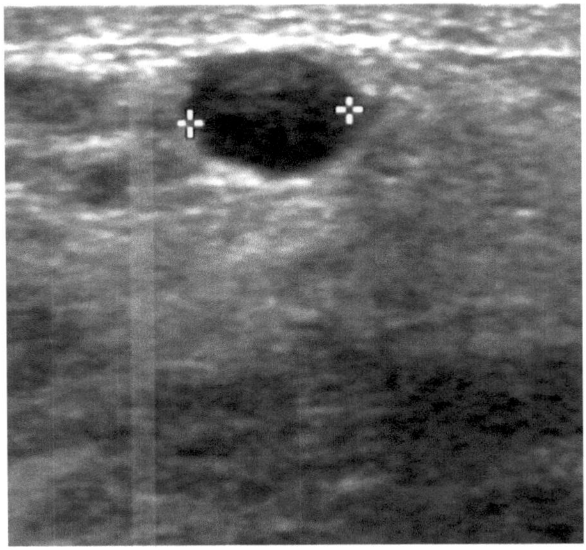

Fig. 2.5 Breast cyst. Breast ultrasound shows a 5-mm anechoic cyst (*calipers*) corresponding to the palpable mass

A 29-year-old woman with a palpable breast mass.

a. US breast
b. Mammogram diagnostic
c. MRI breast with contrast
d. Core biopsy breast
e. No ideal imaging exam

A woman younger than 30 years of age, initial evaluation.

a. *US breast* is the most appropriate (9).
b. Mammogram diagnostic is usually not appropriate. In high-risk patients younger than age 30, mammogram may be used first (3).
c. MRI breast with contrast is usually not appropriate (2).
d. Core biopsy breast is usually not appropriate (1).

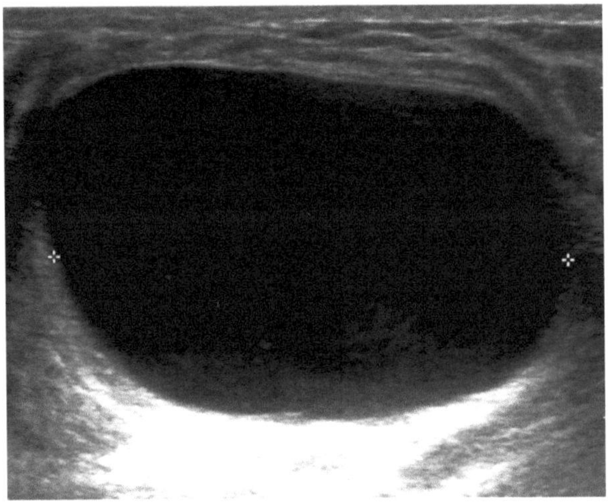

Fig. 2.6 Breast cyst. Breast ultrasound shows a 5-cm anechoic cyst corresponding to the palpable mass

A 27-year-old woman with a palpable breast mass. US shows a finding suspicious for malignancy.

a. Mammogram diagnostic
b. US breast short-interval follow-up
c. MRI breast with contrast
d. PET breast
e. No ideal imaging exam

A woman younger than 30 years of age, US findings suspicious for malignancy.

a. *Mammogram diagnostic* is the most appropriate. Bilateral diagnostic mammogram should be performed immediately after the ultrasound to help characterize the mass and to evaluate for additional lesions that may be occult by ultrasound (9).
b. US breast short-interval follow-up is usually not appropriate (1).
c. MRI breast with contrast is usually not appropriate (2).
d. PET breast is usually not appropriate (1).

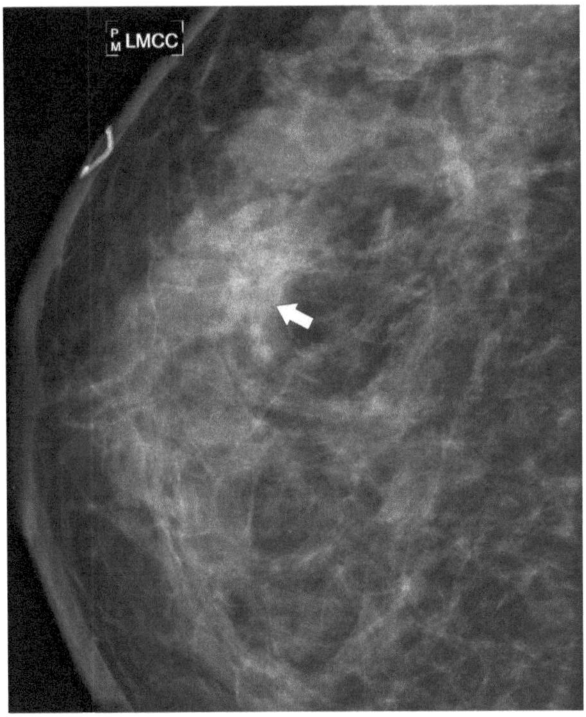

Fig. 2.7 Breast cancer. Mammogram magnified craniocaudal view shows irregular soft tissue density (*arrows*) underlying the skin marker indicating the palpable mass

A 22-year-old woman with a palpable breast mass. US shows a probably benign finding.

a. Mammogram diagnostic
b. US breast short-interval follow-up
c. MRI breast with contrast
d. Core biopsy breast
e. No ideal imaging exam

Woman younger than 30 years of age, US findings probably benign.

a. Mammogram diagnostic may sometimes be appropriate (5).
b. *US breast short-interval follow-up* is the most appropriate (8).
c. MRI breast with contrast is usually not appropriate (2).
d. Core biopsy breast is usually not appropriate. Biopsy may be performed to alleviate patient anxiety (3).

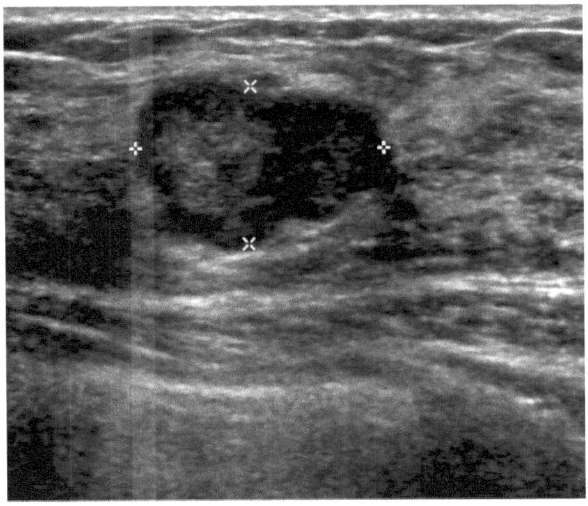

Fig. 2.8 Fibroadenoma. Breast ultrasound shows a solid well-circumscribed hypoechoic lesion corresponding to the palpable mass

A 27-year-old woman with a palpable breast mass. US shows a benign finding.

a. Mammogram diagnostic
b. US breast short-interval follow-up
c. MRI breast with contrast
d. Fine needle aspiration breast
e. No ideal imaging exam

A woman younger than 30 years of age, US findings benign (e.g., simple cyst).

a. Mammogram diagnostic is usually not appropriate (1).
b. US breast short-interval follow-up is usually not appropriate (1).
c. MRI breast with contrast is usually not appropriate (1).
d. Core biopsy breast is usually not appropriate (2).
e. *No ideal imaging exam* is the correct answer.

A 30-year-old woman with a palpable breast mass. US is negative.

a. Mammogram diagnostic
b. US breast short-interval follow-up
c. MRI breast with contrast
d. PET breast
e. No ideal imaging exam

A woman younger than 30 years of age, US findings negative.

a. Mammogram diagnostic may sometimes be appropriate. If clinically suspicious for malignancy, mammogram may be appropriate (5).
b. US breast short-interval follow-up is usually not appropriate (1).
c. MRI breast with contrast is usually not appropriate (1).
d. PET breast is usually not appropriate (1).
e. *No ideal imaging exam* is the correct answer.

2.2 Stage I Breast Carcinoma

A 62-year-old woman newly diagnosed with stage I breast carcinoma. On clinical evaluation for metastatic disease, she is asymptomatic.

a. CT chest
b. CT abdomen
c. Tc-99m bone scan whole body
d. FDG-PET whole body
e. No ideal imaging exam

Rule out metastases – asymptomatic woman.

a. CT chest is usually not appropriate (2).
b. CT abdomen is usually not appropriate (2).
c. Tc-99m bone scan whole body is usually not appropriate (2).
d. FDG-PET whole body is usually not appropriate (2).
e. *No ideal imaging exam* is the correct answer.

Cardiac Imaging

3

3.1 Acute Chest Pain: Low Probability of Coronary Artery Disease

A 25-year-old man with acute chest pain with low probability of coronary artery disease.

a. X-ray chest
b. CTA coronary arteries
c. CTA chest (noncoronary)
d. Myocardial perfusion scan
e. No ideal imaging exam

S.I. Lee, J.H. Thrall, *Choosing the Correct Radiologic Test*,
DOI 10.1007/978-3-642-15772-1_3, © Springer-Verlag Berlin Heidelberg 2013

Low probability of coronary artery disease.

a. *X-ray chest* is the most appropriate. It is useful in ruling out other causes of chest pain such as aortic dissection, pulmonary embolism, pneumothorax, or pneumonia (9).
b. CTA coronary arteries is usually appropriate, but there is a better choice here. Use if a cardiac etiology is suspected (7).
c. CTA chest (noncoronary) may sometimes be appropriate (6).
d. Myocardial perfusion scan is usually appropriate, but there is a better choice here (8).

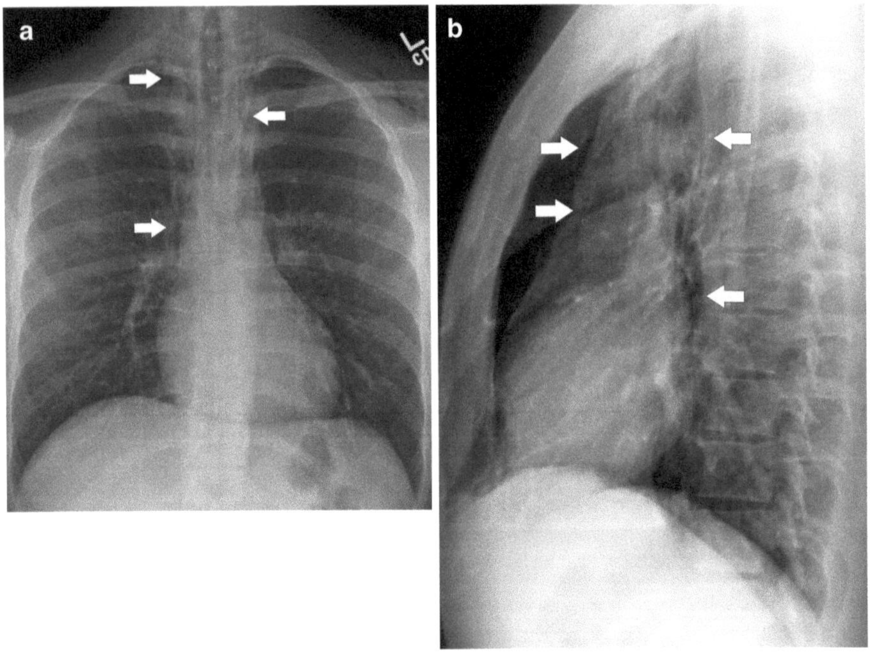

Fig. 3.1 Pneumomediastinum. Chest X-ray posteroanterior (**a**) and lateral (**b**) views demonstrate linear lucencies (*arrows*) corresponding to mediastinal air

3.2 Acute Chest Pain: Suspected Aortic Dissection

A 54-year-old man with acute chest pain. Aortic dissection is suspected.

a. CTA chest and abdomen
b. MRA chest and abdomen
c. US echocardiography transesophageal
d. Angiogram thoracic aorta
e. No ideal imaging exam

Suspected aortic dissection.

a. *CTA chest and abdomen* is the most appropriate. It is recommended as the definitive test in most patients with suspicion of aortic dissection (9).
b. MRA chest and abdomen is usually appropriate, but there is a better choice here. It serves as an alternative to CTA for patients with contraindication to iodinated contrast or multiple prior chest CTA for similar symptoms. Scanner availability and local expertise may limit use as there is potential for delay in diagnosis (8).
c. US echocardiography transesophageal is usually appropriate, but there is a better choice here. It is useful if a skilled operator is readily available (8).
d. Angiogram thoracic aorta may sometimes be appropriate (5).

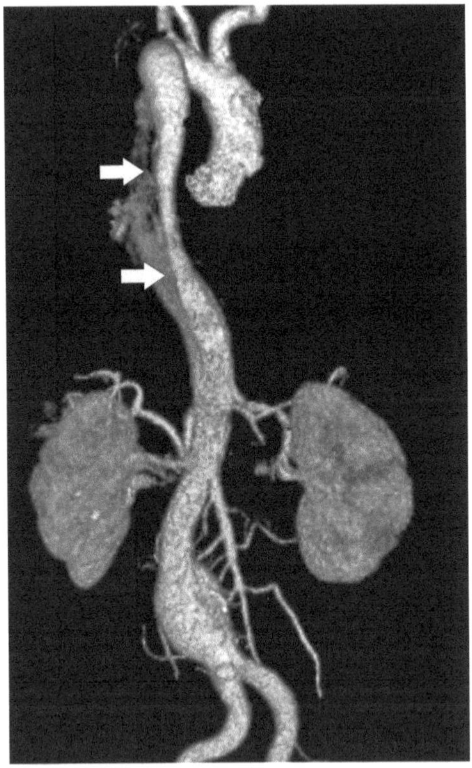

Fig. 3.2 Aortic dissection. Chest and abdomen CTA 3-D reconstruction image shows a dissection flap (*arrows*) separating the two lumens

3.3 Acute Chest Pain: Suspected Pulmonary Embolism

A 57-year-old man with acute chest pain. Pulmonary embolism is suspected.

a. US lower extremity with Doppler
b. CTA chest (noncoronary)
c. Tc-99m ventilation perfusion scan lung
d. Angiogram pulmonary arteries with right heart catheterization
e. No ideal imaging exam

Suspected pulmonary embolism.

a. US lower extremity with Doppler is usually appropriate, but there is a better choice here. Use if chest X-ray is negative and index of suspicion is high (7).
b. *CTA chest* (*noncoronary*) is the most appropriate. It is the current standard of care for detection of pulmonary embolus (9).
c. Tc-99m ventilation perfusion scan lung may sometimes be appropriate. Use if chest X-ray is negative and CTA is contraindicated or nondiagnostic (6).
d. Angiogram pulmonary arteries with right heart catheterization may sometimes be appropriate. Use if suspicion is high and CTA is inconclusive (5).

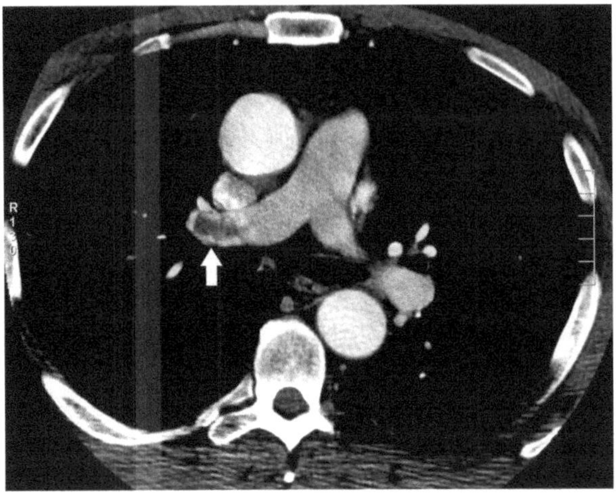

Fig. 3.3 Pulmonary embolus. Chest CTA shows a thrombus (*arrow*) in the right main pulmonary artery

3.4 Chronic Chest Pain: High Probability of Coronary Artery Disease

A 70-year-old man with chronic chest pain and high probability of coronary artery disease.

a. US echocardiography transthoracic
b. CTA coronary arteries
c. Myocardial perfusion scan
d. Angiogram coronary arteries
e. No ideal imaging exam

High probability of coronary artery disease.

a. US echocardiography transthoracic is usually appropriate, but there is a better choice here (7).
b. CTA coronary arteries is usually appropriate, but there is a better choice here. It can be used to demonstrate left ventricular regional dysfunction due to ischemia and is excellent for regional wall motion abnormalities (7).
c. *Myocardial perfusion scan* is the most appropriate (9).
d. Arteriogram coronary arteries is usually appropriate, but there is a better choice here. It is the definitive test for establishing the diagnosis and directing treatment if clinical suspicion of coronary artery disease is high, or if there is an abnormal noninvasive imaging test (7).

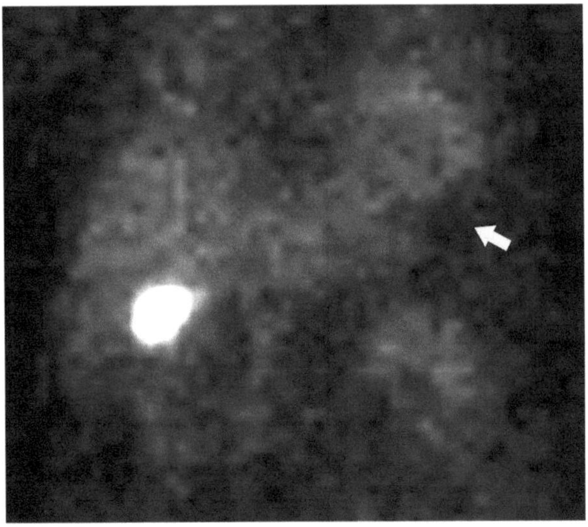

Fig. 3.4 Cardiac ischemia. Myocardial perfusion scan planar frontal image shows a decrease in tracer uptake (*arrow*) in the left ventricular inferolateral wall. Note high levels of tracer excretion into the gallbladder

3.5 Chronic Chest Pain: Low to Intermediate Probability of Coronary Artery Disease

A 74-year-old woman presents with chronic chest pain with low to intermediate probability of coronary artery disease.

a. X-ray chest
b. CTA chest (noncoronary)
c. CTA coronary arteries
d. Myocardial perfusion scan
e. No ideal imaging exam

Low to intermediate probability of coronary artery disease.

a. *X-ray chest* is the most appropriate (9).
b. CTA chest (noncoronary) is usually appropriate, but there is a better choice here. It is an important exam for diagnosing pulmonary embolism and thoracic aortic aneurysm or dissection. It is used to rule out pulmonary embolus and to evaluate for lung pathology. It is also appropriate for chronic anginal chest pain (8).
c. CTA coronary arteries is usually appropriate, but there is a better choice here. It can be used to assess for coronary atherosclerosis, anomalous coronary artery, and pericardial disease. High negative predictive value will exclude coronary artery disease and allow triage to focus on other diagnoses (8).
d. Myocardial perfusion scan is usually appropriate, but there is a better choice here. It eliminates unnecessary catheterizations (8).

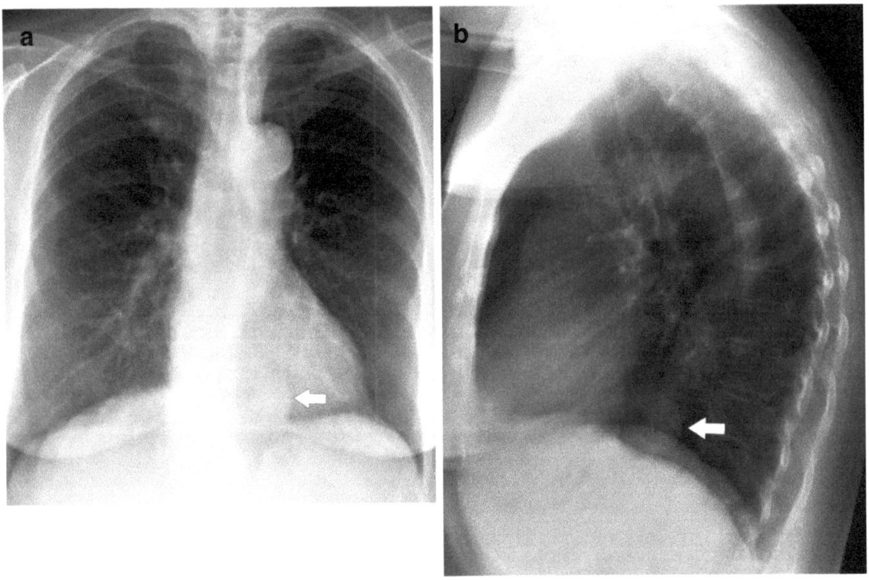

Fig. 3.5 Hiatal hernia. Chest X-ray posteroanterior (**a**) and lateral (**b**) views show a soft tissue density (*arrows*) superior to the esophageal hiatus

3.6 Congestive Heart Failure

A 47-year-old man with suspected new-onset congestive heart failure.

a. X-ray chest
b. US echocardiography transthoracic
c. CT chest
d. MRI chest
e. No ideal imaging exam

New congestive heart failure, suspected based on symptoms and physical examination.

a. *X-ray chest* is the most appropriate (9).
b. US echocardiography transthoracic is not rated in appropriateness.
c. CT chest is usually not appropriate. Congestive heart failure is readily diagnosed on CT obtained for other indications (2).
d. MRI chest is usually not appropriate (2).

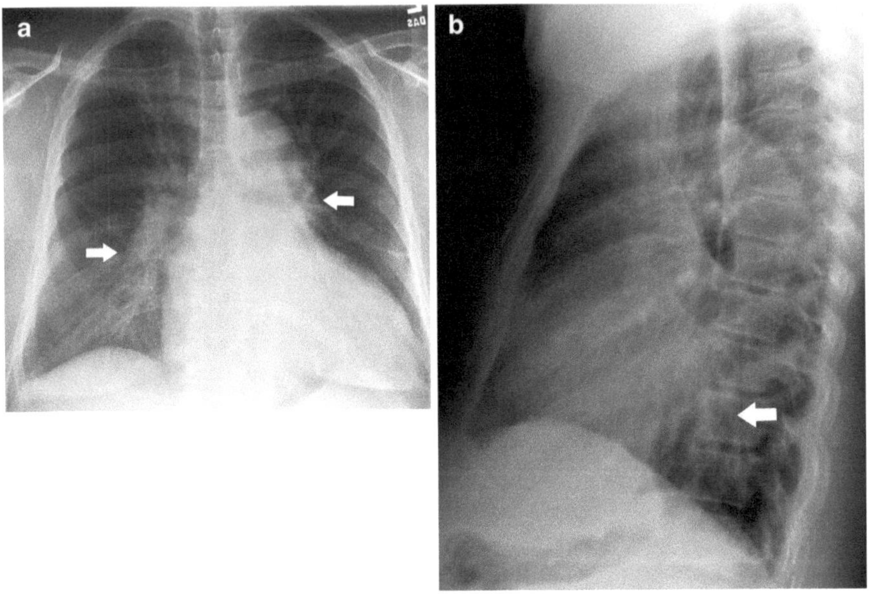

Fig. 3.6 Congestive heart failure. Chest X-ray posteroanterior (**a**) and lateral (**b**) views show bilaterally enlarged pulmonary vessels (*arrows*) and cardiac enlargement

A 78-year-old woman with history of congestive heart failure. She is currently stable.

a. X-ray chest
b. US echocardiography transthoracic
c. CT chest
d. MRI chest
e. No ideal imaging exam

Previous congestive heart failure, currently stable.

a. X-ray chest may sometimes be appropriate (4).
b. US echocardiography transthoracic is not rated in appropriateness.
c. CT chest is usually not appropriate. Congestive heart failure is readily diagnosed on CT obtained for other indications (2).
d. MRI chest is usually not appropriate (2).
e. *No ideal imaging exam* is the correct answer.

A 63-year-old man with history of congestive heart failure. He now presents with new-onset signs and symptoms of failure.

a. X-ray chest
b. US echocardiography transthoracic
c. CT chest
d. MRI chest
e. No ideal imaging exam

Previous congestive heart failure, new-onset signs and symptoms.

a. *X-ray chest* is the most appropriate (9).
b. US echocardiography transthoracic is not rated in appropriateness.
c. CT chest is usually not appropriate. Congestive heart failure is readily diagnosed on CT obtained for other indications (2).
d. MRI chest is usually not appropriate (2).

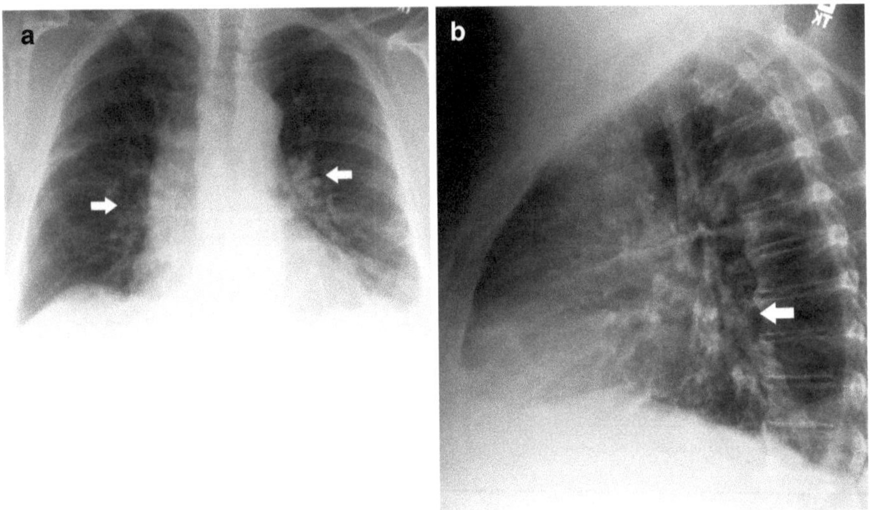

Fig. 3.7 Congestive heart failure. Chest X-ray posteroanterior (**a**) and lateral (**b**) views show bilaterally engorged pulmonary vessels (*arrows*) and cardiac enlargement

3.7 Shortness of Breath: Suspected Cardiac Origin

A 41-year-old woman with shortness of breath suspected to be of cardiac origin.

a. X-ray chest
b. US echocardiography transthoracic
c. Myocardial perfusion scan
d. Angiogram coronary arteries
e. No ideal imaging exam

Shortness of breath: suspected cardiac origin.

a. *X-ray chest* is the most appropriate (9).
b. US echocardiography transthoracic is usually appropriate, but there is a better choice here (8).
c. Myocardial perfusion scan is usually appropriate, but there is a better choice here (7).
d. Angiogram coronary arteries may sometimes be appropriate (6).

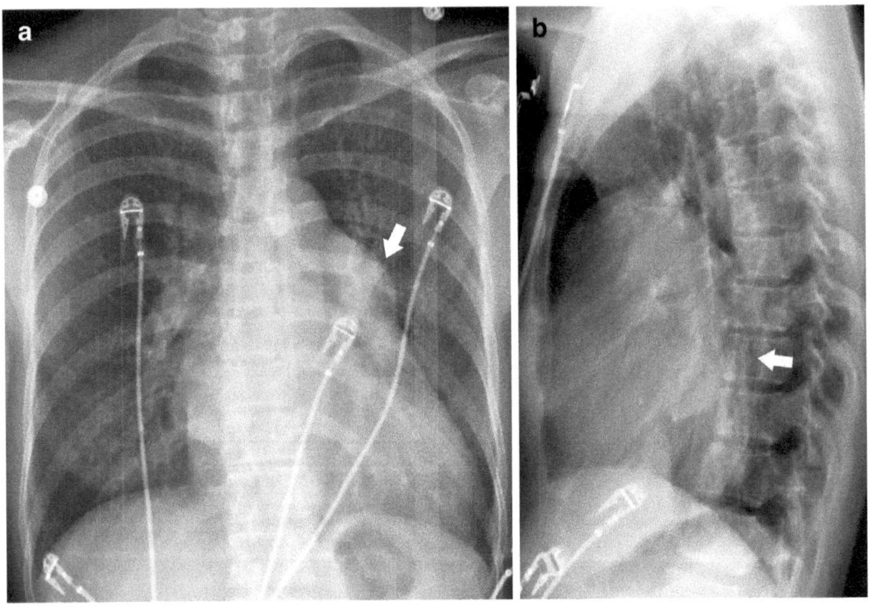

Fig. 3.8 Mitral stenosis. Chest X-ray posteroanterior (**a**) and lateral (**b**) views show an enlarged left atrium (*arrows*)

Gastrointestinal Imaging

4

4.1 Blunt Abdominal Trauma

A 21-year-old man with blunt abdominal trauma. He is hemodynamically unstable.

a. US chest, abdomen, and pelvis for fluid
b. US abdomen and pelvis for organs
c. CT chest, abdomen, and pelvis with contrast
d. Arteriography with possible embolization abdomen and pelvis
e. No ideal imaging exam

S.I. Lee, J.H. Thrall, *Choosing the Correct Radiologic Test*,
DOI 10.1007/978-3-642-15772-1_4, © Springer-Verlag Berlin Heidelberg 2013

Unstable patient.

a. *US chest, abdomen, and pelvis for fluid* is the most appropriate (8).
b. US abdomen and pelvis for organs is usually not appropriate (3).
c. CT chest, abdomen, and pelvis with contrast may sometimes be appropriate (4).
d. Arteriography with possible embolization abdomen and pelvis may sometimes be appropriate (5).

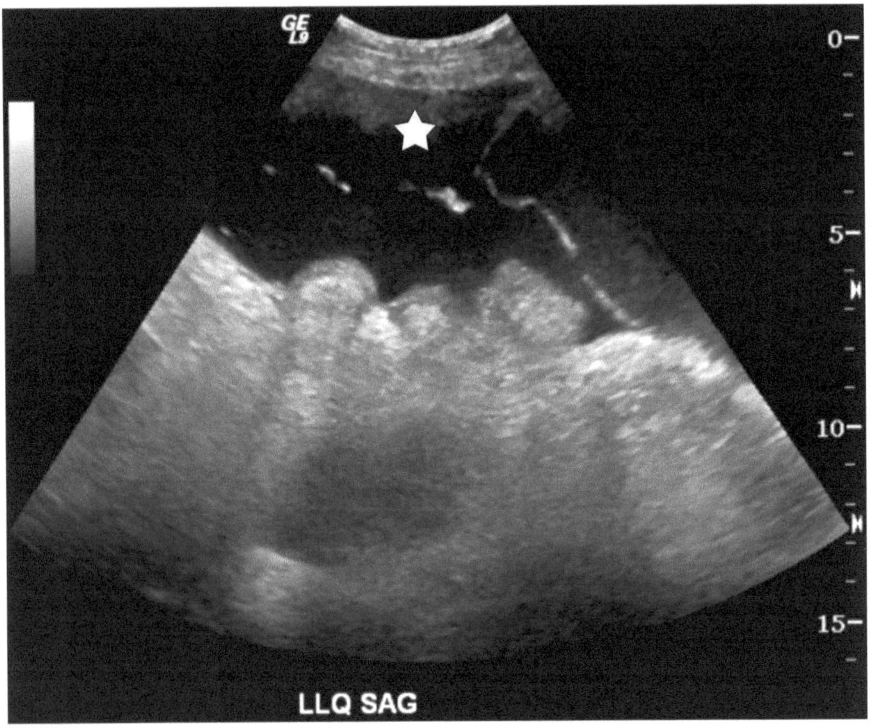

Fig. 4.1 Free abdominal fluid. Abdomen US shows complex free fluid (*star*), likely blood

A 22-year-old man with blunt abdominal trauma. He is hemodynamically stable.

a. X-ray chest
b. US chest, abdomen, and pelvis for fluid
c. CT abdomen and pelvis with contrast
d. Arteriography with possible embolization abdomen and pelvis
e. No ideal imaging exam

Stable patient.

a. X-ray chest is usually appropriate, but there is a better choice here (8).
b. US chest, abdomen, and pelvis for fluid may sometimes be appropriate (5).
c. *CT abdomen and pelvis with contrast* is the most appropriate (9).
d. Arteriography with possible embolization abdomen and pelvis may sometimes be appropriate (5).

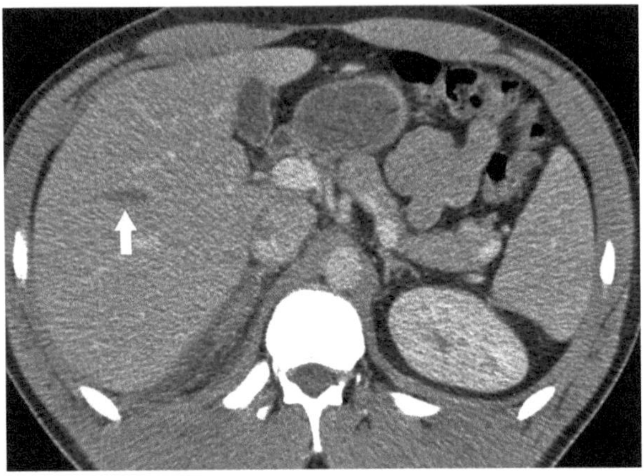

Fig. 4.2 Liver laceration. Abdomen CT with contrast shows a liver laceration (*arrow*) and soft tissue posterior to the liver consistent with a hematoma

A 23-year-old man with blunt abdominal trauma. He has gross hematuria.

a. X-ray chest
b. X-ray cystography
c. CT abdomen and pelvis with contrast
d. CT pelvis with bladder contrast (CT cystography)
e. No ideal imaging exam

Hematuria.

a. X-ray chest is usually appropriate, but there is a better choice here (8).
b. X-ray cystography may sometimes be appropriate. CT cystography is preferred (4).
c. *CT abdomen and pelvis with contrast* is the most appropriate (9).
d. CT pelvis with bladder contrast (CT cystography) may sometimes be appropriate. Indicated in all patients with gross hematuria and pelvic fracture (6).

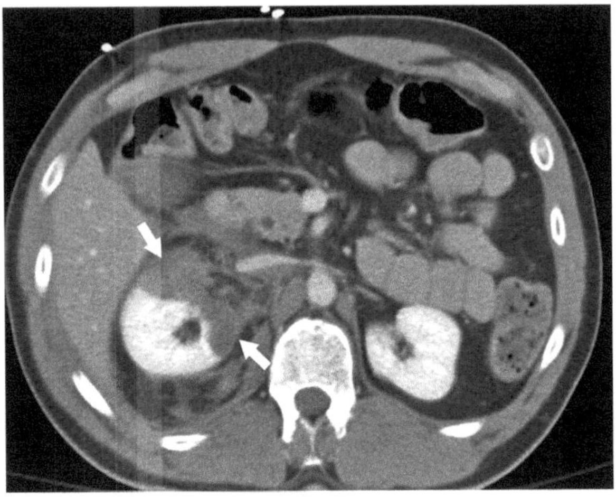

Fig. 4.3 Renal injury. Abdomen CT with contrast shows right renal contusions (*arrows*) and a hematoma around the kidney

4.2 Right Upper Quadrant Pain

A 36-year-old woman with right upper quadrant pain, fever, and leukocytosis. Exam reveals a positive Murphy's sign.

a. X-ray abdomen
b. US abdomen
c. CT abdomen
d. Cholescintigraphy
e. No ideal imaging exam

Fever, elevated white blood cell count, and positive Murphy's sign.

a. X-ray abdomen may sometimes be appropriate (5).
b. *US abdomen* is the most appropriate (9).
c. CT abdomen may sometimes be appropriate (5).
d. Cholescintigraphy may sometimes be appropriate (4).

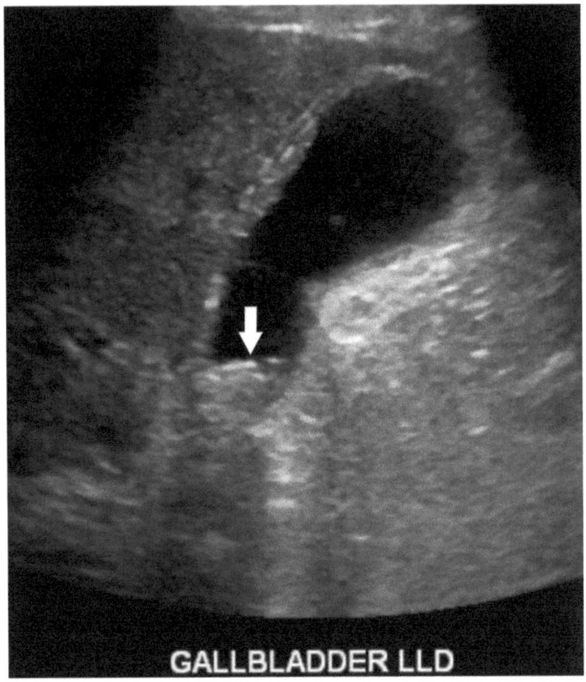

Fig. 4.4 Acute cholecystitis. Abdomen ultrasound shows stone lodged at the neck of the gallbladder (*arrow*). A sonographic Murphy's sign was also elicited

A 45-year-old man with right upper quadrant pain, fever, and leukocytosis. US shows no gallstones. Acalculous cholecystitis is suspected.

a. X-ray abdomen
b. US abdomen (repeated in 24 h)
c. CT abdomen
d. Cholescintigraphy
e. No ideal imaging exam

Suspected acalculous cholecystitis.

a. X-ray abdomen may sometimes be appropriate (6).
b. US abdomen (repeated in 24 h) may sometimes be appropriate (4).
c. CT abdomen may sometimes be appropriate (6).
d. *Cholescintigraphy* is the most appropriate (8).

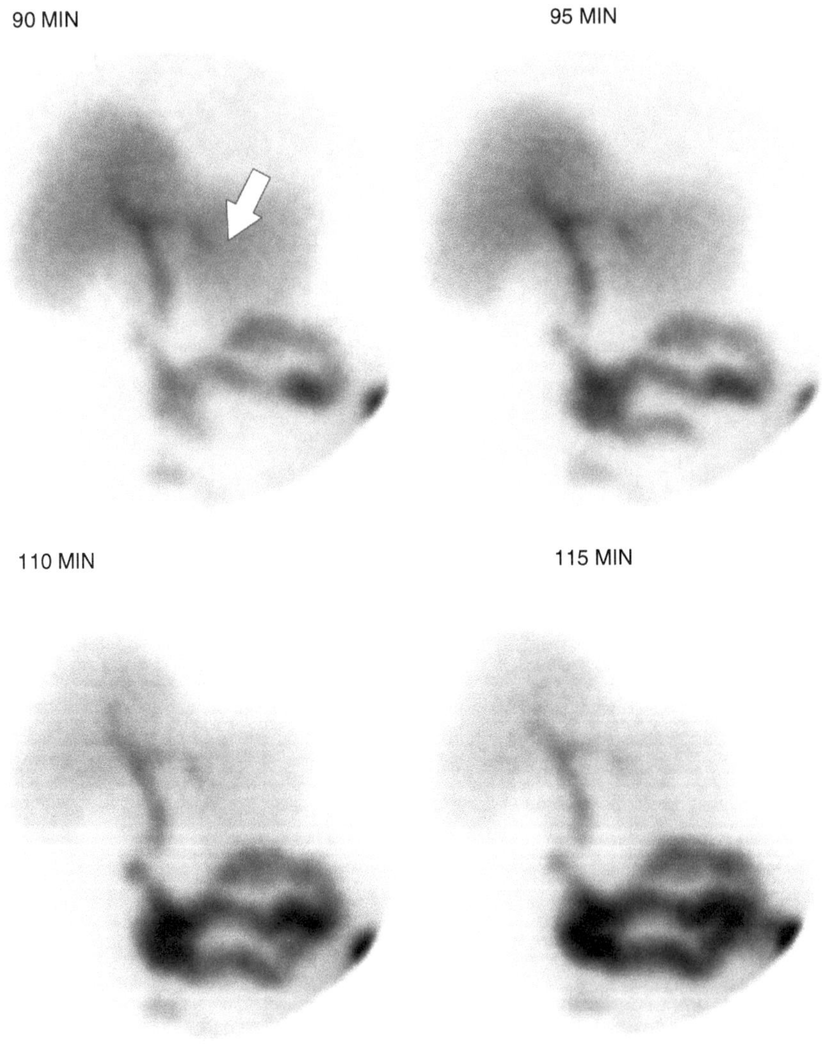

Fig. 4.5 Acalculous cholecystitis. Cholescintigraphy shows tracer uptake in liver (*arrow*) and excretion through the bile ducts into bowel without tracer uptake in the gallbladder

A 46-year-old woman with right upper quadrant pain. She has no fever or leukocytosis.

a. X-ray abdomen
b. US abdomen
c. CT abdomen
d. Cholescintigraphy
e. No ideal imaging exam

No fever, normal white blood cell count.

a. X-ray abdomen may sometimes be appropriate (4).
b. *US abdomen* is the most appropriate (8).
c. CT abdomen is usually appropriate, but there is a better choice here (7).
d. Cholescintigraphy may sometimes be appropriate (6).

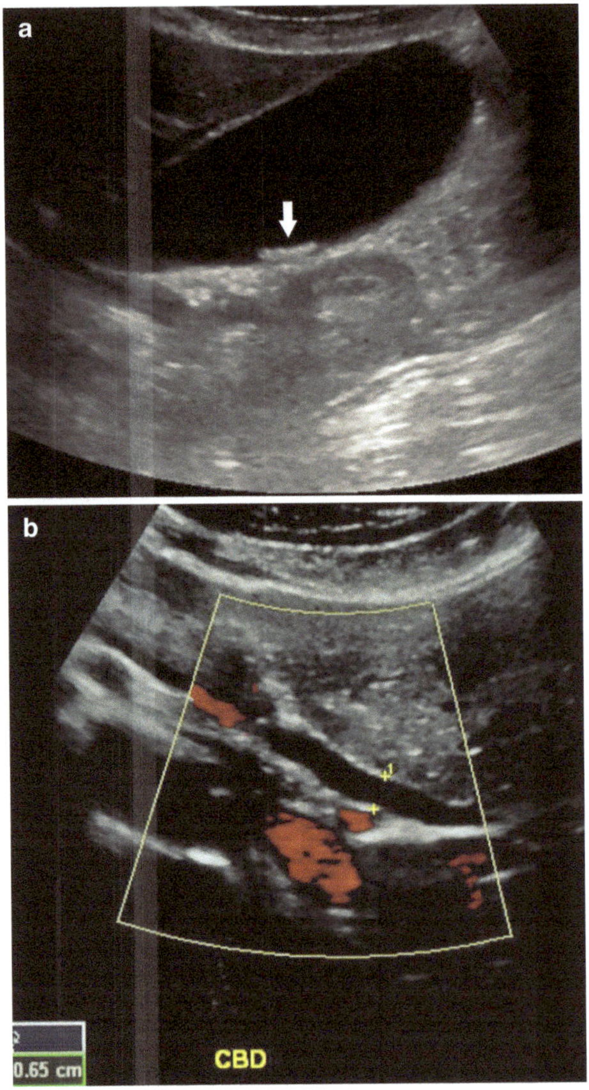

Fig. 4.6 Resolving choledocholithiasis. Abdomen ultrasound of the gallbladder (**a**) and of the common bile duct (**b**) shows stones (*arrow*) and a mildly dilated common bile duct (*calipers*)

A 64-year-old woman with right upper quadrant pain. She has no fever or leukocytosis. US shows gallstones but no other evidence for acute cholecystitis.

a. X-ray abdomen
b. X-ray fluoroscopy upper GI series
c. CT abdomen
d. Cholescintigraphy
e. No ideal imaging exam

No fever or elevated white blood cell count. Ultrasound shows only gallstones.

a. X-ray abdomen may sometimes be appropriate (4).
b. X-ray fluoroscopy upper GI series is usually not appropriate (3).
c. CT abdomen may sometimes be appropriate (6).
d. *Cholescintigraphy* is the most appropriate (8).

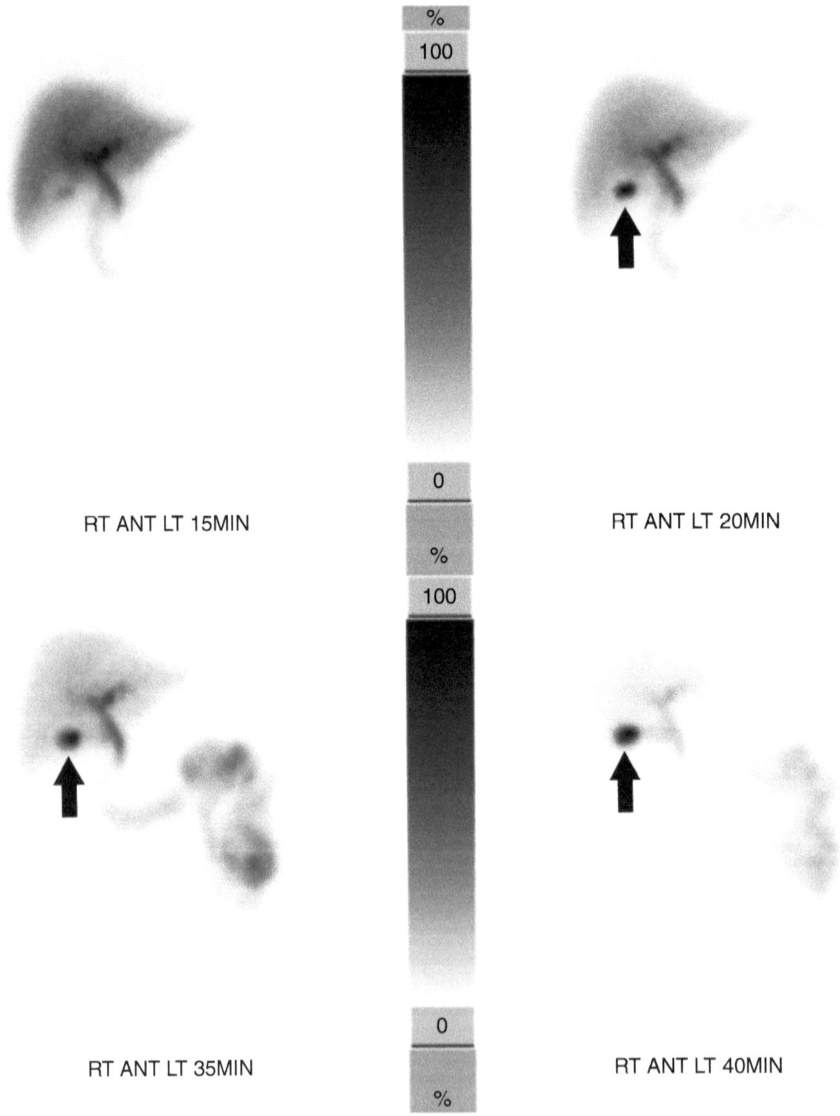

Fig. 4.7 Normal gallbladder. Cholescintigraphy shows tracer uptake in liver, accumulation in the gallbladder (*arrows*), and excretion into bowel

A 38-year-old hospitalized woman with right upper quadrant pain, fever, and leukocytosis. Exam reveals a positive Murphy's sign.

a. X-ray abdomen
b. US abdomen
c. CT abdomen
d. Cholescintigraphy
e. No ideal imaging exam

Hospitalized patient with fever, elevated white blood cell count, and positive Murphy's sign.

a. X-ray abdomen may sometimes be appropriate (6).
b. *US abdomen* is the most appropriate (9).
c. CT abdomen is usually appropriate, but there is a better choice here (7).
d. Cholescintigraphy is usually appropriate, but there is a better choice here (7).

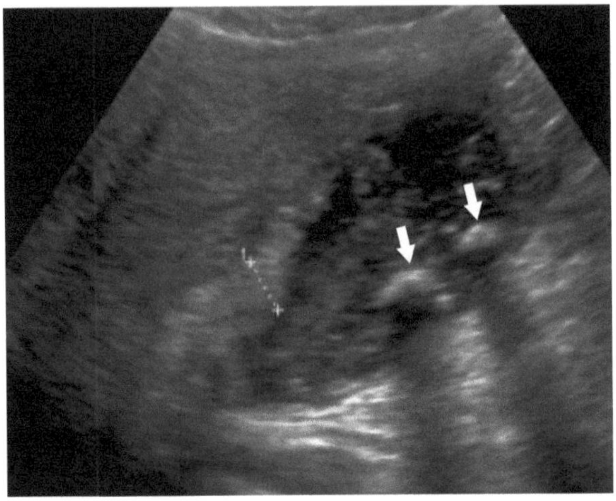

Fig. 4.8 Gangrenous cholecystitis. Abdomen ultrasound shows gallstones (*arrows*) and a thickened gallbladder wall (*calipers*)

4.3 Right Lower Quadrant Pain

A 32-year-old woman with right lower quadrant pain, fever, and leukocytosis. Appendicitis is suspected.

a. X-ray abdomen
b. US abdomen right lower quadrant
c. CT abdomen and pelvis with contrast
d. MRI abdomen and pelvis
e. No ideal imaging exam

Fever, leukocytosis, and classic presentation clinically for appendicitis.

a. X-ray abdomen may sometimes be appropriate (5).
b. US abdomen right lower quadrant may sometimes be appropriate. Exam is performed with graded compression of appendix (6).
c. *CT abdomen and pelvis with contrast* is the most appropriate. Use of oral or rectal contrast depends on institutional preference (8).
d. MRI abdomen and pelvis may sometimes be appropriate (4).

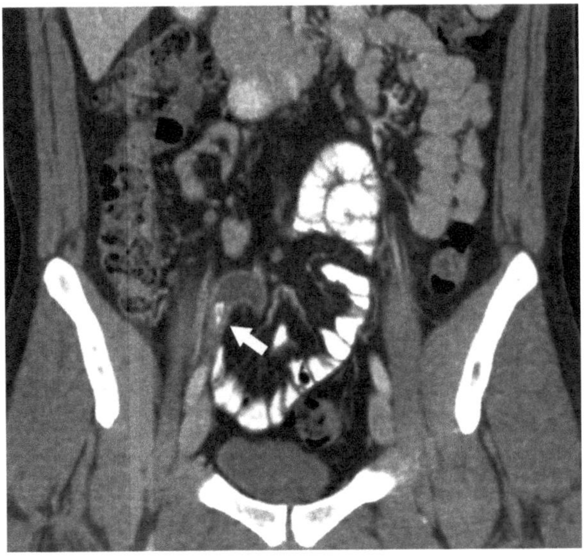

Fig. 4.9 Appendicitis. Abdomen and pelvic CT with contrast coronal reconstruction image shows a dilated appendix containing and appendicolith (*arrow*)

An 18-year-old woman with right lower quadrant pain, fever, and leukocytosis. She is not pregnant. Appendicitis is a possibility.

a. X-ray abdomen
b. US abdomen right lower quadrant
c. CT abdomen and pelvis with contrast
d. MRI abdomen and pelvis
e. No ideal imaging exam

Fever, leukocytosis; possible appendicitis, atypical presentation in adults and adolescents.

a. X-ray abdomen may sometimes be appropriate (6).
b. US abdomen right lower quadrant may sometimes be appropriate. Exam is performed with graded compression of appendix (6).
c. *CT abdomen and pelvis with contrast* is the most appropriate. Use of oral or rectal contrast depends on institutional preference (8).
d. MRI abdomen and pelvis may sometimes be appropriate (5).

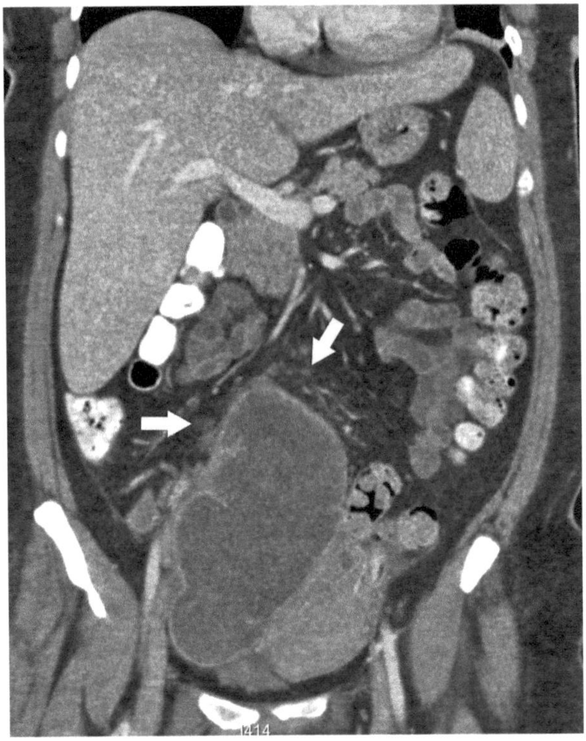

Fig. 4.10 Tubo-ovarian abscess. Abdomen and pelvic CT with contrast coronal reconstruction image shows a right adnexal collection with adjacent fat stranding (*arrows*) consistent with tubo-ovarian abscess

A 32-year-old woman with right lower quadrant pain, fever, and leukocytosis. She is pregnant.

a. X-ray abdomen
b. US pelvis
c. CT abdomen and pelvis with contrast
d. MRI abdomen and pelvis without contrast
e. No ideal imaging exam

Fever, leukocytosis, and pregnant woman.

a. X-ray abdomen is usually not appropriate (2).
b. US pelvis may sometimes be appropriate (6).
c. CT abdomen and pelvis with contrast may sometimes be appropriate. Use of oral or rectal contrast depends on institutional preference (6).
d. *MRI abdomen and pelvis without contrast* is the most appropriate (7).

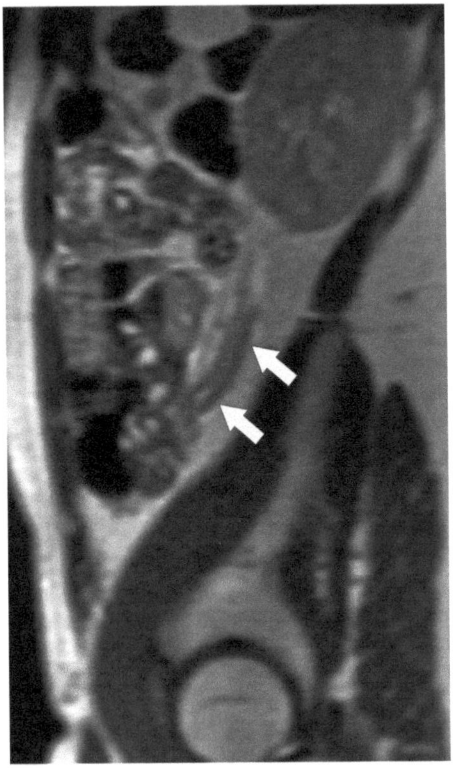

Fig. 4.11 Appendicitis. Abdomen and pelvic MR sagittal image shows a dilated fluid-filled appendix (*arrows*)

4.4 Left Lower Quadrant Pain

A 51-year-old man with left lower quadrant pain. Diverticulitis is suspected.

a. X-ray abdomen and pelvis
b. X-ray contrast enema
c. CT abdomen and pelvis with contrast
d. MRI abdomen and pelvis
e. No ideal imaging exam

Older patient with typical clinical presentation for diverticulitis.

a. X-ray abdomen and pelvis may sometimes be appropriate (4).
b. X-ray contrast enema may sometimes be appropriate (5).
c. *CT abdomen and pelvis with contrast* is the most appropriate. Oral and/or colonic contrast may be helpful for visualizing the bowel lumen (8).
d. MRI abdomen and pelvis may sometimes be appropriate (4).

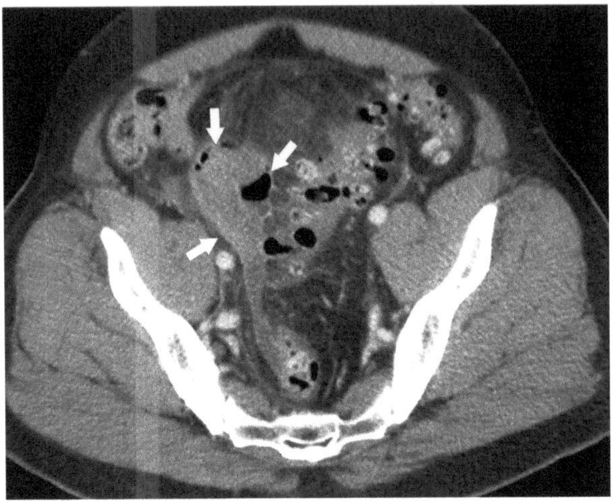

Fig. 4.12 Diverticulitis with perforation. Pelvic CT with intravenous contrast shows sigmoid colon diverticuli, adjacent fat stranding indicating inflammation, and an extraluminal collection of fluid and air (*arrows*)

A 59-year-old woman with acute severe left lower quadrant pain.

a. X-ray abdomen and pelvis
b. X-ray contrast enema
c. CT abdomen and pelvis with contrast
d. MRI abdomen and pelvis
e. No ideal imaging exam

Acute, severe, with or without fever.

a. X-ray abdomen and pelvis may sometimes be appropriate (5).
b. X-ray contrast enema may sometimes be appropriate (4).
c. *CT abdomen and pelvis with contrast* is the most appropriate. Oral and/or colonic contrast may be helpful for visualizing the bowel lumen (9).
d. MRI abdomen and pelvis is usually not appropriate (3).

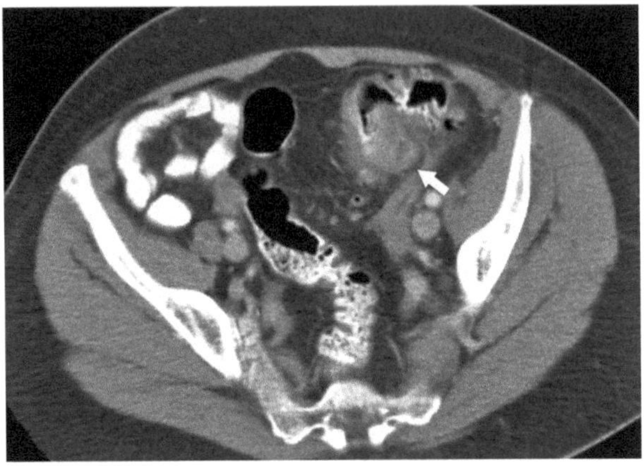

Fig. 4.13 Diverticulitis without perforation. Pelvic CT with contrast shows diverticuli and thickening of the sigmoid colon (*arrow*) with soft tissue stranding of the adjacent mesenteric fat indicating inflammation

An 83-year-old woman with chronic intermittent left lower quadrant pain.

a. X-ray abdomen and pelvis
b. X-ray contrast enema
c. CT abdomen and pelvis with contrast
d. MRI abdomen and pelvis
e. No ideal imaging exam

Chronic, intermittent, or low grade.

a. X-ray abdomen and pelvis may sometimes be appropriate (5).
b. X-ray contrast enema may sometimes be appropriate (6).
c. *CT abdomen and pelvis with contrast* is the most appropriate. Oral and/or colonic contrast may be helpful for visualizing the bowel lumen (8).
d. MRI abdomen and pelvis may sometimes be appropriate (4).

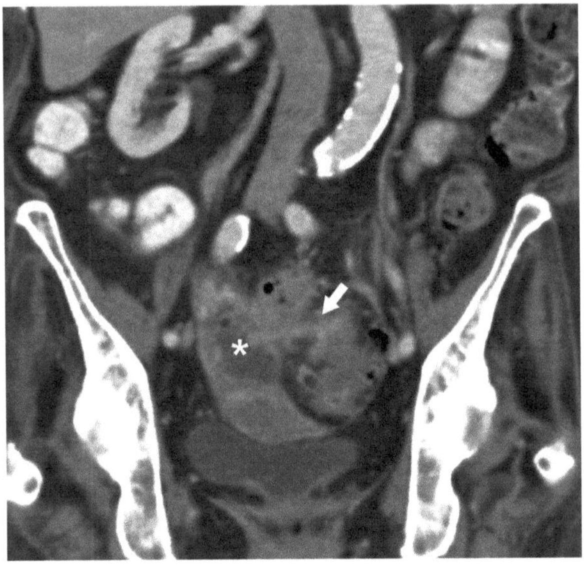

Fig. 4.14 Chronic diverticulitis. Abdomen and pelvic CT with contrast coronal reconstruction image shows an extraluminal collection of air, fluid, and soft tissue (*asterisk*) that communicates with the sigmoid colon through a fistula (*arrow*)

A 34-year-old woman with left lower quadrant pain.

a. X-ray abdomen and pelvis
b. US pelvis transvaginal
c. CT abdomen and pelvis with contrast
d. MRI abdomen and pelvis
e. No ideal imaging exam

Woman of childbearing age.

a. X-ray abdomen and pelvis may sometimes be appropriate (5).
b. *US pelvis transvaginal* is the most appropriate. This is done first to evaluate for gynecologic abnormality (8).
c. CT abdomen and pelvis with contrast is usually appropriate, but there is a better choice here. Oral and/or colonic contrast may be helpful for visualizing bowel lumen (7).
d. MRI abdomen and pelvis may sometimes be appropriate (5).

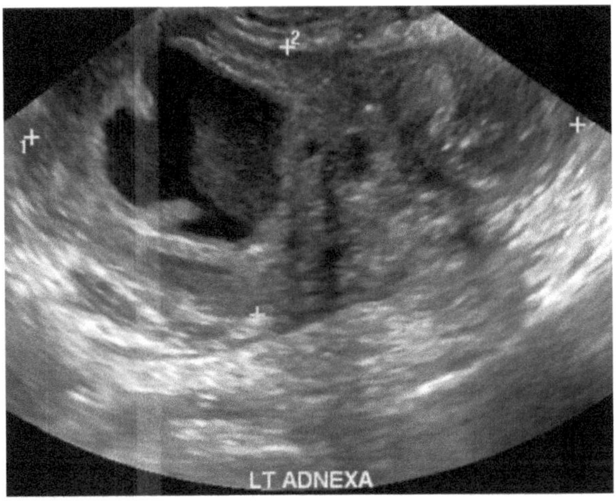

Fig. 4.15 Tubo-ovarian abscess. Pelvic transvaginal ultrasound shows a 7-cm mixed solid and cystic left adnexal lesion (*calipers*)

4.5 Acute Abdominal Pain and Fever or Suspected Abdominal Abscess

A 57-year-old man status post recent abdominal surgery with pain and fever. Abscess is suspected.

a. X-ray abdomen and pelvis
b. US abdomen
c. CT abdomen and pelvis with contrast
d. MRI abdomen and pelvis
e. No ideal imaging exam

Postoperative patient with fever.

a. X-ray abdomen and pelvis may sometimes be appropriate (5).
b. US abdomen may sometimes be appropriate (6).
c. *CT abdomen and pelvis with contrast* is the most appropriate (8).
d. MRI abdomen and pelvis may sometimes be appropriate (5).

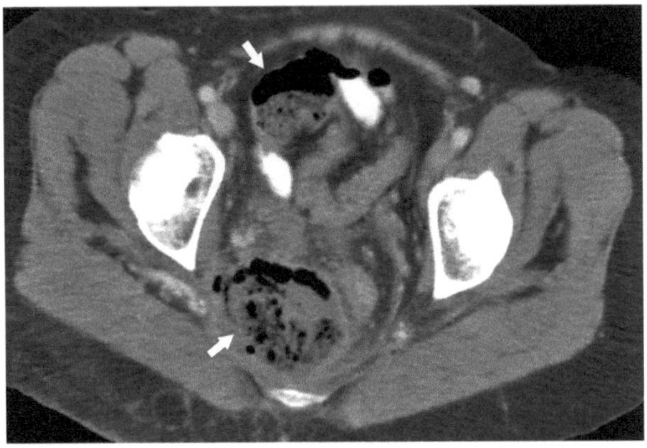

Fig. 4.16 Postoperative abscess. Pelvic CT with contrast shows two extraluminal collections (*arrows*) containing air and fluid

A 46-year-old woman status post recent pelvic surgery with persistent pain and fever. No abscess was seen on CT scan 7 days ago.

a. X-ray abdomen and pelvis
b. US abdomen
c. CT abdomen and pelvis with contrast
d. MRI abdomen and pelvis
e. No ideal imaging exam

Postoperative patient with persistent fever and no abscess seen on CT scan within the last 7 days.

a. X-ray abdomen and pelvis may sometimes be appropriate (5).
b. US abdomen may sometimes be appropriate (6).
c. *CT abdomen and pelvis with contrast* is the most appropriate (8).
d. MRI abdomen and pelvis may sometimes be appropriate (5).

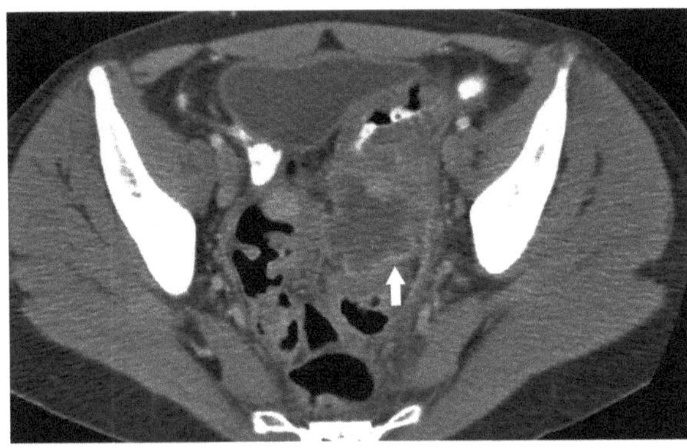

Fig. 4.17 Postoperative abscess. Pelvic CT with contrast shows a rim-enhancing extraluminal fluid collection (*arrow*)

A 52-year-old man with nonlocalizing abdominal pain and fever. He has no history of recent surgery.

a. X-ray abdomen and pelvis
b. US abdomen
c. CT abdomen and pelvis with contrast
d. MRI abdomen and pelvis
e. No ideal imaging exam

Patient presenting with fever, nonlocalizing abdominal pain, and no recent operation.

a. X-ray abdomen and pelvis may sometimes be appropriate (6).
b. US abdomen may sometimes be appropriate (6).
c. *CT abdomen and pelvis with contrast* is the most appropriate (8).
d. MRI abdomen and pelvis may sometimes be appropriate (5).

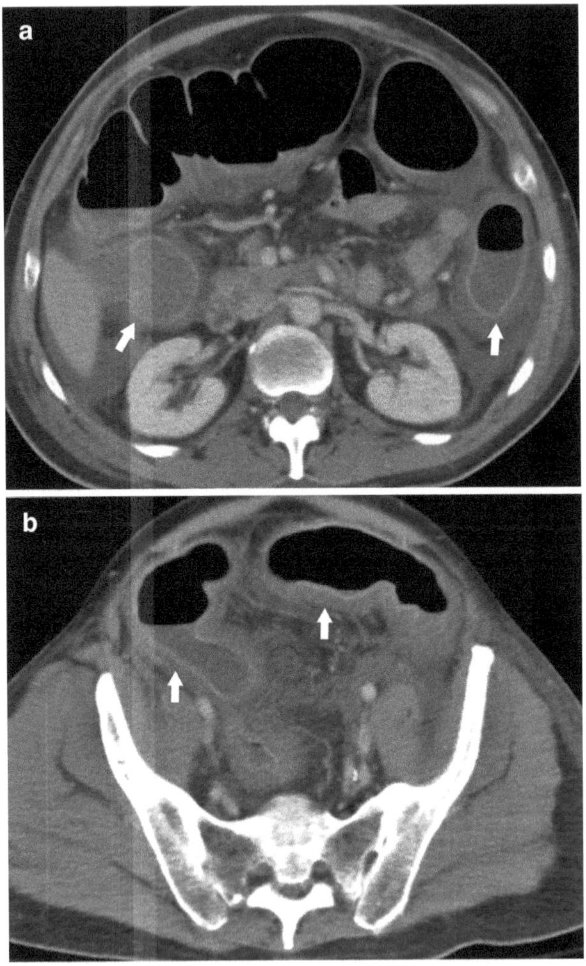

Fig. 4.18 Pseudomembranous colitis. Abdomen (**a**) and pelvic (**b**) CT with contrast shows diffuse colonic wall thickening (*arrows*)

A 19-year-old pregnant woman with abdominal pain and fever.

a. X-ray abdomen and pelvis
b. US abdomen
c. CT abdomen and pelvis with contrast
d. MRI abdomen and pelvis
e. No ideal imaging exam

Pregnant patient.

a. X-ray abdomen and pelvis may sometimes be appropriate (4).
b. *US abdomen* is the most appropriate (8).
c. CT abdomen and pelvis with contrast may sometimes be appropriate. Use only after other studies without radiation has been utilized (5).
d. MRI abdomen and pelvis is usually appropriate, but there is a better choice here (7).

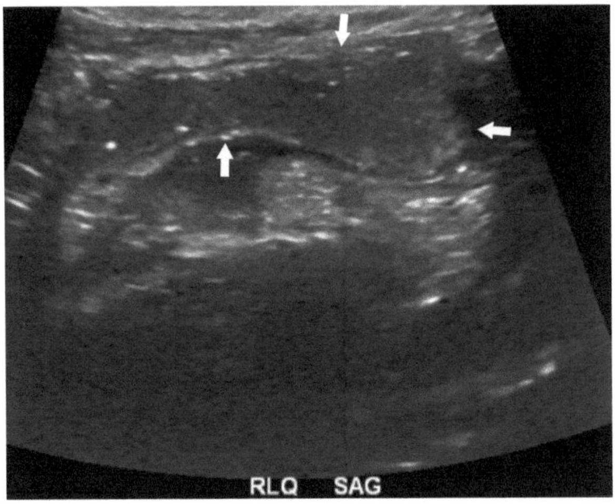

Fig. 4.19 Abscess. Abdomen ultrasound shows a loculated collection (*arrows*) in the right lower quadrant

4.6 Suspected Small Bowel Obstruction

An 84-year-old woman with suspected complete or high-grade small bowel obstruction.

a. X-ray abdomen
b. X-ray small bowel follow-through
c. CT abdomen and pelvis with contrast (routine)
d. CT abdomen and pelvis with contrast (enterocolysis)
e. No ideal imaging exam

Suspected complete or high-grade partial small bowel obstruction.

a. X-ray abdomen is usually appropriate, but there is a better choice here (7).
b. X-ray small bowel follow-through may sometimes be appropriate (4).
c. *CT abdomen and pelvis with contrast* (*routine*) is the most appropriate. Oral contrast should not be used. Additional fluid from oral contrast is not well tolerated with bowel obstruction (8).
d. CT abdomen and pelvis with contrast (enterocolysis) may sometimes be appropriate (4).

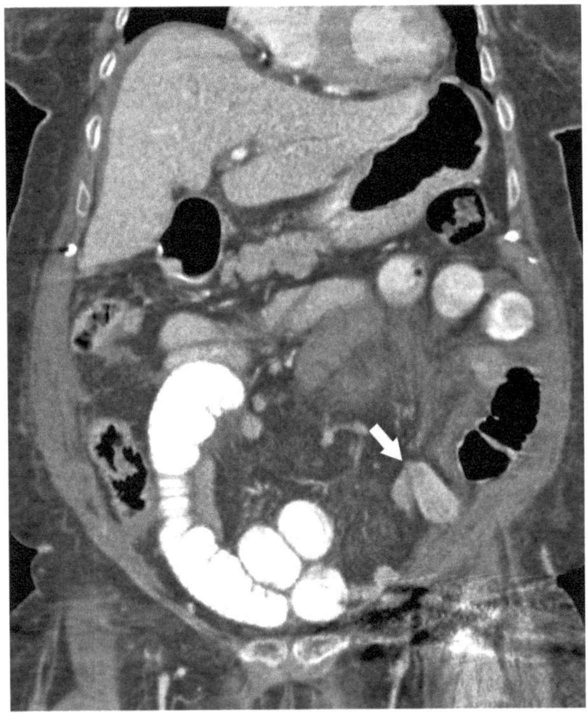

Fig. 4.20 Small bowel obstruction. Abdomen and pelvic CT with contrast coronal reconstruction image shows distended markedly dilated loops of proximal small bowel and decompressed colon with a transition in bowel caliber (*arrow*) in the jejunum

A 70-year-old woman with intermittent or low-grade small bowel obstruction.

a. X-ray abdomen and pelvis
b. X-ray small bowel follow-through
c. CT abdomen and pelvis with contrast (routine)
d. CT abdomen and pelvis with contrast (enterocolysis)
e. No ideal imaging exam

Suspected intermittent or low-grade small bowel obstruction.

a. X-ray abdomen and pelvis may sometimes be appropriate (4).
b. X-ray small bowel follow-through is not rated in appropriateness.
c. CT abdomen and pelvis with contrast (routine) may sometimes be appropriate (5).
d. *CT abdomen and pelvis with contrast (enterocolysis)* is the most appropriate (8).

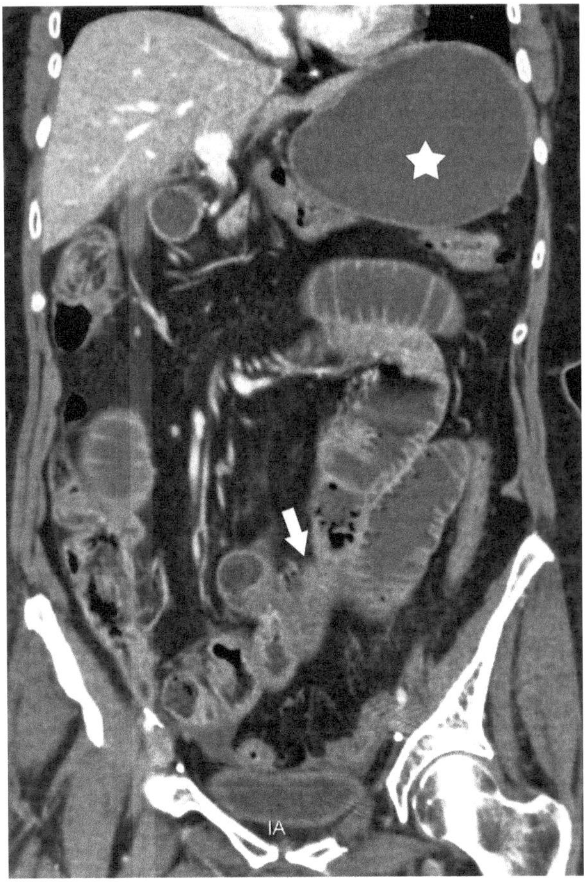

Fig. 4.21 Small bowel obstruction. Abdomen and pelvic CT with contrast coronal reconstruction image shows a distended stomach (*star*), dilated proximal small bowel, and decompressed colon with a transition in bowel caliber (*arrow*) in the jejunum

4.7 Jaundice

A 52-year-old woman with jaundice, fever, and acute abdominal pain. She has a known history of gallstones.

a. US abdomen
b. CT abdomen without and with contrast
c. MRI abdomen with MRCP
d. ERCP
e. No ideal imaging exam

Acute abdominal pain and at least one of the following: fever, history of biliary surgery, and known cholelithiasis.

a. *US abdomen* is the most appropriate (9).
b. CT abdomen without and with contrast is usually appropriate, but there is a better choice here (7).
c. MRI abdomen with MRCP may sometimes be appropriate. If cholangitis or hepatic abscess is suspected, with contrast is preferred (5).
d. ERCP may sometimes be appropriate. For high suspicion of common bile duct stones, some would advocate doing ERCP initially (4).

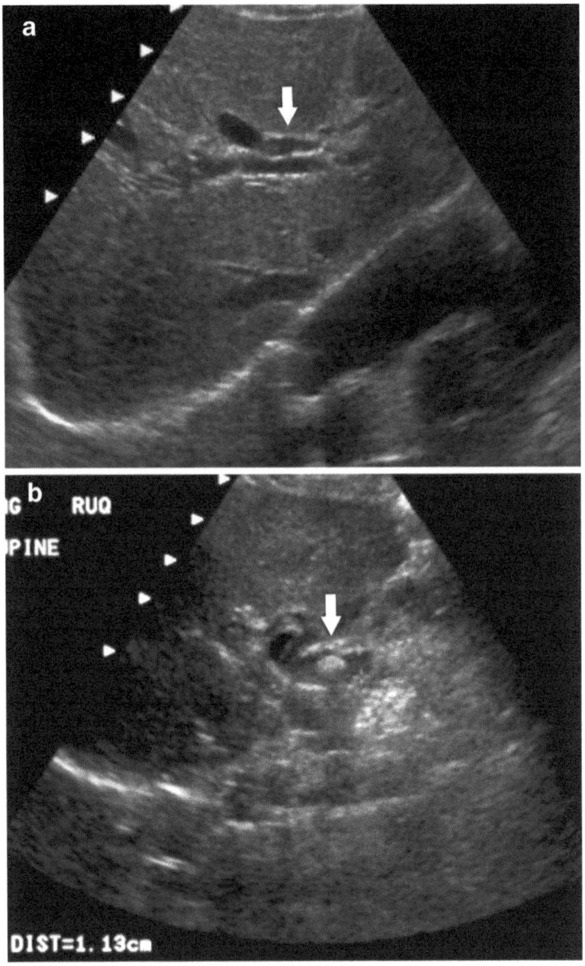

Fig. 4.22 Biliary obstruction from choledocholithiasis. Abdomen US of the liver (**a**) shows dilated intrahepatic ducts (*arrow*). The common bile duct (**b**) is dilated and contains a stone (*arrow*)

A 60-year-old man with painless jaundice and a history of unexplained weight loss over the past 4 months.

a. US abdomen
b. CT abdomen without and with contrast
c. MRI abdomen with contrast and with MRCP
d. ERCP
e. No ideal imaging exam

Painless and one or more of the following: weight loss, fatigue, and anorexia, duration of symptoms greater than 3 months. Patient otherwise healthy.

a. US abdomen is usually appropriate, but there is a better choice here (8).
b. *CT abdomen without and with contrast* is the most appropriate (9).
c. MRI abdomen with contrast and with MRCP is usually appropriate, but there is a better choice here (7).
d. ERCP may sometimes be appropriate (6).

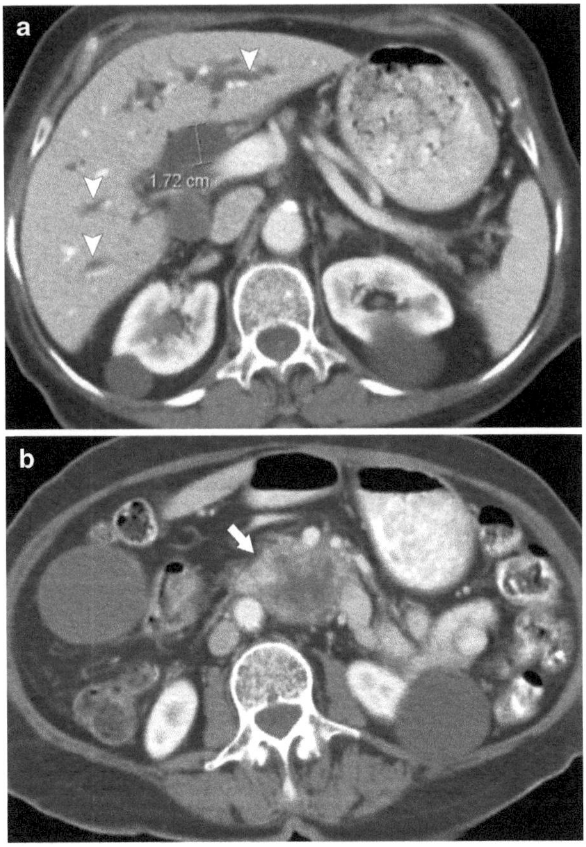

Fig. 4.23 Biliary obstruction from pancreatic cancer. Abdomen CT with contrast (**a**, **b**) shows intrahepatic biliary ductal dilatation (*arrowheads*), a dilated common bile duct (*calipers*), and a pancreatic mass (*arrow*)

A 27-year-old man with jaundice. Clinical evaluation and laboratory values are not consistent with mechanical biliary obstruction.

a. US abdomen
b. CT abdomen
c. MRI abdomen with MRCP
d. ERCP
e. No ideal imaging exam

Clinical condition and laboratory examination makes mechanical obstruction unlikely.

a. *US abdomen* is the most appropriate (8).
b. CT abdomen may sometimes be appropriate (5).
c. MRI abdomen with MRCP may sometimes be appropriate (6).
d. ERCP is usually not appropriate (3).

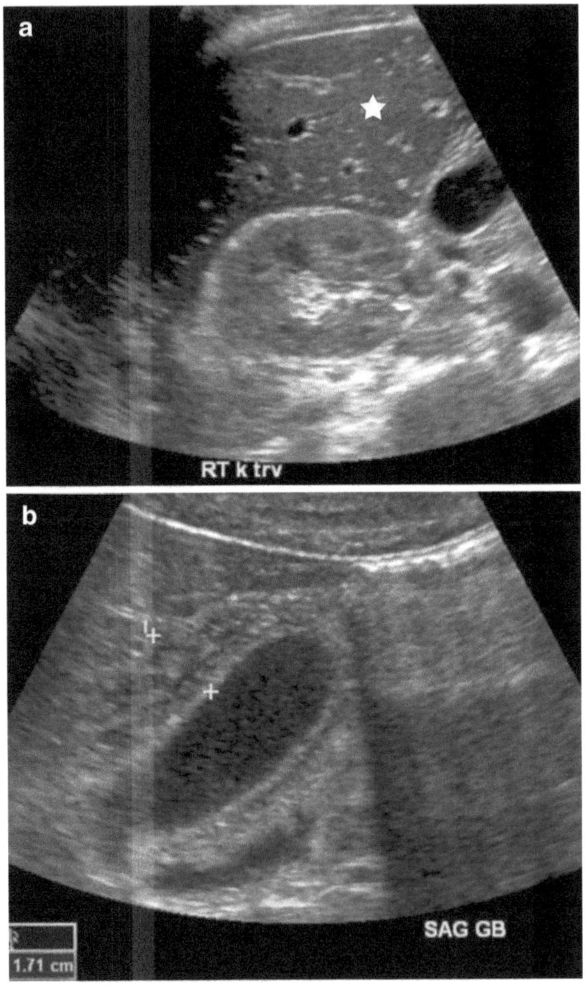

Fig. 4.24 Hepatitis. Abdomen ultrasound shows a hypoechoic liver (**a**) (*star*) and thick gallbladder wall (**b**) (*calipers*), findings consistent with hepatitis

4.8 Acute Pancreatitis

A 41-year-old previously healthy man presents with acute pancreatitis.

a. US abdomen
b. CT abdomen
c. MRI abdomen with MRCP
d. US abdomen endoscopic
e. No ideal imaging exam

Etiology unknown, first episode of pancreatitis.

a. *US abdomen* is the most appropriate (8).
b. CT abdomen may sometimes be appropriate (6).
c. MRI abdomen with MRCP may sometimes be appropriate (6).
d. US abdomen endoscopic may sometimes be appropriate (5).

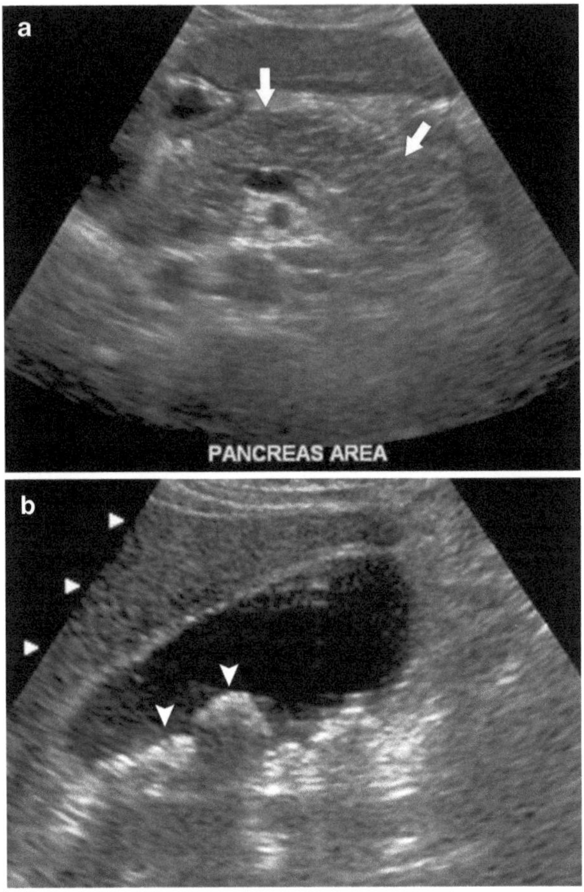

Fig. 4.25 Pancreatitis from gallstones. Abdomen ultrasound shows a hypoechoic diffusely enlarged pancreas (**a**) (*arrows*) consistent with pancreatitis and gallstones (**b**) (*arrowheads*)

An 82-year-old man with acute pancreatitis. Clinical condition unimproved after 48 h of medical management.

a. US abdomen
b. CT abdomen
c. MRI abdomen with MRCP
d. US abdomen endoscopic
e. No ideal imaging exam

Severe abdominal pain, elevated amylase and lipase, and no improvement or degradation over 48 h. Assuming no prior imaging.

a. US abdomen is usually appropriate, but there is a better choice here (7).
b. *CT abdomen* is the most appropriate (8).
c. MRI abdomen is usually appropriate, but there is a better choice here (7).
d. US abdomen endoscopic is not rated in appropriateness.

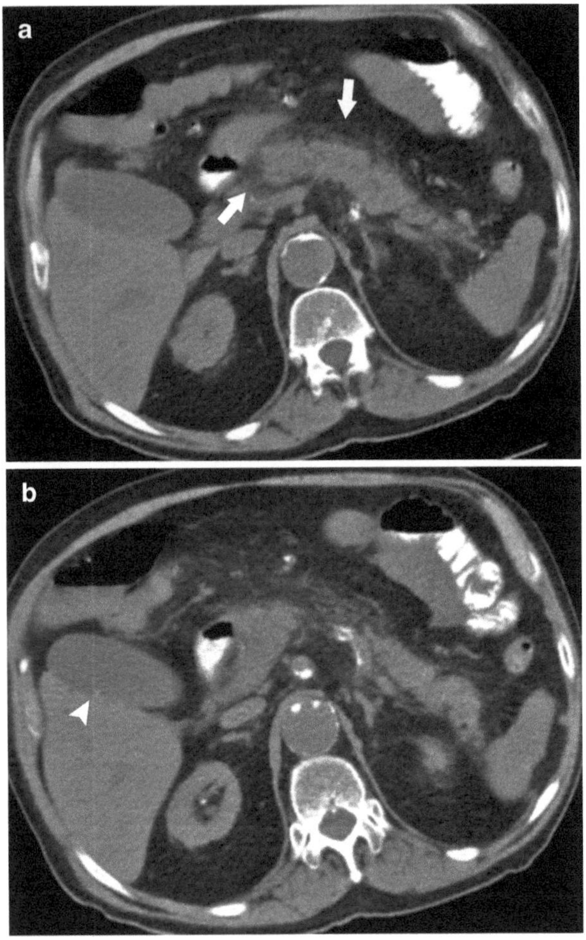

Fig. 4.26 Pancreatitis. Abdomen CT (**a**, **b**) shows peripancreatic fat stranding (*arrows*) consistent with pancreatitis and gallstones (*arrowhead*)

A 49-year-old woman with acute pancreatitis, fever, and leukocytosis.

a. US abdomen
b. CT abdomen
c. MRI abdomen with MRCP
d. US abdomen endoscopic
e. No ideal imaging exam

Severe abdominal pain, fever, elevated amylase, lipase, and white blood cell count.

a. US abdomen is usually appropriate, but there is a better choice here (7).
b. *CT abdomen* is the most appropriate (8).
c. MRI abdomen is usually appropriate, but there is a better choice here (7).
d. US abdomen endoscopic is not rated in appropriateness.

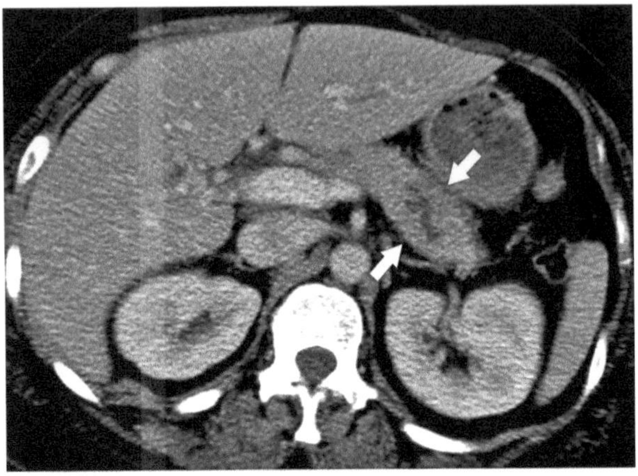

Fig. 4.27 Pancreatitis. Abdomen CT with contrast shows pancreatic ductal dilatation and peripancreatic fat stranding. Focal lack of enhancement (*arrows*) indicates necrosis

A 36-year-old man with acute pancreatitis now with hemoconcentration, oliguria, and tachycardia.

a. US abdomen
b. CT abdomen
c. MRI abdomen with MRCP
d. US abdomen endoscopic
e. No ideal imaging exam

Severe abdominal pain, elevated amylase and lipase, hemoconcentration, oliguria, and tachycardia.

a. US abdomen is usually appropriate, but there is a better choice here (7).
b. *CT abdomen* is the most appropriate (9).
c. MRI abdomen is usually appropriate, but there is a better choice here (7).
d. US abdomen endoscopic is not rated in appropriateness.

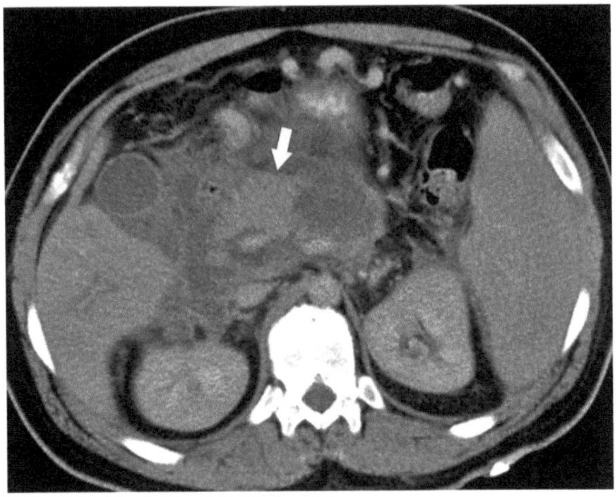

Fig. 4.28 Pancreatitis with pancreatic necrosis. Abdomen CT with contrast shows a mixed fluid and soft tissue density collection surrounding and replacing much of the pancreas. Residual-enhancing normal tissue at the pancreatic head (*arrow*) is seen

4.9 Dysphagia

A 69-year-old man status post recent stroke now with oropharyngeal dysphagia.

a. X-ray pharynx dynamic and static imaging
b. X-ray barium swallow
c. X-ray barium swallow modified
d. Tc-99m transit scintigraphy esophagus
e. No ideal imaging exam

Oropharyngeal dysphagia with an attributable cause.

a. X-ray pharynx dynamic and static imaging may sometimes be appropriate (6).
b. X-ray barium swallow may sometimes be appropriate. Perform biphasic esophagogram with air contrast then single contrast (4).
c. *X-ray barium swallow modified* is the most appropriate (8).
d. Tc-99m transit scintigraphy esophagus is usually not appropriate (2).

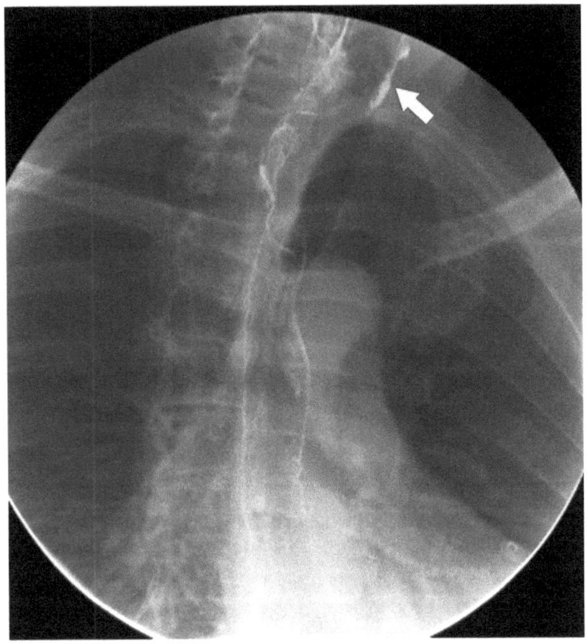

Fig. 4.29 Aspiration. X-ray modified barium swallow spot image shows contrast in the upper trachea (*arrow*)

A 49-year-old woman with unexplained oropharyngeal dysphagia.

a. X-ray barium swallow
b. X-ray barium swallow modified
c. Tc-99m transit scintigraphy esophagus
d. Manometry esophagus
e. No ideal imaging exam

Unexplained oropharyngeal dysphagia.

a. *X-ray barium swallow* is the most appropriate. Perform biphasic esophagogram with air contrast then single contrast. Both pharyngeal and esophageal exams are needed, since patient may have referred dysphagia (8).
b. X-ray barium swallow modified may sometimes be appropriate.(6).
c. Tc-99m transit scintigraphy esophagus may sometimes be appropriate (4).
d. Manometry esophagus is not rated in appropriateness.

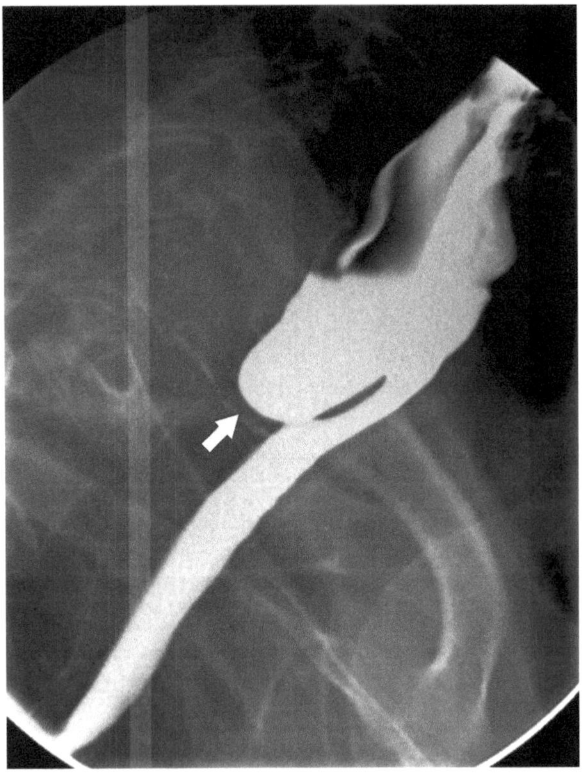

Fig. 4.30 Zenker's diverticulum. X-ray barium swallow spot image shows a large outpouching (*arrow*) of the posterior hypopharynx

A 74-year-old man with substernal dysphagia.

a. X-ray pharynx dynamic and static imaging
b. X-ray barium swallow
c. X-ray barium swallow modified
d. Tc-99m transit scintigraphy esophagus
e. No ideal imaging exam

Substernal dysphagia in immunocompetent patients.

a. X-ray pharynx dynamic and static imaging may sometimes be appropriate (4).
b. *X-ray barium swallow* is the most appropriate. Perform biphasic esophagogram with air contrast then single contrast. Endoscopy and biphasic esophagogram are both excellent diagnostic tests in this setting (8).
c. X-ray barium swallow modified may sometimes be appropriate (4).
d. Tc-99m transit scintigraphy esophagus may sometimes be appropriate (4).

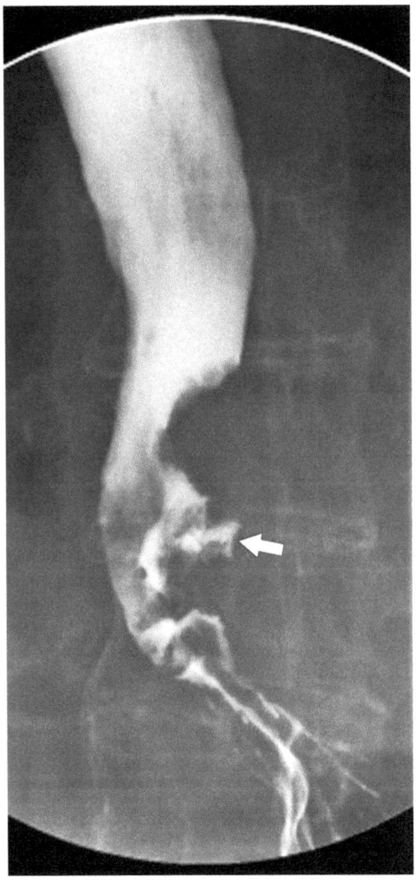

Fig. 4.31 Esophageal cancer. X-ray barium swallow spot image shows irregular narrowing in the distal esophagus with ulceration (*arrow*)

A 55-year-old woman with substernal dysphagia. She is immunocompromised.

a. X-ray pharynx dynamic and static imaging
b. X-ray barium swallow
c. X-ray barium swallow modified
d. Tc-99m transit scintigraphy esophagus
e. No ideal imaging exam

Substernal dysphagia in immunocompromised patients.

a. X-ray pharynx dynamic and static imaging is usually not appropriate (3).
b. *X-ray barium swallow* is the most appropriate. Perform biphasic esophagogram with air contrast then single contrast. Endoscopy and biphasic esophagogram are both excellent diagnostic tests in this setting (8).
c. X-ray barium swallow modified may sometimes be appropriate (4).
d. Tc-99m transit scintigraphy esophagus is usually not appropriate (2).

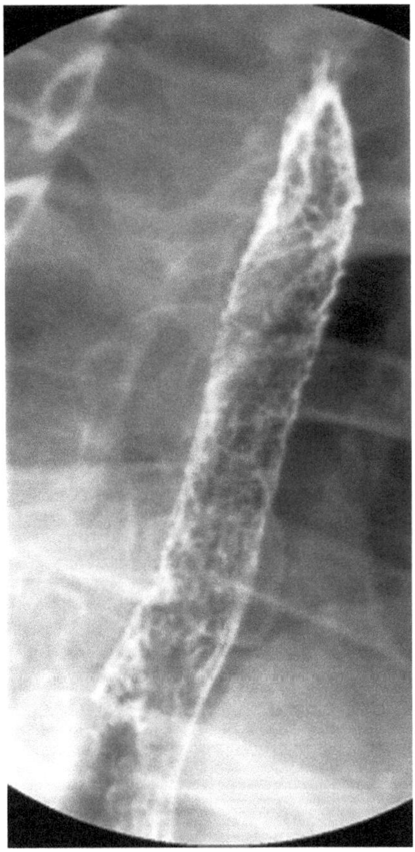

Fig. 4.32 Candida esophagitis. X-ray barium swallow spot image shows a "shaggy" esophagus caused by multiple confluent mucosal plaques and ulcers

4.10 Colorectal Cancer Screening

A 51-year-old woman presents for colorectal cancer screening. She is at average risk.

a. X-ray barium enema single-contrast every 5 years after negative screen
b. X-ray barium enema double-contrast every 5 years after negative screen
c. CT colonography every 5 years after negative screen
d. MR colonography every 5 years after negative screen
e. No ideal imaging exam

Average risk, age > 50 years.

a. X-ray barium enema single-contrast every 5 years after negative screen may sometimes be appropriate. Use if double-contrast barium enema or CT colonography cannot be performed (4).
b. X-ray barium enema double-contrast every 5 years after negative screen is usually appropriate, but there is a better choice here (7).
c. *CT colonography every 5 years after negative screen* is the most appropriate (8).
d. MR colonography every 5 years after negative screen may sometimes be appropriate (4).

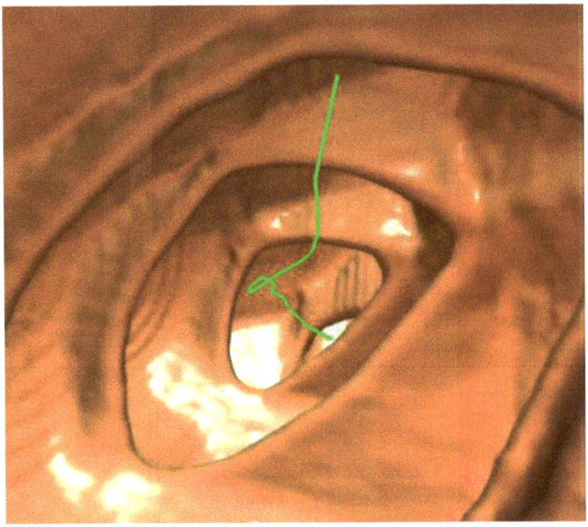

Fig. 4.33 Normal colon. CT colonography 3-D "fly through" reconstruction image shows no polyps or masses. *Line* indicates the course of the lumen

A 54-year-old man presents for colorectal cancer screening. He is at average risk, but fecal occult blood test is positive.

a. X-ray barium enema single-contrast
b. X-ray barium enema double-contrast
c. CT colonography
d. MR colonography
e. No ideal imaging exam

Average-risk individual after positive fecal occult blood test indicating a relative elevation in risk.

a. X-ray barium enema single-contrast may sometimes be appropriate. Use if double-contrast barium enema or CT colonography cannot be performed (4).
b. X-ray barium enema double-contrast is usually appropriate, but there is a better choice here (7).
c. *CT colonography* is the most appropriate (8).
d. MR colonography may sometimes be appropriate (4).

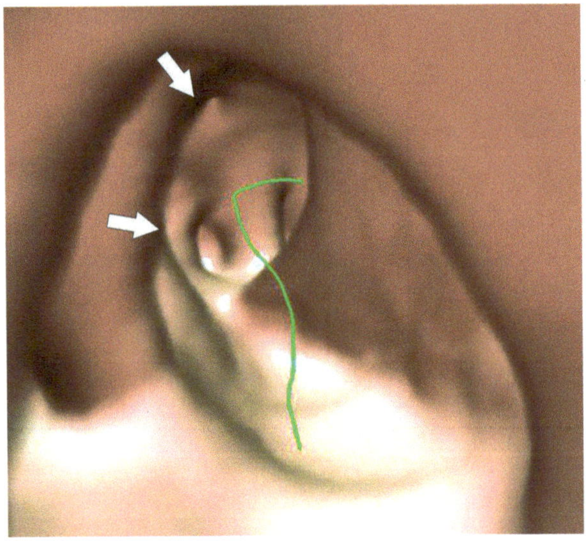

Fig. 4.34 Colonic diverticuli. CT colonography 3-D "fly through" reconstruction image shows diverticuli (*arrows*) but no polyps or masses. *Line* indicates the course of the lumen

A 60-year-old woman with incomplete screening colonoscopy. She is at moderate risk with a family history of colon cancer.

a. X-ray barium enema single-contrast
b. X-ray barium enema double-contrast
c. CT colonography
d. MR colonography
e. No ideal imaging exam

Average-, moderate-, or high-risk individual after incomplete colonoscopy.

a. X-ray barium enema single-contrast may sometimes be appropriate. Use if double-contrast barium enema or CT colonography cannot be performed (4).
b. X-ray barium enema double-contrast is usually appropriate, but there is a better choice here (7).
c. *CT colonography* is the most appropriate (9).
d. MR colonography is usually not appropriate (3).

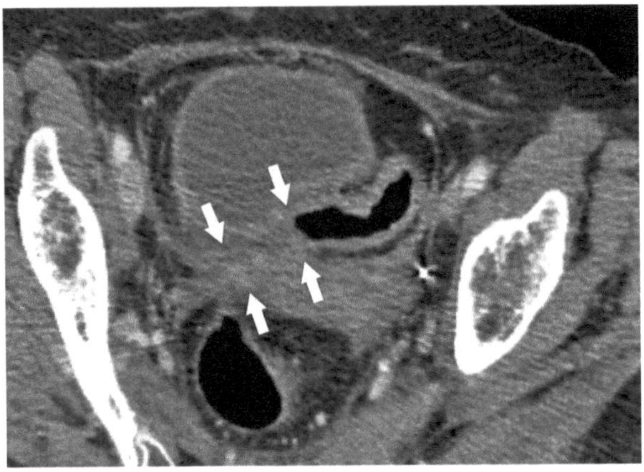

Fig. 4.35 Colonic stricture. CT colonography axial image shows luminal narrowing (*arrows*) in the sigmoid colon through which the colonoscope could not pass. Remainder of the colon was otherwise unremarkable

A 54-year-old man presents for colon cancer screening. He is at moderate risk with a history of an adenomatous polyp.

a. X-ray barium enema single-contrast
b. X-ray barium enema double-contrast
c. CT colonography
d. MR colonography
e. No ideal imaging exam

Moderate risk: personal history or first-degree family history of cancer or adenoma.

a. X-ray barium enema single-contrast may sometimes be appropriate. Use if double-contrast barium enema or CT colonography cannot be performed (4).
b. X-ray barium enema double-contrast is usually appropriate, but there is a better choice here (7).
c. *CT colonography* is the most appropriate (8).
d. MR colonography may sometimes be appropriate (4).

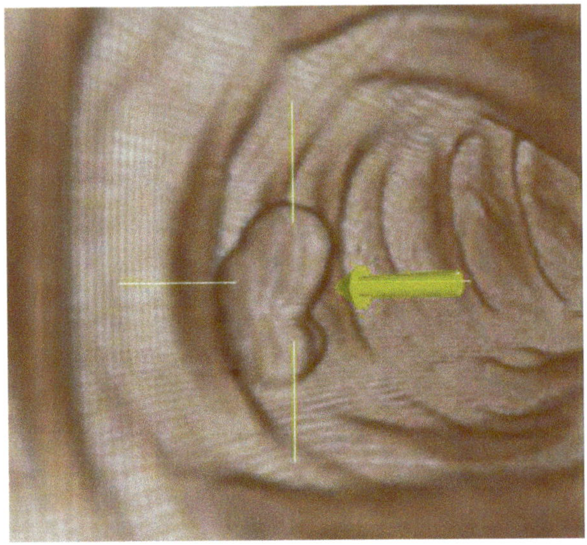

Fig. 4.36 Colonic adenoma. CT colonography 3-D "fly through" reconstruction image shows a 2.1-cm polyp (*arrow*)

A 30-year-old man presents for colon cancer screening. He is at high risk with hereditary nonpolyposis colorectal cancer syndrome.

a. X-ray barium enema single-contrast
b. X-ray barium enema double-contrast
c. CT colonography
d. MR colonography
e. No ideal imaging exam

High-risk individual: hereditary nonpolyposis colorectal cancer.

a. X-ray barium enema single-contrast is usually not appropriate. Colonoscopy is preferred (2).
b. X-ray barium enema double-contrast is usually not appropriate. Colonoscopy is preferred (3).
c. CT colonography is usually not appropriate. Colonoscopy is preferred (3).
d. MR colonography is usually not appropriate. Colonoscopy is preferred (2).
e. *No ideal imaging exam* is the correct answer.

A 43-year-old woman presents for colon cancer screening. She is at high risk with a diagnosis of ulcerative colitis.

a. X-ray barium enema single-contrast
b. X-ray barium enema double-contrast
c. CT colonography
d. MR colonography
e. No ideal imaging exam

High-risk individual: ulcerative colitis or Crohn's colitis.

a. X-ray barium enema single-contrast is usually not appropriate. Colonoscopy is preferred for ability to obtain biopsies and to look for dysplasia (2).
b. X-ray barium enema double-contrast is usually not appropriate. Colonoscopy is preferred for ability to obtain biopsies and to look for dysplasia (3).
c. CT colonography is usually not appropriate. Colonoscopy is preferred for ability to obtain biopsies and to look for dysplasia (3).
d. MR colonography is usually not appropriate. Colonoscopy is preferred for ability to obtain biopsies and to look for dysplasia (2).
e. *No ideal imaging exam* is the correct answer.

5 Musculoskeletal Imaging

5.1 Suspected Spine Trauma

NEXUS Criteria
C-Spine imaging is recommended in trauma patients unless they meet all of the following criteria.

- No posterior midline cervical spine tenderness
- No evidence of intoxication
- Normal level of alertness
- No focal neurological deficit
- No clinically apparent painful injuries that might distract from pain of a cervical spine injury

S.I. Lee, J.H. Thrall, *Choosing the Correct Radiologic Test*,
DOI 10.1007/978-3-642-15772-1_5, © Springer-Verlag Berlin Heidelberg 2013

Canadian C-Spine Rules (CCR)

No imaging is necessary if the following criteria are met.
Absence of high-risk factors:

- Age >65 years
- Dangerous mechanism – fall from an elevation of 3 ft or 5 stairs, axial load to the head (e.g., diving), motor vehicle collision at high speed or with rollover or ejection, collision involving a motorized recreational vehicle, or bicycle collision
- Paresthesias in the extremities

Low-risk factors that allow safe assessment of range of motion:

- Simple rear-end motor vehicle collision – excludes being pushed into oncoming traffic, being hit by a bus, a large truck, or a high speed vehicle, or a rollover
- Sitting position
- Ambulatory at any time
- Delayed onset of neck pain
- No midline cervical tenderness
  Able to actively rotate neck 45° left and right

A 23-year-old man with suspected cervical spine trauma after a low-speed motor vehicle collision complaining of neck pain. He is alert and sitting upright. On exam, no point tenderness over posterior midline of spine or focal neurologic deficit is elicited.

a. X-ray cervical spine lateral view only
b. X-ray cervical spine lateral, anteroposterior, and open mouth views
c. CT cervical spine with sagittal and coronal reformats
d. MRI cervical spine
e. No ideal imaging exam

Cervical spine imaging not indicated by NEXUS or CCR clinical criteria. Patient meets low-risk criteria.

a. X-ray cervical spine lateral views only is usually not appropriate (1).
b. X-ray cervical spine lateral, anteroposterior, and open mouth views is usually not appropriate (1).
c. CT cervical spine with sagittal and coronal reformats is usually not appropriate (1).
d. MRI cervical spine is usually not appropriate (1).
e. *No ideal imaging exam* is the correct answer.

A 33-year-old man with suspected cervical spine trauma after a high-speed motor vehicle accident complaining of neck pain. On exam, point tenderness over posterior midline of spine is elicited.

a. X-ray cervical spine lateral view only
b. X-ray cervical spine anteroposterior, lateral, and open mouth views
c. CT cervical spine with sagittal and coronal reformats
d. MRI cervical spine
e. No ideal imaging exam

Suspected acute cervical spine trauma. Imaging indicated by clinical criteria (NEXUS or CCR), not otherwise specified.

a. X-ray cervical spine lateral only may sometimes be appropriate. It may be useful if CT reconstructions are not optimal (6).
b. X-ray cervical spine anteroposterior, lateral, and open mouth views is usually not appropriate. It may be used in addition to CT, but not instead of CT (2).
c. *CT cervical spine with sagittal and coronal reformats* is the most appropriate (9).
d. MRI cervical spine is usually not appropriate (1).

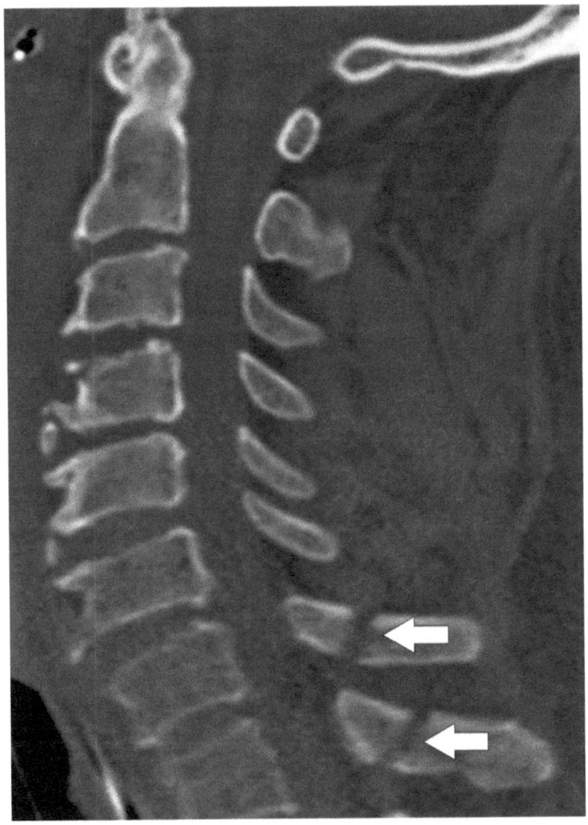

Fig. 5.1 Cervical spine fracture. Cervical spine CT sagittal reconstruction shows C7 and T1 spinous process fractures (*arrows*)

A 33-year-old man with suspected cervical spine trauma after a high-speed motor vehicle accident complaining of neck pain. Exam reveals myelopathy.

a. X-ray cervical spine lateral view only
b. X-ray cervical spine anteroposterior, lateral, and open mouth views
c. CT myelography cervical spine
d. MRI cervical spine
e. No ideal imaging exam

Suspected acute cervical spine trauma. Imaging indicated by clinical criteria (NEXUS or CCR). Myelopathy.

a. X-ray cervical spine lateral view only may sometimes be appropriate. It may be useful if CT reconstructions are not optimal (6).
b. X-ray cervical spine anteroposterior, lateral, and open mouth views is usually not appropriate (1).
c. CT myelography cervical spine may sometimes be appropriate. Use if MRI is contraindicated or inconclusive (5).
d. *MRI cervical spine* is the most appropriate. MRI and CT provide complementary information and both can sometimes be used (9).

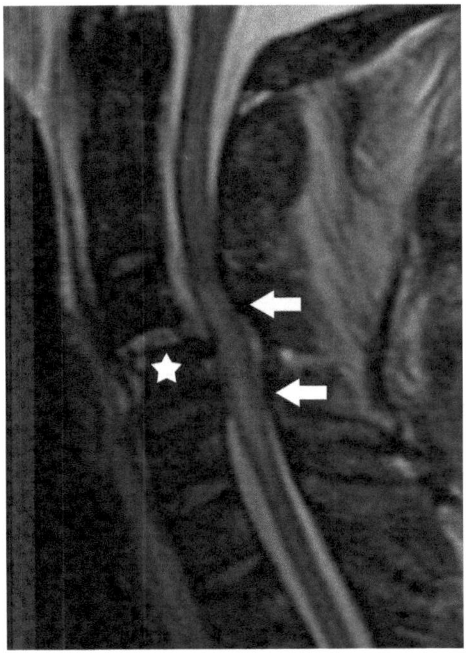

Fig. 5.2 Spinal cord injury. Cervical spine MR sagittal T2-weighted image shows cord compression and edema (*arrows*) secondary to a C5 fracture (*star*)

A 47-year-old man with suspected cervical spine trauma after a high-speed motor vehicle accident complaining of neck pain. Treatment for mechanically unstable spine is required.

a. X-ray cervical spine lateral view only
b. X-ray cervical spine anteroposterior, lateral, and open mouth views
c. CT cervical spine with sagittal and coronal reformats
d. MRI cervical spine
e. No ideal imaging exam

Acute cervical spine trauma. Imaging indicated by clinical criteria (NEXUS or CCR). Treatment planning for mechanically unstable spine.

a. X-ray cervical spine lateral view only may sometimes be appropriate (6).
b. X-ray cervical spine anteroposterior, lateral, and open mouth views may sometimes be appropriate (6).
c. *CT cervical spine with sagittal and coronal reformats* is the most appropriate (9).
d. MRI cervical spine is usually appropriate, but there is a better choice here (8).

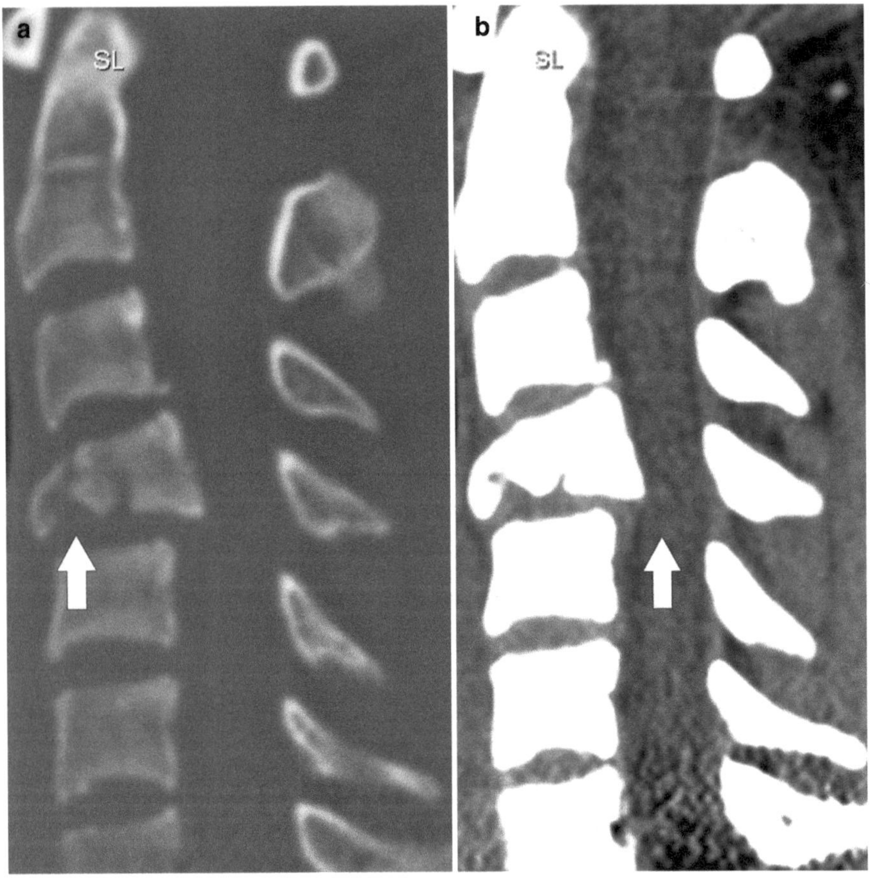

Fig. 5.3 Unstable cervical spine fracture with cord compression. Cervical spine CT sagittal (*SL*) reconstruction images in bone window (**a**) reveals a C4 fracture (*arrow*). Corresponding image in soft tissue window (**b**) reveals cord compression (*arrow*)

A 20-year-old woman with suspected cervical spine trauma after a high-speed motor vehicle accident. Patient has been unresponsive for >48 h and cannot be examined.

a. X-ray cervical spine lateral view only
b. X-ray cervical spine anteroposterior, lateral, and open mouth views
c. CT cervical spine with sagittal and coronal reformats
d. CT myelography cervical spine
e. No ideal imaging exam

Suspected acute cervical spine trauma. Imaging indicated by clinical criteria (NEXUS or CCR). Patient is persistently clinically unevaluable for >48 h.

a. X-ray cervical spine lateral view only is usually not appropriate (1).
b. X-ray cervical spine anteroposterior, lateral, and open mouth views is usually not appropriate (1).
c. *CT cervical spine with sagittal and coronal reformats* is the most appropriate. Another CT is not needed if already done on initial evaluation (9).
d. CT myelography cervical spine is usually not appropriate (2).

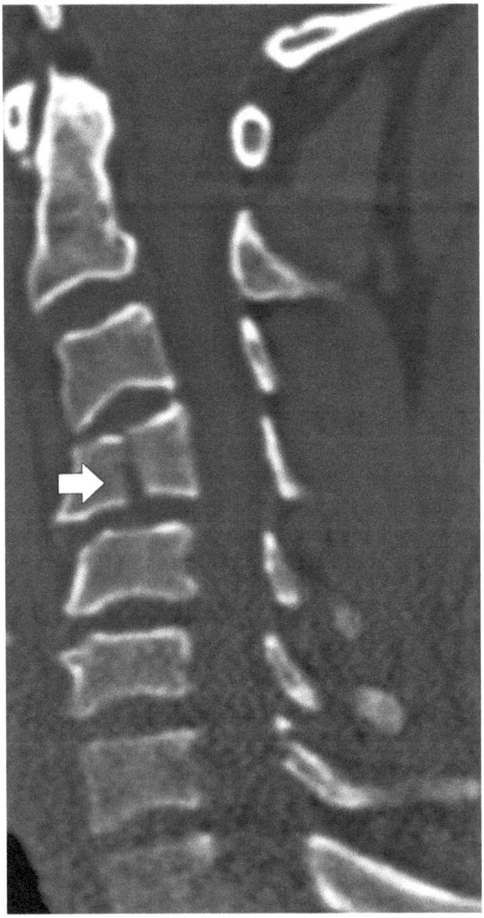

Fig. 5.4 Cervical spine fracture. Cervical spine CT sagittal reconstruction image shows an unstable C4 vertebral fracture (*arrow*)

A 54-year-old man with suspected cervical spine trauma after a motor vehicle accident. Clinical exam and cervical spine CT raises concern for arterial injury.

a. X-ray cervical spine anteroposterior, lateral, and open mouth views
b. MRI cervical spine
c. MRA neck
d. Angiography of the head and neck
e. No ideal imaging exam

Suspected acute cervical spine trauma. Imaging indicated by clinical criteria (NEXUS or CCR). Clinical or imaging findings suggest arterial injury.

a. X-ray cervical spine anteroposterior, lateral, and open mouth views is usually not appropriate (1).
b. MRI cervical spine is usually appropriate, but there is a better choice here. Use if neurological deficit is present (8).
c. *MRA neck* is the most appropriate. Either CTA or MRA can be performed depending on institutional preference (9).
d. Angiography of the head and neck may sometimes be appropriate (5).

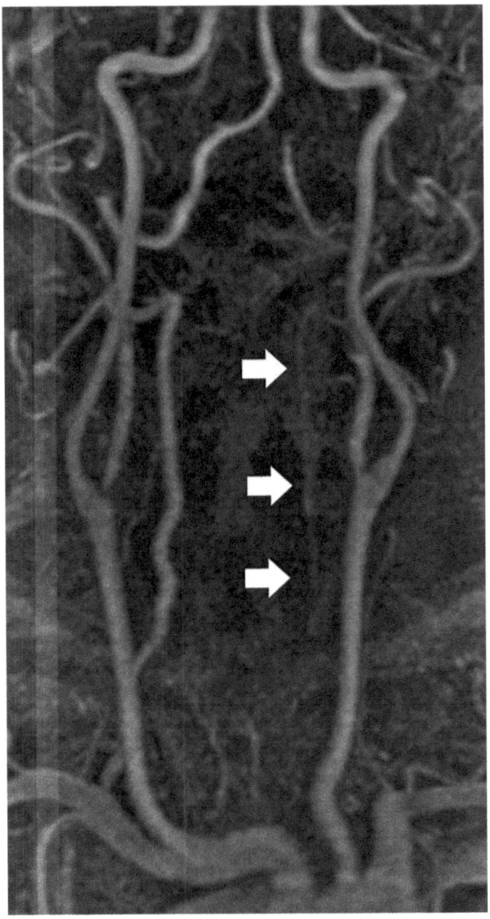

Fig. 5.5 Vertebral artery dissection. Neck MRA 3-D reconstruction coronal image reveals significant narrowing of the left vertebral artery (*arrows*)

A 32-year-old man with suspected cervical spine trauma after a motor vehicle accident. Clinical exam and cervical spine CT raises concern for ligamentous injury.

a. X-ray cervical spine anteroposterior, lateral, and open mouth views
b. X-ray cervical spine anteroposterior, lateral, open mouth, oblique, flexion, and extension
c. CT myelography cervical spine
d. MRI cervical spine
e. No ideal imaging exam

Suspected acute cervical spine trauma. Imaging indicated by clinical criteria (NEXUS or CCR). Clinical or imaging findings suggest ligamentous injury.

a. X-ray cervical spine anteroposterior, lateral, and open mouth views is usually not appropriate. Exam can be performed if needed for surgical planning (1).
b. X-ray cervical spine anteroposterior, lateral, open mouth, oblique, flexion, and extension views is usually not appropriate. Flexion and extension views are contraindicated (1).
c. CT myelography cervical spine is usually not appropriate (1).
d. *MRI cervical spine* is the most appropriate. Both CT and MRI are often needed to evaluate for soft tissue and ligamentous damage (8).

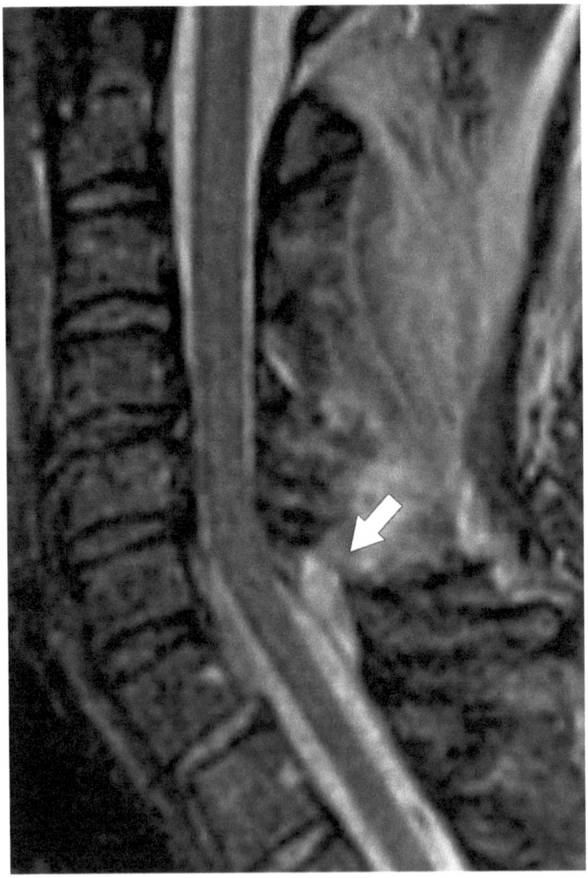

Fig. 5.6 Ligamentous injury. Cervical spine MR sagittal T2-weighted image shows disruption of the posterior longitudinal ligament (*arrow*) at the C7–T1 level

A 49-year-old woman with suspected cervical spine trauma after a high-speed motor vehicle accident. CT revealed no unstable injury but the collar has been left on due to neck pain. Patient now returns for further evaluation.

a. X-ray cervical spine anteroposterior, lateral, open mouth, and oblique views
b. X-ray cervical spine anteroposterior, lateral, open mouth, oblique, flexion, and extension views
c. CT cervical spine with sagittal and coronal reformats
d. MRI cervical spine
e. No ideal imaging exam

Suspected cervical spine trauma. Imaging indicated by clinical criteria (NEXUS or CCR). Follow-up imaging on patient with no unstable injury demonstrated initially, but kept in collar for neck pain. Patient now returns for evaluation.

a. X-ray cervical spine anteroposterior, lateral, open mouth, and oblique views is usually not appropriate (1).
b. *X-ray cervical spine anteroposterior, lateral, open mouth, oblique, flexion, and extension views* is the most appropriate. Exam can be individualized based on clinical findings (7).
c. CT cervical spine with sagittal and coronal reformats is usually not appropriate. Exam is not indicated unless follow-up radiographs or clinical examination suggest an abnormality (1).
d. MRI cervical spine is usually not appropriate. Exam is not indicated unless follow-up radiographs or clinical examination suggest an abnormality (1).

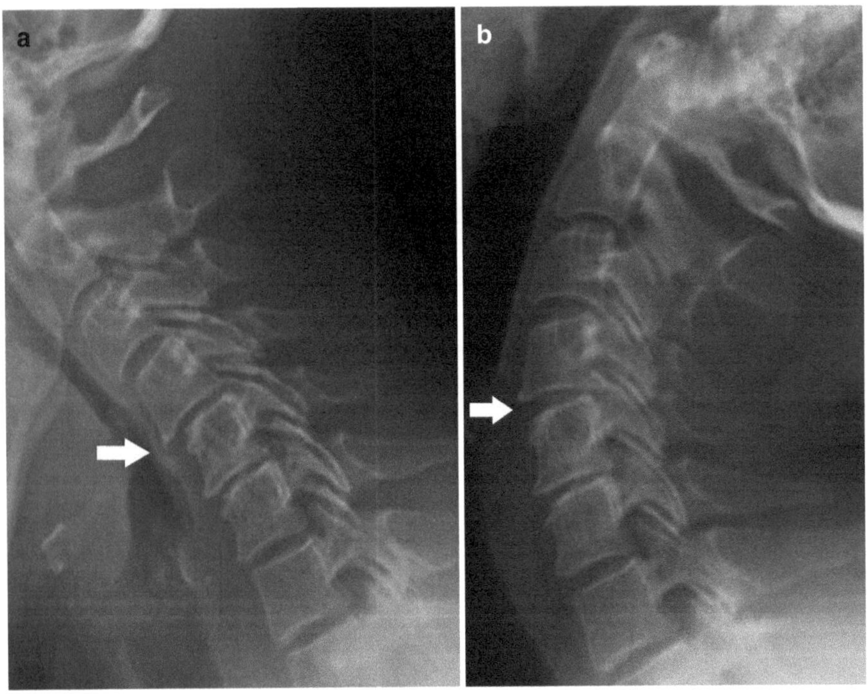

Fig. 5.7 Cervical spine instability. Cervical spine X-ray lateral flexion (**a**) and extension (**b**) views show anterolisthesis of C4 on C5 (*arrows*) with flexion but not extension, suggesting ligamentous injury

A 19-year-old woman with suspected thoracolumbar spine trauma following a high-speed motor vehicle accident.

a. X-ray thoracic or lumbar spine anteroposterior and lateral
b. CT thoracic or lumbar spine with sagittal and coronal reformats
c. CT myelography thoracic or lumbar spine
d. MRI thoracic or lumbar spine
e. No ideal imaging exam

Blunt trauma meeting criteria for thoracic or lumbar imaging with or without localizing signs.

a. X-ray thoracic or lumbar spine anteroposterior and lateral is usually not appropriate. It can be useful for localizing signs (3).
b. *CT thoracic or lumbar spine with sagittal and coronal reformats* is the most appropriate. Source images can be obtained from a dedicated spine CT or derived from abdominopelvic CT (9).
c. CT myelography thoracic or lumbar spine is usually not appropriate. Use if MRI is contraindicated (3).
d. MRI thoracic or lumbar spine may sometimes be appropriate (5).

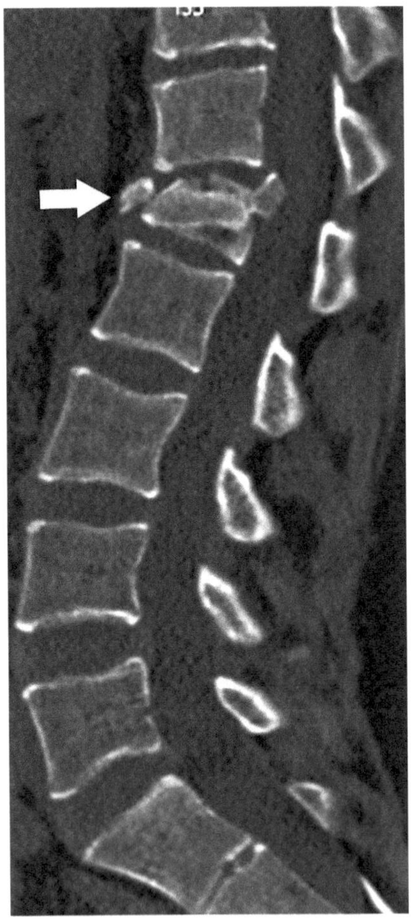

Fig. 5.8 Lumbar spine fracture. Lumbar spine CT sagittal reformation image shows an L1 fracture (*arrow*)

A 55-year-old man with suspected thoracolumbar spine trauma following a high-speed motor vehicle accident. Exam reveals neurologic abnormalities.

a. X-ray thoracic or lumbar spine lateral view only
b. X-ray thoracic or lumbar spine anteroposterior and lateral views
c. CT myelography thoracic or lumbar spine
d. MRI thoracic or lumbar spine
e. No ideal imaging exam

Blunt trauma meeting criteria for thoracic or lumbar imaging with neurologic abnormalities.

a. X-ray thoracic or lumbar spine lateral view only is usually not appropriate (NA).
b. X-ray thoracic or lumbar spine anteroposterior and lateral views is usually not appropriate (NA).
c. CT myelography thoracic or lumbar spine is usually appropriate, but there is a better choice here (7).
d. *MRI thoracic or lumbar spine* is the most appropriate. It is useful for detecting cord abnormalities (9).

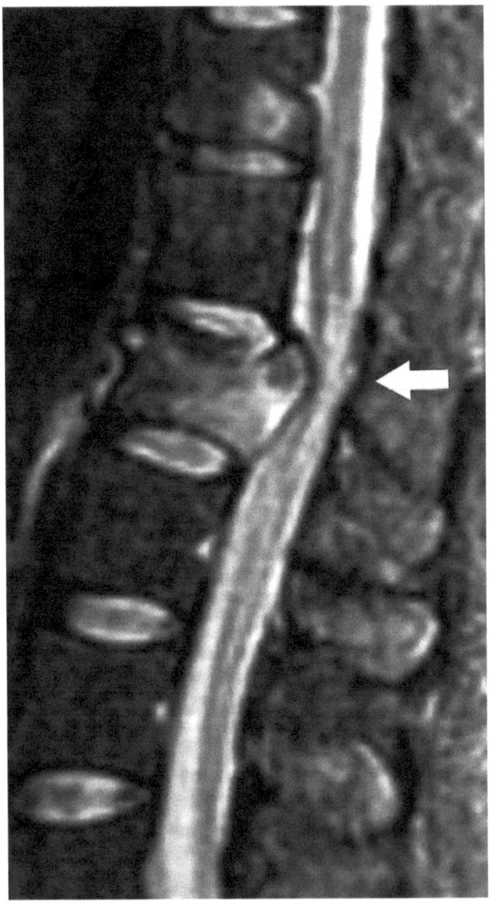

Fig. 5.9 Lumbar cord compression. Lumbar spine MR sagittal T2-weighted image reveals an L1 vertebral fracture resulting in cord compression (*arrow*)

5.2 Shoulder Trauma

A 20-year-old presents after shoulder trauma.

a. X-ray shoulder
b. X-ray arthrography shoulder
c. CT shoulder
d. MRI shoulder
e. No ideal imaging exam

Rule out fracture or dislocation.

a. *X-ray shoulder* is the most appropriate. Exams should include anteroposterior and axillary lateral or scapular Y views. Grashey views with internal and external humeral rotation are also recommended (9).
b. X-ray arthrography shoulder is usually not appropriate (1).
c. CT shoulder is usually not appropriate (1).
d. MRI shoulder is usually not appropriate (1).

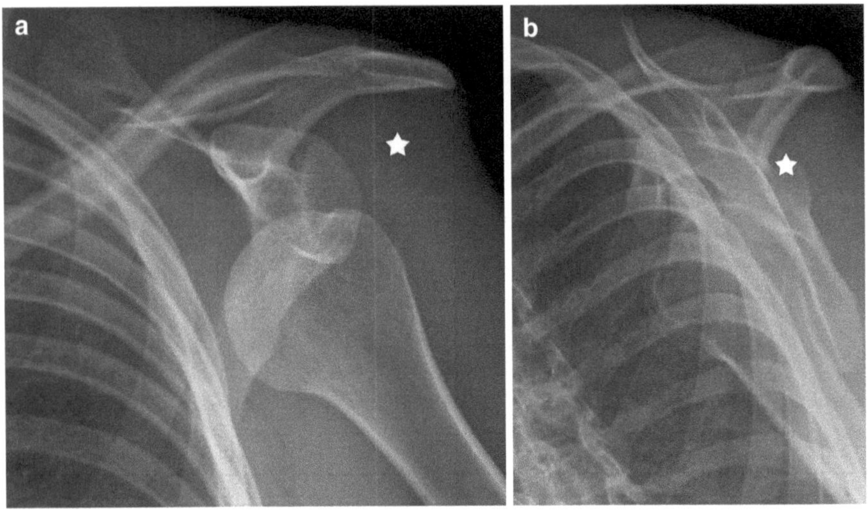

Fig. 5.10 Anterior dislocation. Shoulder X-ray anteroposterior (**a**) and scapular Y (**b**) views reveal inferior and anterior dislocation of the humeral head from its expected location (*star*)

A 50-year-old presents after shoulder trauma. Radiographs are negative.

a. X-ray arthrography shoulder
b. US shoulder
c. CT shoulder
d. MRI shoulder
e. No ideal imaging exam

Acute or recent trauma, normal recent radiographs, and significant clinical symptoms.

a. X-ray arthrography shoulder is usually not appropriate (1).
b. US shoulder is usually not appropriate (1).
c. CT shoulder is usually not appropriate (1).
d. MRI shoulder may sometimes be appropriate (5).
e. *No ideal imaging exam* is the correct answer.

A 73-year-old presents with 3-month history of shoulder pain. No history of trauma.

a. X-ray arthrography shoulder
b. US shoulder
c. CT shoulder
d. MRI shoulder
e. No ideal imaging exam

Subacute shoulder pain and suspected rotator cuff tear injury or impingement. Patient age ≥35. Normal radiographs or radiographs that demonstrate coracoacromial arch osteophytes or syndesmophytes.

a. X-ray arthrography shoulder may sometimes be appropriate. It can serve as an alternative if MR is contraindicated or if US expertise is not available (5).
b. US shoulder is usually appropriate, but there is a better choice here. Choice depends on the availability of expertise (7).
c. CT shoulder is usually not appropriate (1).
d. *MRI shoulder* is the most appropriate (9).

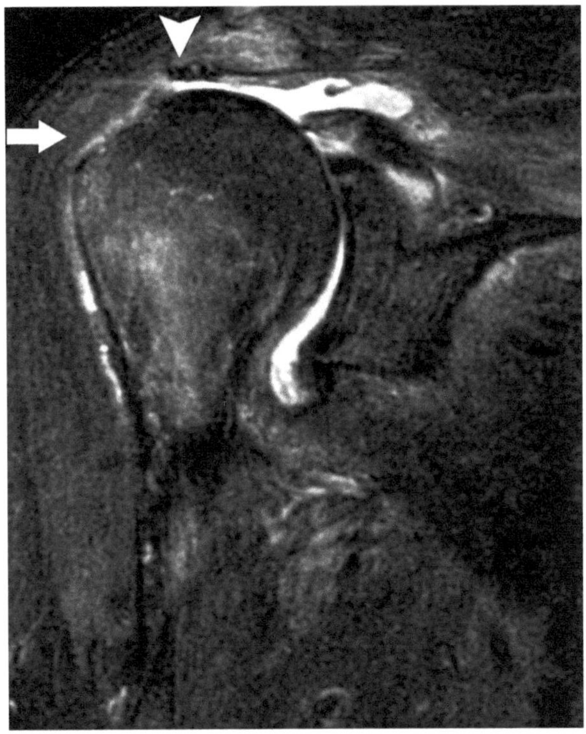

Fig. 5.11 Rotator cuff tear. Shoulder MR coronal inversion recovery image shows that the supraspinatus tendon is missing from its insertion site on the humeral head (*arrow*). The free flap of the tendon (*arrowhead*) is seen retracted medially

A 22-year-old presents with 3-month history of shoulder pain.

a. X-ray arthrography shoulder
b. US shoulder
c. CT arthrography shoulder
d. MRI shoulder
e. No ideal imaging exam

Subacute shoulder pain. Patient age <35.

a. X-ray arthrography shoulder is usually not appropriate (1).
b. US shoulder is usually not appropriate. Exam utility is limited in patients with a low likelihood of rotator cuff disease (1).
c. CT arthrography shoulder may sometimes be appropriate. This is the procedure of choice if MR is contraindicated or not available (4).
d. *MRI shoulder* is the most appropriate. Either routine MR or MR arthrography is appropriate. Choice depends on availability of expertise (9).

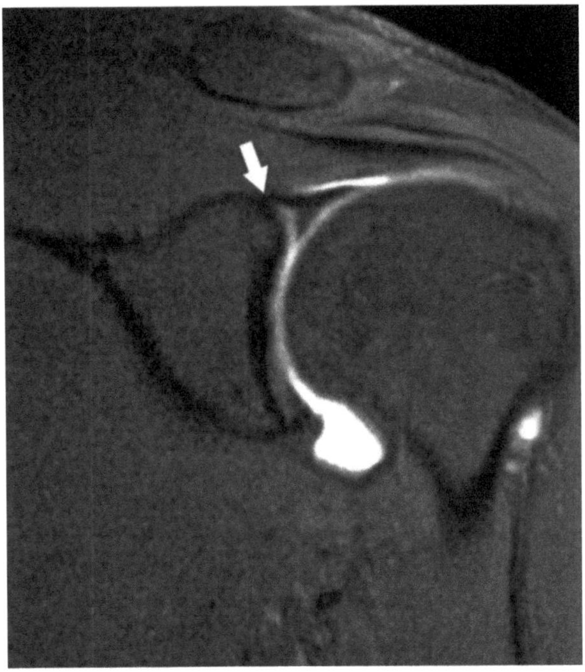

Fig. 5.12 Labral tear. Shoulder MR arthrogram coronal T2-weighted image reveals a superior labral tear (*arrow*)

5.3 Acute Hand and Wrist Trauma

A 57-year-old woman reports wrist pain after trauma.

a. X-ray wrist
b. CT wrist without contrast
c. MRI wrist without contrast
d. Tc-99m bone scan wrist
e. No ideal imaging exam

Wrist trauma, first exam.

a. *X-ray wrist* is the most appropriate. Exams should include at least a posteroanterior, lateral, and semipronated oblique views (9).
b. CT wrist without contrast is usually not appropriate (2).
c. MRI wrist without contrast is usually not appropriate (2).
d. Tc-99m bone scan wrist is usually not appropriate (2).

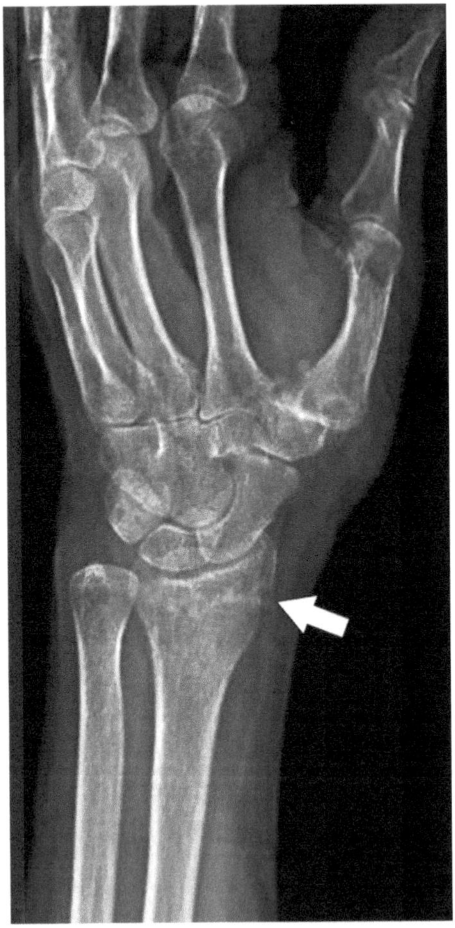

Fig. 5.13 Distal radial fracture. Wrist X-ray semipronated oblique view reveals a nondisplaced fracture of the distal radius (*arrow*)

A 31-year-old woman reports wrist pain after trauma. Exam reveals focal tenderness at the distal radius. Radiographs are normal.

a. US wrist
b. CT wrist without contrast
c. MRI wrist without contrast
d. Tc-99m bone scan wrist
e. No ideal imaging exam

Suspected acute distal radius fracture. Radiographs are normal. Next procedure.

a. US wrist is usually not appropriate (2).
b. CT wrist without contrast may sometimes be appropriate. Use only if casted and repeat radiographs are negative (5).
c. *MRI wrist without contrast* is the most appropriate. Use if immediate confirmation or exclusion of fracture is required (8).
d. Tc-99m bone scan wrist is usually not appropriate (2).

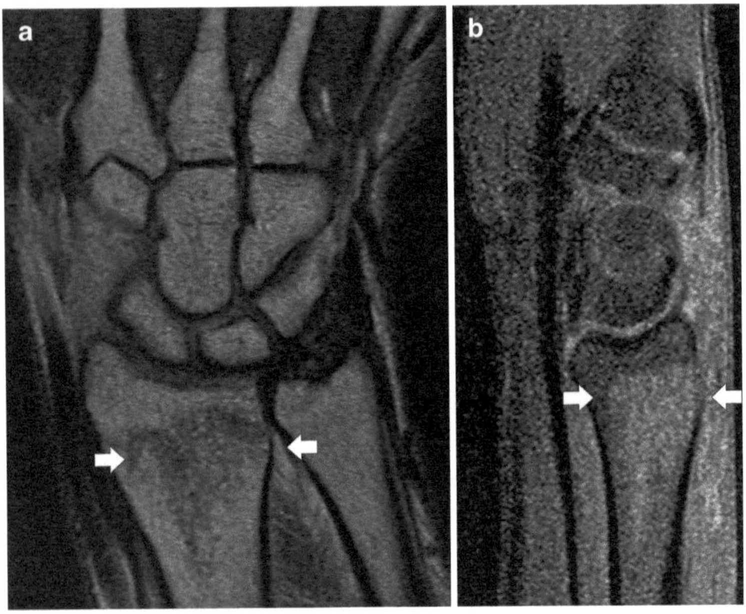

Fig. 5.14 Distal radial fracture. Wrist MR anteroposterior T1-weighted (**a**) and lateral T2-weighted (**b**) images reveal abnormal signal intensity indicating a fracture

A 59-year-old man reports wrist pain after trauma. Radiographs reveal a distal radius fracture requiring surgery.

a. US wrist
b. CT wrist without contrast
c. MRI wrist without contrast
d. Tc-99m bone scan wrist
e. No ideal imaging exam

Comminuted, intra-articular distal radius fracture on radiographs. Surgical planning.

a. US wrist is usually not appropriate (1).
b. *CT wrist without contrast* is the most appropriate (9).
c. MRI wrist without contrast is usually not appropriate (2).
d. Tc-99m bone scan wrist is usually not appropriate (1).

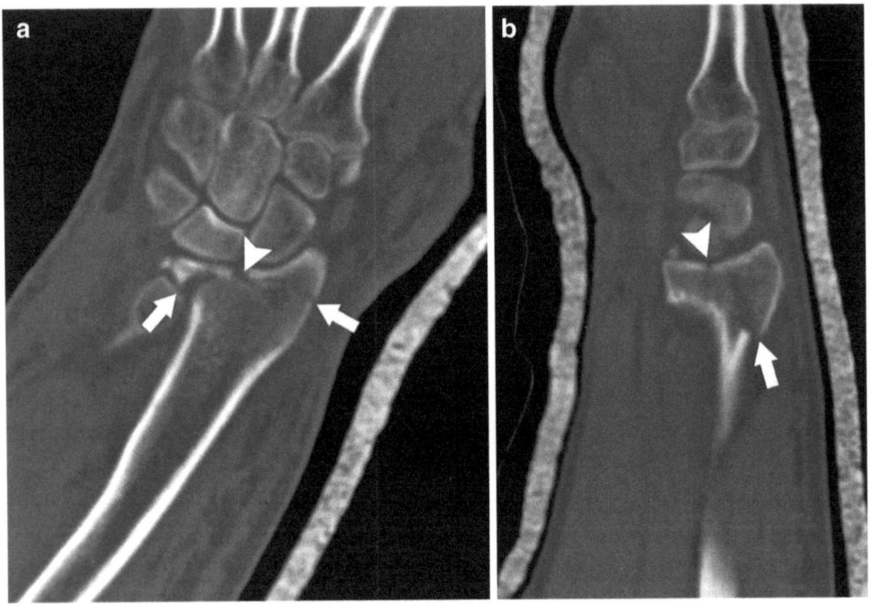

Fig. 5.15 Intra-articular distal radius fracture. Wrist CT with anteroposterior (**a**) and lateral (**b**) reconstructions reveals a comminuted fracture of the distal radius (*arrows*) extending into the radiocarpal joint (*arrowhead*)

A 62-year-old man reports wrist pain after trauma. Exam reveals scaphoid tenderness.

a. X-ray wrist
b. CT wrist without contrast
c. MRI wrist without contrast
d. Tc-99m bone scan wrist
e. No ideal imaging exam

Suspected acute scaphoid fracture, first exam.

a. *X-ray wrist* is the most appropriate. Exams should include at least posteroanterior, lateral, and semipronated oblique views. Posteroanterior view with ulnar deviation or a scaphoid view is also recommended if a scaphoid fracture is suspected (9).
b. CT wrist without contrast is usually not appropriate (1).
c. MRI wrist without contrast is usually not appropriate (1).
d. Tc-99m bone scan wrist is usually not appropriate (1).

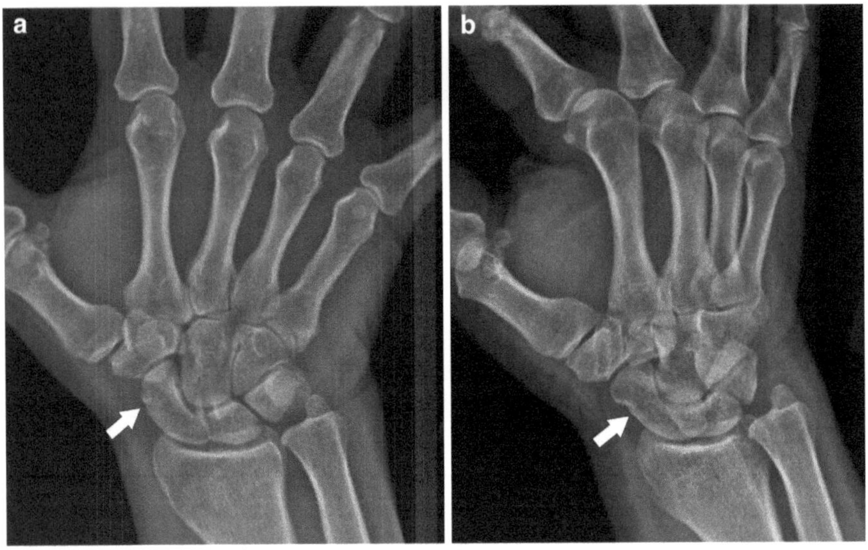

Fig. 5.16 Scaphoid fracture. Wrist X-ray reveals a scaphoid fracture (*arrows*) that is subtle on the posteroanterior (**a**) and more obvious on the semipronated oblique (**b**) view

A 20-year-old man reports wrist trauma after a fall. Exam reveals scaphoid tenderness. Radiographs are normal.

a. X-ray wrist repeated 10–14 days after casting
b. US wrist
c. CT wrist without contrast
d. Tc-99m bone scan wrist
e. No ideal imaging exam

Suspected acute scaphoid fracture. Radiographs are normal. Next procedure.

a. *X-ray wrist repeated 10–14 days after casting* is the most appropriate. MRI is equally appropriate depending on the clinical circumstances (8).
b. US wrist is usually not appropriate (1).
c. CT wrist without contrast may sometimes be appropriate (4).
d. Tc-99m bone scan wrist is usually not appropriate (1).

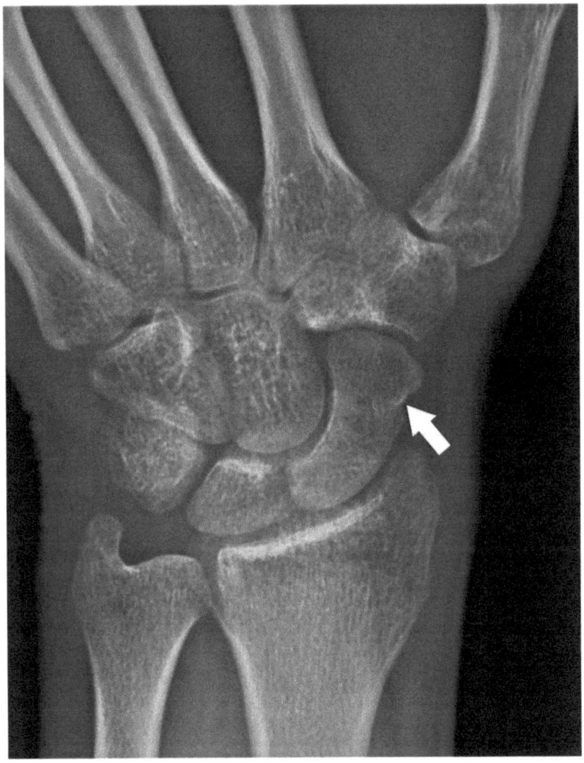

Fig. 5.17 Scaphoid fracture, partially healed. Wrist X-ray in a patient with trauma 12 days ago reveals a healing scaphoid fracture (*arrow*)

A 25-year-old woman reports wrist pain after trauma. Exam reveals scaphoid tenderness. Radiographs have been normal after 12 days of casting.

a. US wrist
b. CT wrist without contrast
c. MRI wrist without contrast
d. Tc-99m bone scan wrist
e. No ideal imaging exam

Suspected occult scaphoid fracture. Initial radiographs and repeat radiographs after 10–14 days of casting normal. There is continued clinical suspicion of a scaphoid fracture.

a. US wrist is usually not appropriate (1).
b. CT wrist without contrast is usually appropriate, but there is a better choice here. Use if MRI cannot be performed (7).
c. *MRI wrist without contrast* is the most appropriate (9).
d. Tc-99m bone scan wrist may sometimes be appropriate. Use if MRI or CT cannot be performed (5).

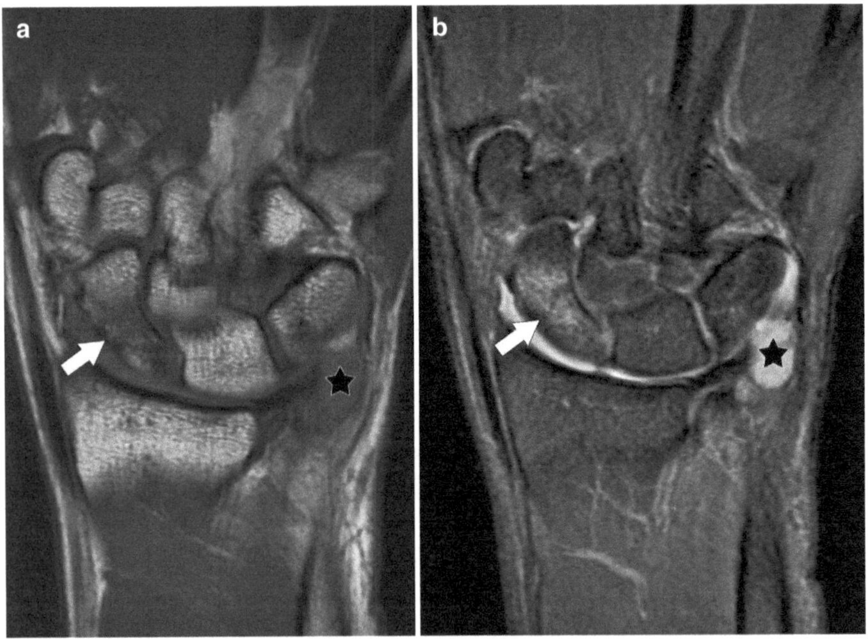

Fig. 5.18 Scaphoid fracture. Wrist MR T1- (**a**) and T2-weighted (**b**) images in a patient with negative wrist X-rays reveals abnormal linear signal in the scaphoid (*arrows*). A joint effusion (*star*) is also noted

A 54-year-old man reports wrist pain after trauma. Exam reveals instability at the radioulnar joint.

a. US wrist
b. CT wrist without contrast
c. MRI wrist without contrast
d. Tc-99m bone scan wrist
e. No ideal imaging exam

Suspected distal radioulnar joint subluxation.

a. US wrist is usually not appropriate (1).
b. *CT wrist without contrast* is the most appropriate. Bilateral wrist CT pronated and supinated is indicated in addition to radiographs of the affected side (9).
c. MRI wrist without contrast is usually not appropriate. Exams should include contralateral wrist for comparison and scan in both supinated and prone positions (2).
d. Tc-99m bone scan wrist is usually not appropriate (1).

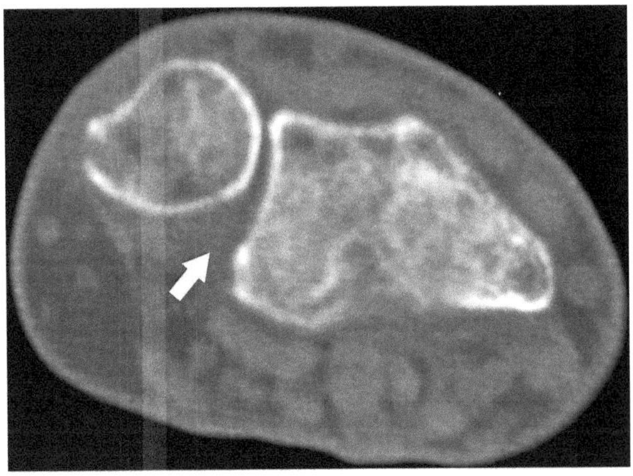

Fig. 5.19 Radioulnar joint subluxation. Wrist CT reveals misalignment of the distal radioulnar joint (*arrow*)

A 67-year-old man reports wrist pain after trauma. Exam reveals tenderness over the hook of the hamate. Radiographs are equivocal.

a. X-ray wrist
b. US wrist
c. MRI wrist without contrast
d. Tc-99m bone scan wrist
e. No ideal imaging exam

Suspected hook of the hamate fracture. Initial radiographs normal or equivocal.

a. *X-ray wrist* is the most appropriate. Exams should include semisupinated and carpal tunnel views (9).
b. US wrist is usually not appropriate (1).
c. MRI wrist without contrast is usually not appropriate (2).
d. Tc-99m bone scan wrist is usually not appropriate (2).

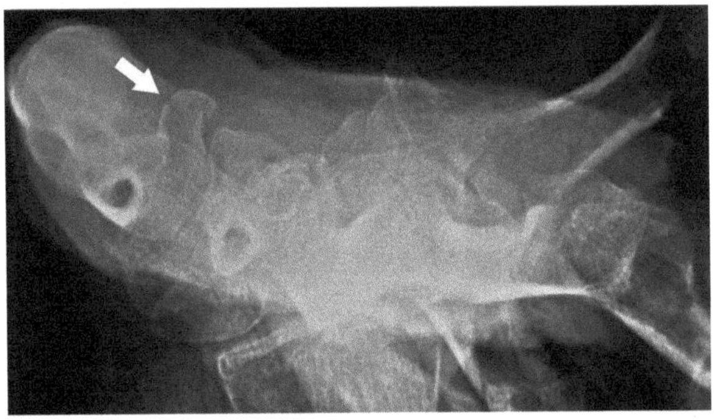

Fig. 5.20 Hook of the hamate of the fracture. Wrist X-ray carpal tunnel view reveals a nondisplaced fracture (*arrow*) of the hook of the hamate

A 37-year-old man reports hand pain after trauma. Exam reveals tenderness over the 5th metacarpal.

a. X-ray hand
b. CT hand without contrast
c. MRI hand without contrast
d. Tc-99m bone scan hand
e. No ideal imaging exam

Suspected metacarpal fracture or dislocation.

a. *X-ray hand* is the most appropriate. Exam should include at least a posteroanterior, lateral, and semipronated oblique views (9).
b. CT hand without contrast is usually appropriate, but there is a better choice here. Use if strong clinical concern exists following negative or equivocal radiographs (7).
c. MRI hand without contrast is usually not appropriate (3).
d. Tc-99m bone scan hand is usually not appropriate (1).

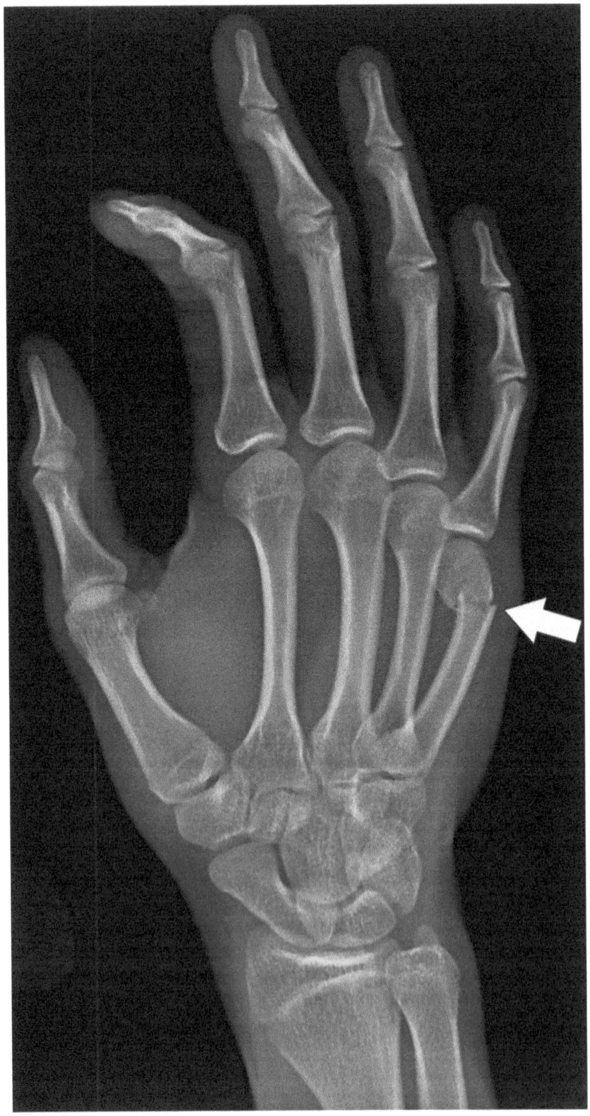

Fig. 5.21 Hand X-ray posteroanterior view demonstrates a intra-articular fracture (*arrow*) of the 5th metacarpal

A 21-year-old man reports hand pain after trauma. Exam reveals tenderness over the 3rd proximal phalanx.

a. X-ray hand or finger
b. CT hand or finger without contrast
c. MRI hand or finger without contrast
d. Tc-99m bone scan hand
e. No ideal imaging exam

Suspected phalangeal fracture or dislocation.

a. *X-ray hand or finger* is the most appropriate. Exam should include at least a posteroanterior, lateral, and externally rotated oblique view. Internally rotated oblique can also be useful but not always routine (9).
b. CT hand or finger without contrast is usually not appropriate (2).
c. MRI hand or finger without contrast is usually not appropriate (1).
d. Tc-99m bone scan hand is usually not appropriate (1).

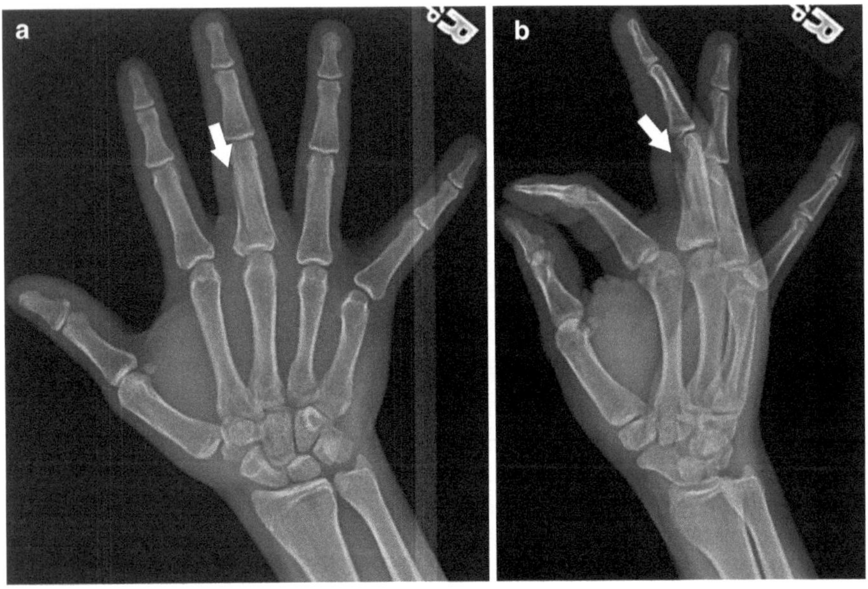

Fig. 5.22 Phalangeal fracture. Hand X-ray posteroanterior (**a**) and semipronated oblique (**b**) views reveal a comminuted fracture (*arrows*) of the third proximal phalanx

A 51-year-old woman reports hand pain after trauma. Exam reveals tenderness over the thumb.

a. X-ray thumb
b. CT thumb without contrast
c. MRI thumb without contrast
d. Tc-99m bone scan hand
e. No ideal imaging exam

Suspected thumb fracture or dislocation.

a. *X-ray thumb* is the most appropriate. Exam should include at least anteroposterior or posteroanterior, lateral, and rotated oblique views (9).
b. CT thumb without contrast may sometimes be appropriate. It may be useful for surgical planning for complex, intra-articular fractures of the first metacarpal base (5).
c. MRI thumb without contrast may sometimes be appropriate (4).
d. Tc-99m bone scan hand is usually not appropriate (1).

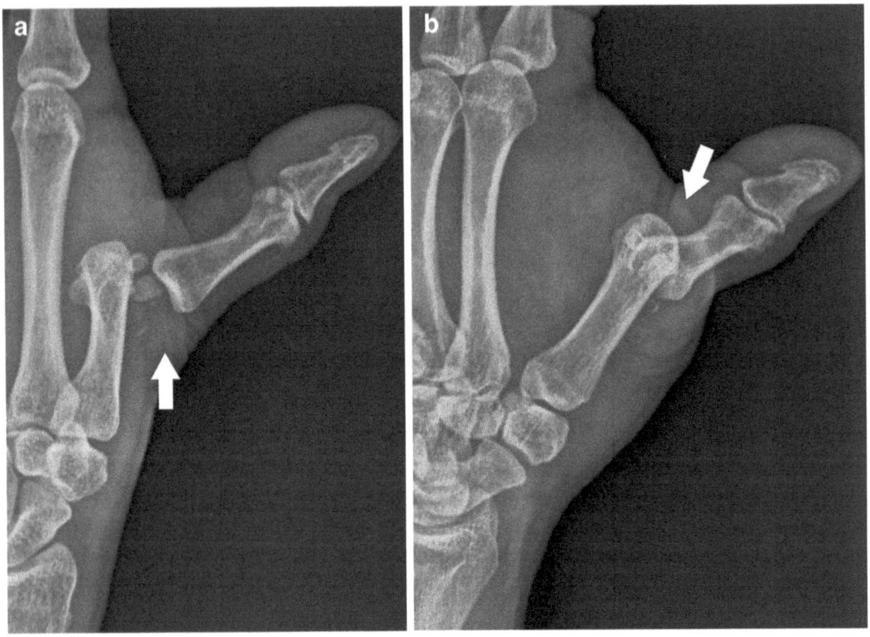

Fig. 5.23 Thumb dislocation. Thumb X-ray posteroanterior (**a**) and semipronated oblique (**b**) views reveal abnormal alignment of the metacarpophalangeal joint (*arrows*)

A 45-year-old man reports thumb pain after trauma. Exam reveals tenderness over the medial aspect of the metacarpophalangeal joint.

a. X-ray thumb
b. X-ray thumb with valgus stress and contralateral comparison
c. X-ray arthrography thumb
d. MRI thumb without contrast
e. No ideal imaging exam

Suspected gamekeeper injury (thumb ulnar metacarpophalangeal collateral ligament injury).

a. *X-ray thumb* is the most appropriate (9).
b. X-ray thumb with valgus stress and contralateral comparison may sometimes be appropriate (6).
c. X-ray arthrography thumb is usually not appropriate (2).
d. MRI thumb without contrast is usually appropriate, but there is a better choice here (8).

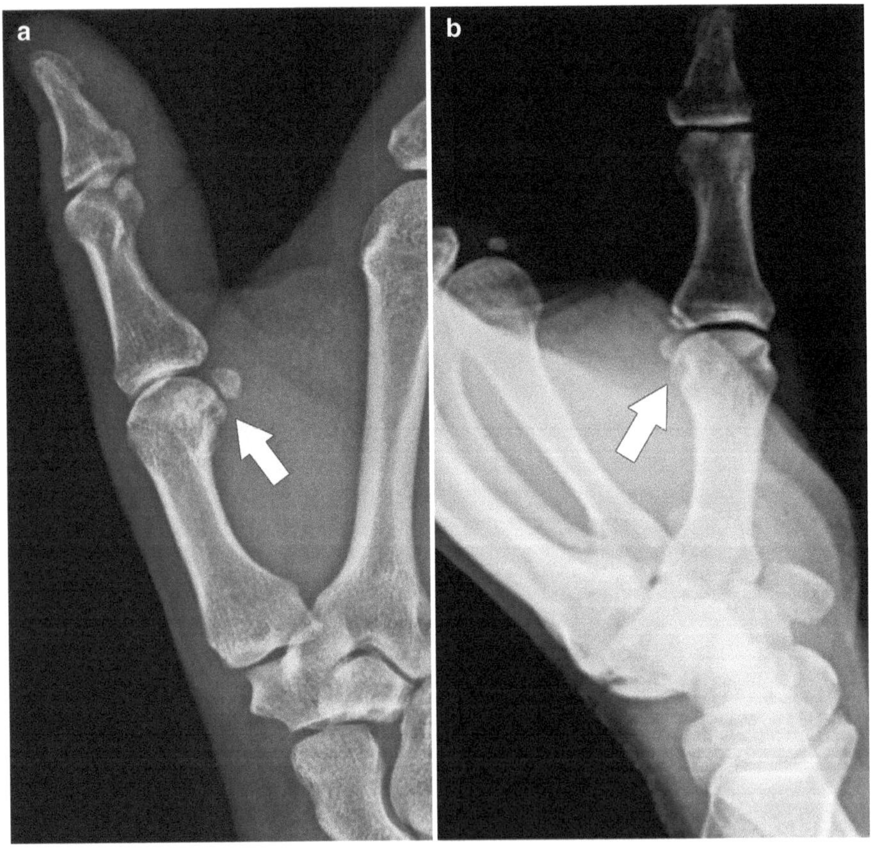

Fig. 5.24 Gamekeeper's thumb fracture. Thumb X-ray posteroanterior (**a**) and lateral (**b**) views reveal bony avulsion of the ulnar aspect of the base of the 1st metacarpal

5.4 Acute Trauma to the Knee

A 55-year-old man reports knee pain after trauma. He is able to walk. Exam reveals no focal tenderness or effusion.

a. X-ray knee
b. US knee
c. CT knee
d. MRI knee
e. No ideal imaging exam

Patient at any age except infants. Fall or twisting injury with no focal tenderness or effusion. Patient is able to walk.

a. X-ray knee is usually not appropriate (2).
b. US knee is usually not appropriate (2).
c. CT knee is usually not appropriate (2).
d. MRI knee is usually not appropriate (2).
e. *No ideal imaging exam* is the correct answer.

A 42-year-old man reports knee pain after a fall. Exam reveals focal tenderness and effusion.

a. X-ray knee
b. US knee
c. CT knee
d. MRI knee
e. No ideal imaging exam

Patient at any age except infants. Fall or twisting injury with one or more of the following: focal tenderness, effusion, or inability to bear weight.

a. *X-ray knee* is the most appropriate (9).
b. US knee is usually not appropriate (2).
c. CT knee is usually not appropriate (2).
d. MRI knee may sometimes be appropriate (5).

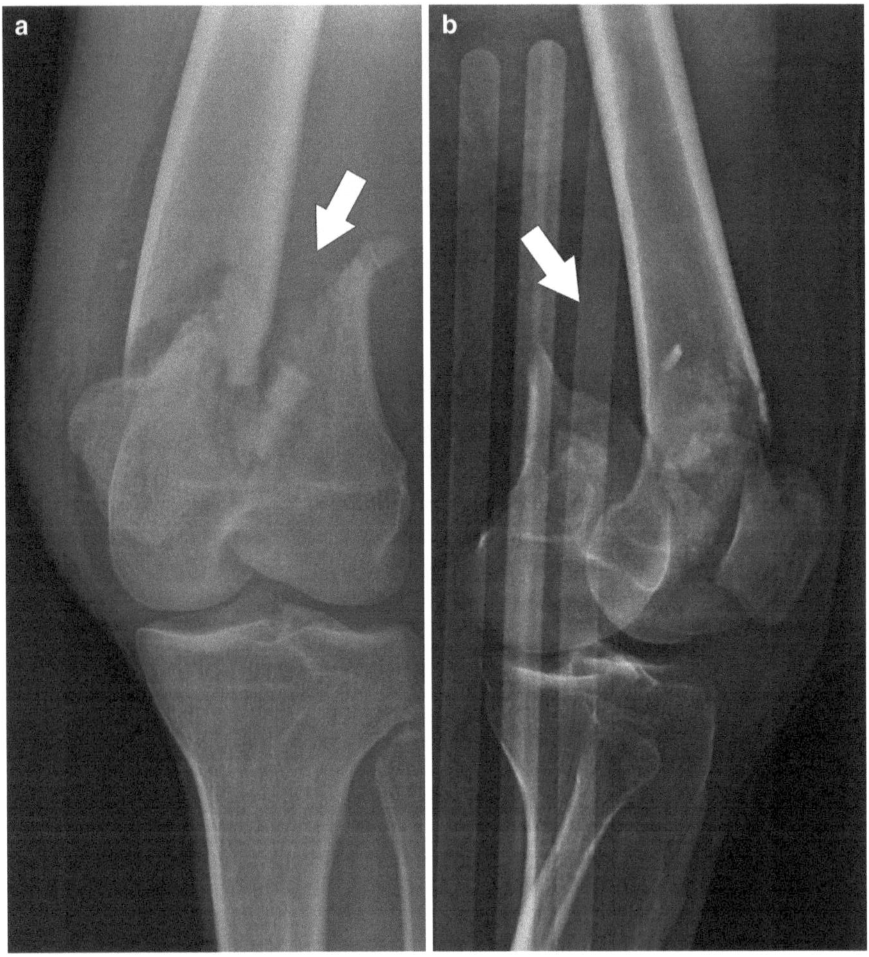

Fig. 5.25 Distal tibial fracture. Knee X-ray anteroposterior (**a**) and lateral (**b**) views of a patient in splint reveals a comminuted displaced tibial fracture (*arrows*)

A 72-year-old woman reports knee pain after trauma. She is able to walk. Exam reveals focal patellar tenderness.

a. X-ray knee
b. US knee
c. CT knee
d. MRI knee
e. No ideal imaging exam

Injury to knee, mechanism unknown. Focal patellar tenderness. Patient is able to walk.

a. *X-ray knee* is the most appropriate (9).
b. US knee is usually not appropriate (2).
c. CT knee is usually not appropriate (2).
d. MRI knee may sometimes be appropriate (5).

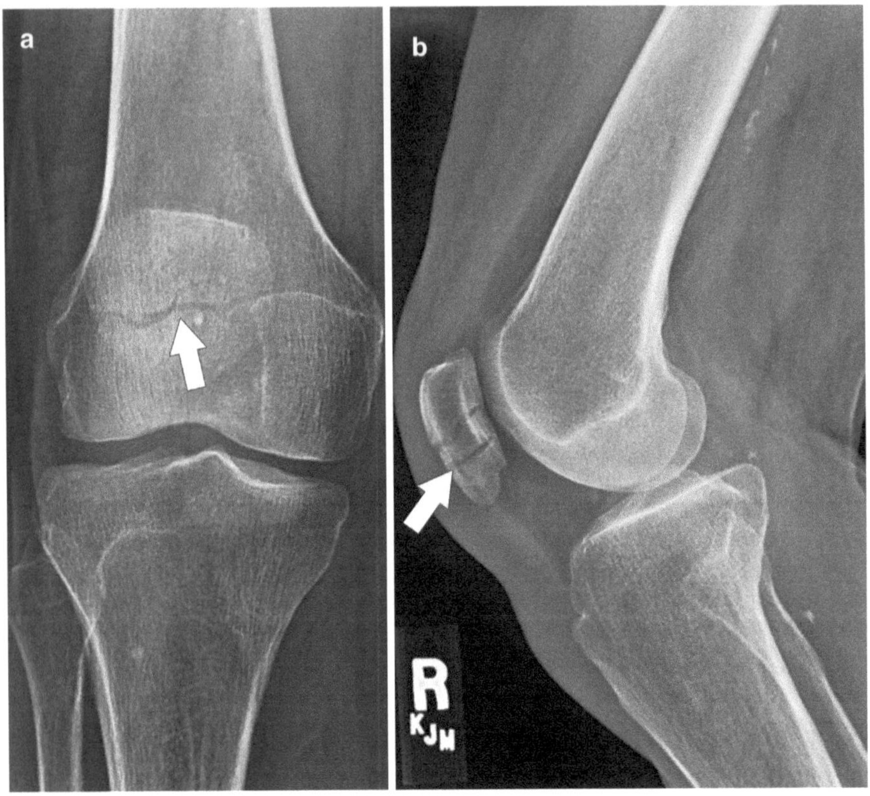

Fig. 5.26 Patellar fracture. Knee X-ray posteroanterior (**a**) and lateral (**b**) views reveal a transverse patellar fracture (*arrows*)

A 55-year-old man reports knee pain after trauma. Exam is suspicious for knee dislocation.

a. X-ray knee
b. US knee
c. CT knee
d. MRA lower extremity
e. No ideal imaging exam

Significant trauma to knee from motor vehicle accident. Suspected knee dislocation.

a. *X-ray knee* is the most appropriate (9).
b. US knee is usually not appropriate (2).
c. CT knee is usually not appropriate (2).
d. MRA lower extremity is usually appropriate, but there is a better choice here. If MRA is chosen, MRI will be performed at same time (7).

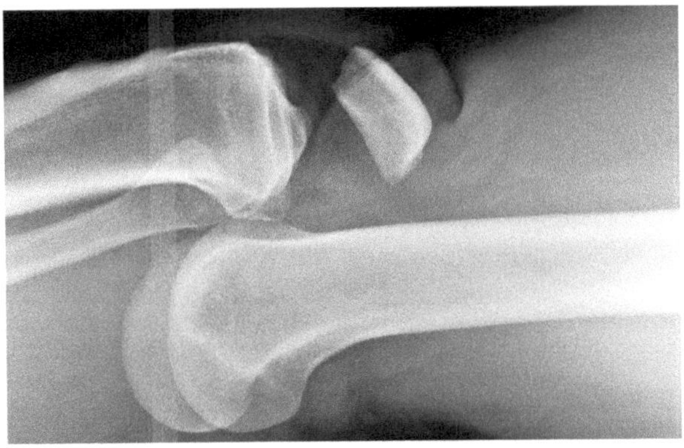

Fig. 5.27 Anterior knee dislocation. Knee X-ray shoot-through lateral view shows anterior dislocation of the tibia and fibula relative to the femur

5.5 Suspected Ankle Fracture

Ottawa Ankle Rules

In patients with acute ankle injury, radiographs are indicated only if there is pain in the malleolar area and one of the following are present.

1. Bone tenderness along the posterior edge or tip of the lateral malleolus
2. Bone tenderness along the posterior edge or tip of the medial malleolus
3. Inability to bear weight both immediately after injury and in the emergency department

A 52-year-old woman with suspected ankle fracture. Patient is unable to bear weight on the injured ankle.

a. X-ray ankle
b. CT ankle
c. MRI ankle
d. Tc-99m bone scan ankle
e. No ideal imaging exam

Patient meeting Ottawa Rules.

a. *X-ray ankle* is the most appropriate. Exam should include anteroposterior lateral and mortise views (9).
b. CT ankle is usually not appropriate (NA).
c. MRI ankle is usually not appropriate (NA).
d. Tc-99m bone scan ankle is usually not appropriate (NA).

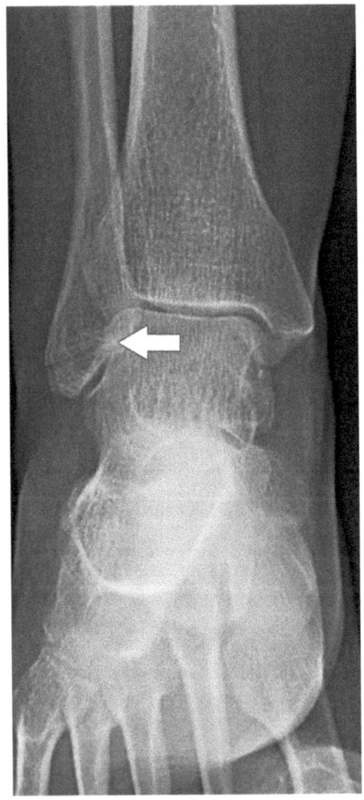

Fig. 5.28 Ankle fracture. Ankle X-ray mortis view demonstrates a fracture through the distal fibula (*arrow*) with overlying soft tissue swelling

A 55-year-old man with suspected ankle fracture. Patient is able to ambulate for >4 steps.

a. X-ray ankle
b. CT ankle
c. MRI ankle
d. Tc-99m bone scan ankle
e. No ideal imaging exam

Patient not meeting Ottawa Rules.

a. X-ray ankle is usually not appropriate (3).
b. CT ankle is usually not appropriate (NA).
c. MRI ankle is usually not appropriate (NA).
d. Tc-99m bone scan ankle is usually not appropriate (NA).
e. *No ideal imaging exam* is the correct answer.

5.6 Stress or Insufficiency Fracture

A 51-year-old woman with suspected stress fracture of the hip.

a. X-ray area of interest
b. CT area of interest without contrast
c. MRI area of interest without contrast
d. Tc-99m bone scan with SPECT area of interest
e. No ideal imaging exam

Suspected stress or insufficiency fracture. Initial imaging.

a. *X-ray area of interest* is the most appropriate. Radiograph is a required first step before consideration of other imaging (9).
b. CT area of interest without contrast is usually not appropriate (1).
c. MRI area of interest without contrast is usually not appropriate (1).
d. Tc-99m bone scan with SPECT area of interest is usually not appropriate (1).

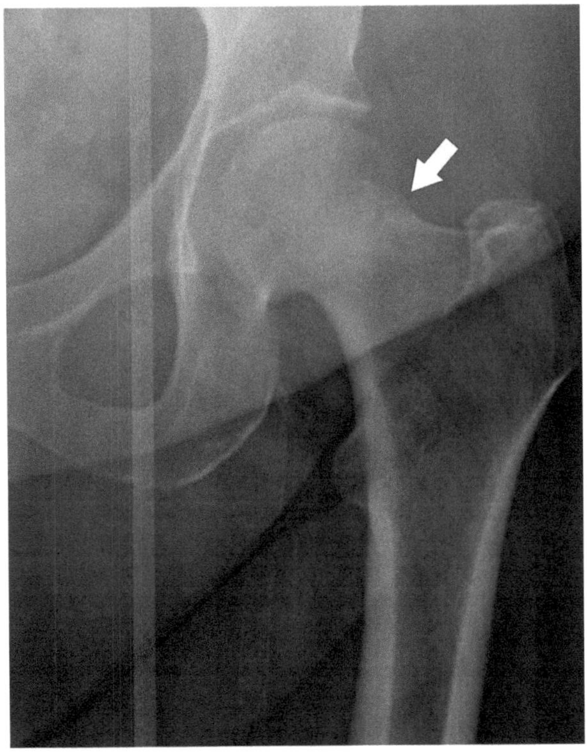

Fig. 5.29 Stress fracture. Hip X-ray anteroposterior view shows a linear lucency of the femoral neck (*arrow*)

A 30-year-old woman with suspected stress fracture of the heel. Radiographs are negative.

a. X-ray area of interest repeated in 10–14 days
b. CT area of interest without contrast
c. Tc-99m bone scan with SPECT area of interest
d. FDG-PET area of interest
e. No ideal imaging exam

Suspected stress fracture (not hip or sacrum). Radiographs are normal.

a. *X-ray area of interest repeated in 10–14 days* is the most appropriate. Many patients will recover in the interim and not return. If the immediate imaging is desired, MR or bone scan can be performed (9).
b. CT area of interest without contrast is usually not appropriate (1).
c. Tc-99m bone scan with SPECT area of interest is usually not appropriate (1).
d. FDG-PET area of interest is usually not appropriate (NA).

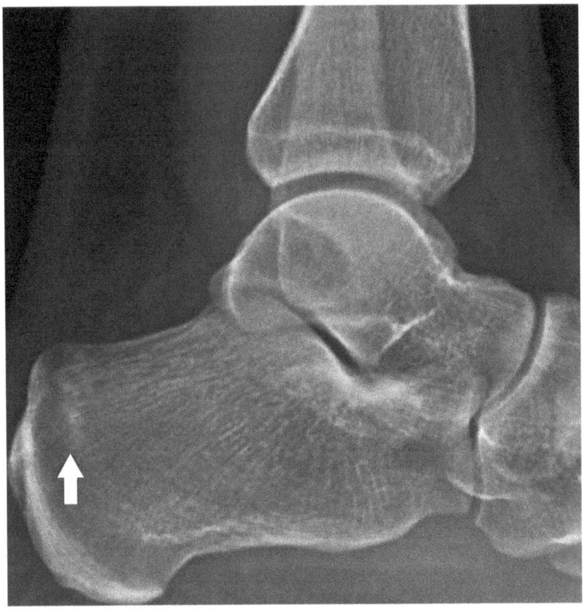

Fig. 5.30 Stress fracture. Ankle X-ray lateral view shows linear sclerosis of the calcaneus (*arrow*)

A 77-year-old woman with suspected stress fracture of the knee. Radiographs are negative. Bone scan shows increased tracer uptake in symptomatic knee.

a. X-ray area of interest repeated in 10–14 days
b. CT area of interest without contrast
c. MRI area of interest without contrast
d. FDG-PET area of interest
e. No ideal imaging exam

Suspected stress fracture, not hip or sacrum. Radiographs are normal. Bone scan is positive and nonspecific.

a. X-ray area of interest repeated in 10–14 days is usually appropriate, but there is a better choice here. Use to confirm bone scan findings or for question of a complication (7).
b. CT area of interest without contrast if MRI contraindicated (5)
c. *MRI area of interest* without contrast is the most appropriate (9).
d. FDG-PET area of interest is usually not appropriate (NA).

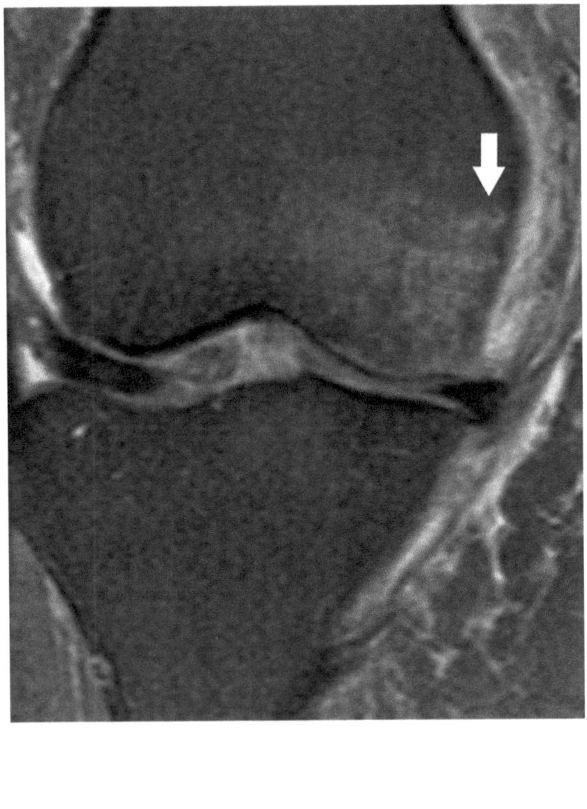

Fig. 5.31 Stress fracture. Knee MR coronal T2-weighted image reveals linear hyperintensity of the medial femoral condyle (*arrow*). Extensive edema of the surrounding soft tissue is also seen

A 55-year-old woman with suspected stress fracture of hip. Radiographs and MRI are normal.

a. X-ray area of interest repeated in 10–14 days
b. CT area of interest without contrast
c. MRI area of interest without contrast
d. Tc-99m bone scan with SPECT area of interest
e. No ideal imaging exam

Suspected stress fracture in otherwise normal patient. Radiographs and bone scan or MRI are normal.

a. X-ray area of interest repeated in 10–14 days is usually not appropriate (1).
b. CT area of interest without contrast is usually not appropriate (1).
c. MRI area of interest without contrast is usually not appropriate (2).
d. Tc-99m bone scan with SPECT area of interest (1)
e. *No ideal imaging exam* is the correct answer.

A 33-year-old woman with suspected fracture versus metastasis to the femur. Radiographs are normal. Bone scan shows increased focal uptake in symptomatic bone.

a. X-ray area of interest repeated in 10–14 days
b. CT area of interest without contrast
c. MRI area of interest without contrast
d. Tc-99m bone scan with SPECT area of interest repeated in 10–14 days
e. No ideal imaging exam

Clinical differential diagnosis of fracture versus metastasis in long bone. Radiographs are normal; bone scan hot but nonspecific.

a. X-ray area of interest repeated in 10–14 days is usually not appropriate (1).
b. CT area of interest without contrast is usually not appropriate (1).
c. *MRI area of interest without contrast* is the most appropriate (9).
d. Tc-99m bone scan with SPECT area of interest repeated in 10–14 days is usually not appropriate (NA).

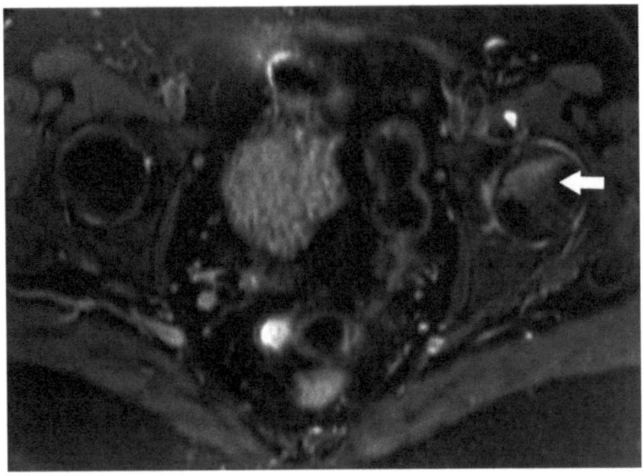

Fig. 5.32 Femoral head fracture. Hip MR axial T2-weighted image demonstrates linear abnormal signal (*arrow*) in the left femoral head

A 83-year-old woman with suspected insufficiency fracture versus bone metastasis of the sacrum. Radiographs are negative. Bone scan demonstrates increased focal tracer uptake in sacrum.

a. X-ray sacrum repeated in 10–14 days
b. CT sacrum without contrast
c. MRI sacrum without contrast
d. Tc-99m bone scan with SPECT of sacrum repeated in 10–14 days
e. No ideal imaging exam

Clinical differential diagnosis is insufficiency fracture versus metastasis in sacrum. Radiographs are normal. Bone scan hot but nonspecific.

a. X-ray sacrum repeated in 10–14 days is usually not appropriate (1).
b. *CT sacrum without contrast* is the most appropriate. Exam is definitive for diagnosing fracture (8).
c. MRI sacrum without contrast may sometimes be appropriate. Exam may show the fracture or other causes for pain (6).
d. Tc-99m bone scan with SPECT of sacrum repeated in 10–14 days is usually not appropriate (NA).

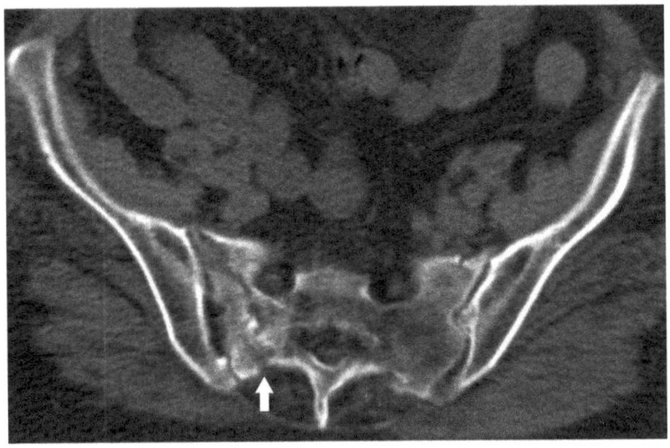

Fig. 5.33 Insufficiency fracture. Pelvic CT demonstrates linear lucency (*arrow*) through the right sacral ala

A 70-year-old woman with suspected insufficiency fracture of the sacrum. Radiographs are negative. Bone scan demonstrates increased focal linear uptake in sacrum.

a. X-ray area of interest repeated in 10–14 days
b. CT area of interest without contrast
c. MRI area of interest without contrast
d. Tc-99m bone scan with SPECT of sacrum repeated in 10–14 days
e. No ideal imaging exam

Suspected insufficiency fracture in sacrum or pelvis in elderly patient. Radiographs are normal. Bone scan hot in linear pattern typical for fracture.

a. X-ray area of interest repeated in 10–14 days is usually not appropriate (1).
b. CT area of interest without contrast may sometimes be appropriate (4).
c. MRI area of interest without contrast may sometimes be appropriate (6).
d. Tc-99m bone scan with SPECT of sacrum repeated in 10–14 days is usually not appropriate (NA).
e. *No ideal imaging exam* is the correct answer.

A 65-year-old woman with known osteoporosis with suspected insufficiency fracture of the knee. Radiographs and bone scan are negative.

a. X-ray arthrography area of interest
b. US area of interest
c. CT area of interest without contrast
d. MRI area of interest without contrast
e. No ideal imaging exam

Suspected insufficiency fracture in a patient with osteoporosis or on long-term corticosteroid therapy. Any location except the hip. Radiographs are normal.

a. X-ray arthrography area of interest is usually not appropriate (NA).
b. US area of interest is usually not appropriate (NA).
c. CT area of interest without contrast is usually not appropriate (1).
d. *MRI area of interest without contrast* is the most appropriate (9).

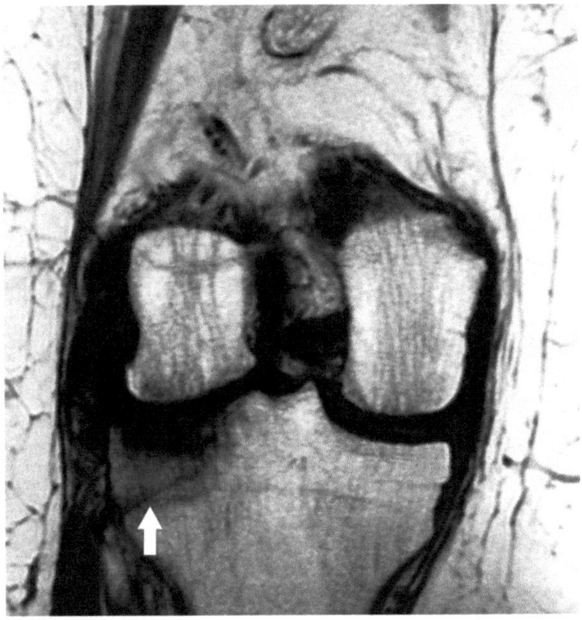

Fig. 5.34 Insufficiency fracture. Knee MR coronal T1-weighted image reveals linear hypointense signal (*arrow*) through the lateral tibial plateau

A 56-year-old man on long-term corticosteroid therapy now with suspected sacral insufficiency fracture. Radiographs are negative.

a. X-ray area of interest repeated in 10–14 days
b. CT area of interest without contrast
c. Tc-99m bone scan with SPECT area of interest
d. FDG-PET area of interest
e. No ideal imaging exam

Suspected insufficiency fracture in a patient with osteoporosis or on long-term corticosteroid therapy. Any location except the hip. Radiographs and bone scan or MRI are normal at 48 hours.

a. *X-ray area of interest repeated in 10–14 days* is the most appropriate. If diagnosis is urgent, MRI can be performed. Bone scan may be falsely negative in this patient population (9).
b. CT area of interest without contrast is usually not appropriate (1).
c. Tc-99m bone scan with SPECT area of interest is usually not appropriate (NA).
d. FDG-PET area of interest is usually not appropriate (NA).

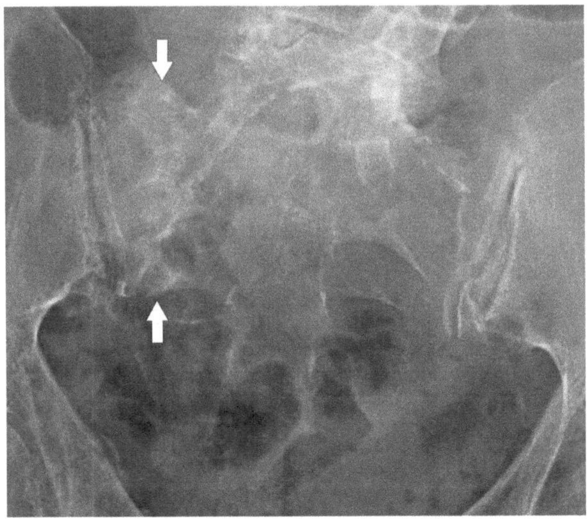

Fig. 5.35 Insufficiency fracture. Pelvic X-ray anteroposterior view shows linear sclerosis (*arrows*) of the right sacral ala

A 40-year-old woman on long-term corticosteroid therapy with suspected insufficiency fracture of the hip. Radiographs are negative.

a. X-ray hip repeated in 10–14 days
b. CT hip without contrast
c. MRI hip without contrast
d. Tc-99m bone scan with SPECT hip
e. No ideal imaging exam

Suspected insufficiency hip fracture in a patient with osteoporosis or on long-term corticosteroid therapy. Radiographs are normal.

a. X-ray hip repeated in 10–14 days is usually not appropriate (1).
b. CT hip without contrast is usually not appropriate (1).
c. *MRI hip without contrast* is the most appropriate (9).
d. Tc-99m bone scan with SPECT hip is usually appropriate, but there is a better choice here. Use if MRI contraindicated (8).

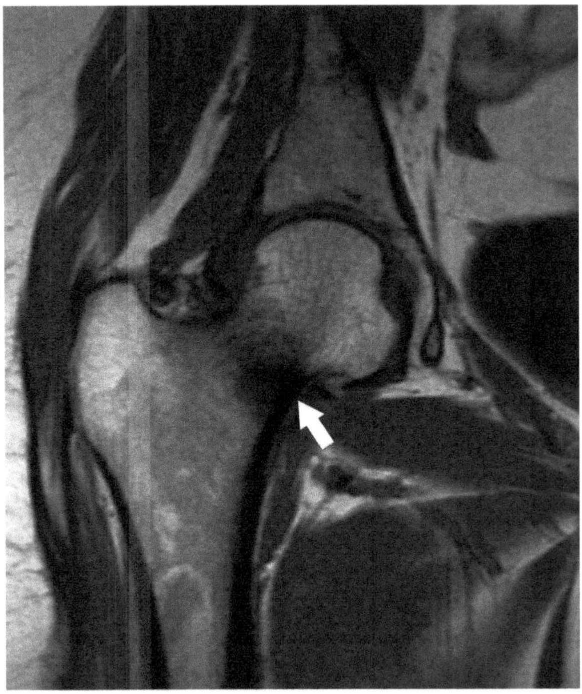

Fig. 5.36 Insufficiency fracture. Hip MR coronal T1-weighted image shows abnormal linear hypointense signal through the femoral neck (*arrow*)

5.7 Osteoporosis and Bone Mineral Density

A 57-year-old postmenopausal female presents for assessment of bone density and fracture risk.

a. X-ray thoracic or lumbar spine
b. DXA posteroanterior spine and total hip
c. QUS heel
d. QCT spine
e. No ideal imaging exam

Identification of low bone density and fracture risk. Postmenopausal females, greater than 50 years old, and males greater than 50 years old with risk factors. All races.

a. X-ray thoracic or lumbar spine is usually not appropriate. Exam is useful for diagnosing stress fractures but not osteoporosis (2).
b. *DXA posteroanterior spine and total hip* is the most appropriate (9).
c. QUS heel may sometimes be appropriate. This can be used for preliminary evaluation of patients at risk for fracture (4).
d. QCT spine is usually appropriate, but there is a better choice here. This is the preferred method of evaluation if DXA not available or cannot be performed (8).

DXA PA spine
Bone mass is low (*T* score = −3.50). At this patient's age, 1% have lower bone mineral density in this region (*Z* score = −2.30).

DXA hip
Bone mass is low (*T* score = −3.20). At this patient's age, 1% have lower bone mineral density in this region (*Z* score = −2.10).

Fig. 5.37 DXA report

A 57-year-old postmenopausal female presents for assessment of bone density and fracture risk. She has a past history of low bone mineral density.

a. DXA posteroanterior spine and total hip
b. DXA forearm
c. QCT spine
d. QCT proximal femur
e. No ideal imaging exam

Follow-up of patients with demonstrated risk for fracture or low bone mineral density.

a. *DXA posteroanterior spine and total hip* is the most appropriate (9).
b. DXA forearm is usually not appropriate. However, this is the primary site for evaluating patients with hyperparathyroidism (3).
c. QCT spine is usually appropriate, but there is a better choice here (8).
d. QCT proximal femur is usually not appropriate (3).

DXA PA spine:
Bone mass is low (*T* score = −2.60) and at this patient's age, 34% have lower bone mineral density in this region (*Z* score = −0.30).

DXA hip:
Bone mass is low (*T* score = −2.20) and at this patient's age, 34% have lower bone mineral density in this region (*Z* score = −0.30).

Fig. 5.38 DXA report

A 21-year-old man on long-term corticosteroid therapy who is at risk for low bone mineral density and fracture.

a. DXA posteroanterior spine and total hip
b. DXA forearm
c. QUS heel
d. QCT spine
e. No ideal imaging exam

Identify low bone mineral density. Premenopausal females and males 20–50 years old with risk factors. All races.

a. *DXA posteroanterior spine and total hip* is the most appropriate (9).
b. DXA forearm is usually not appropriate. Use only if spine or hip exam cannot be performed. However, this is the primary site for evaluating patients with hyperparathyroidism (2).
c. QUS heel is usually not appropriate (2).
d. QCT spine is usually appropriate, but there is a better choice here (8).

DXA PA spine:

Bone mass is low (*T* score = −2.90) and at this patient's age, 34 % have lower bone mineral density in this region (*Z* score = −0.30).

DXA hip:

Bone mass is normal (*T* score = −1.10) and at this patient's age, 11 % have lower bone mineral density in this region (*Z* score = −1.10).

Fig. 5.39 DXA report

A 42-year-old woman on long-term corticosteroid therapy known to be at risk for fracture from low bone mineral density now presents for follow-up.

a. DXA posteroanterior spine and total hip
b. DXA forearm
c. QCT spine
d. QCT proximal femur
e. No ideal imaging exam

Follow-up to known low bone mineral density. Premenopausal females and males 20–50 years old with risk factors. All races.

a. *DXA posteroanterior spine and total hip* is the most appropriate (9).
b. DXA forearm is usually not appropriate. However, this is the primary site for evaluating patients with hyperparathyroidism (1).
c. QCT spine is usually appropriate, but there is a better choice here (8).
d. QCT proximal femur is usually not appropriate (3).

DXA PA spine:

Bone mass is normal (*T* score = −0.40) and at this patient's age, 42 % have lower bone mineral density in this region (*Z* score = −0.10).

DXA hip:

Bone mass is borderline low (*T* score = −1.50) and at this patient's age, 9 % have lower bone mineral density in this region (*Z* score = −1.20).

Fig. 5.40 DXA report

A 52-year-old female with severe degenerative spine changes due to scoliosis presents for assessment of bone density and fracture risk.

a. DXA proximal femur and femoral neck and total hip
b. DXA forearm
c. QCT spine
d. QCT proximal femur
e. No ideal imaging exam

Males and females greater than 50 years old with advanced degenerative changes of the spine with or without scoliosis.

a. *DXA proximal femur and femoral neck and total hip* is the most appropriate. When posteroanterior spine cannot be assessed, bilateral hip scans should be performed. If only one hip is available for assessment, hip and forearm can be used (9).
b. DXA forearm is usually not appropriate. However, this is the primary site for evaluating patients with hyperparathyroidism (3).
c. QCT spine is usually appropriate, but there is a better choice here (8).
d. QCT proximal femur is usually not appropriate (3).

DXA Bilateral Hip:

Bone mass is low (*T* score = −2.30 and at this patient's age, 9 % have lower bone mineral density in this region (*Z* score = −1.30).

Fig. 5.41 DXA report

A 83-year-old woman with known vertebral body fractures presents for bone mineral density assessment.

a. X-ray thoracic and lumbar spine
b. DXA vertebral fracture assessment
c. CT thoracic and lumbar spine
d. Height by stadiometer
e. No ideal imaging exam

Suspected vertebral body fracture, incident or prevalent, based on clinical history or height loss.

a. X-ray thoracic and lumbar spine is usually appropriate, but there is a better choice here (8).
b. *DXA vertebral fracture assessment* is the most appropriate (9).
c. CT thoracic and lumbar spine is usually not appropriate (NA).
d. Height by stadiometer may sometimes be appropriate (4).
e. No ideal imaging exam

> DXA PA spine:
> Bone mass is low (*T* score = −3.70) and at this patient's age, 0 % have lower bone mineral density in this region (*Z* score = −0.90).
> Severe compression fracture of L1 is noted.

Fig. 5.42 DXA report

5.8 Imaging After Total Hip Arthroplasty

A 79-year-old woman with total hip replacement presenting for routine follow-up. She is asymptomatic.

a. X-ray hip
b. DXA total hip
c. CT hip
d. Tc-99m bone scan and Ga-67 scan
e. No ideal imaging exam

Follow-up of the asymptomatic patient with a total hip arthroplasty.

a. *X-ray hip* is the most appropriate (9).
b. DXA total hip is usually not appropriate (1).
c. CT hip is usually not appropriate (1).
d. Tc-99m bone scan and Ga-67 scan is usually not appropriate (1).

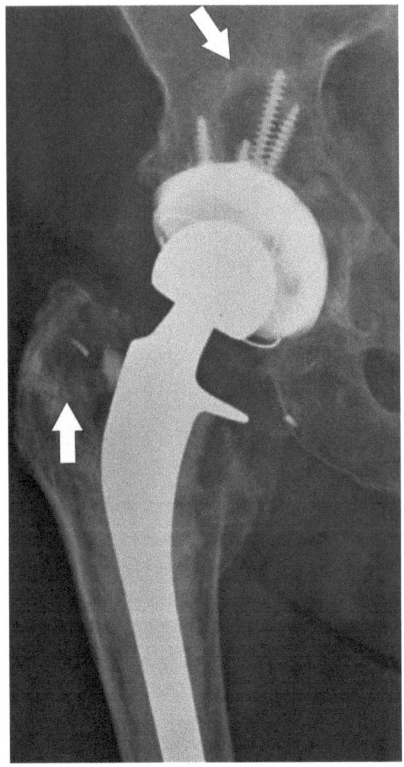

Fig. 5.43 Particle disease. Hip X-ray anteroposterior view reveals lucencies (*arrows*) adjacent to the acetabular and proximal femoral components

A 76-year-old woman with painful primary total hip arthroplasty. Hardware loosening or wear is suspected.

a. X-ray hip
b. CT hip
c. Tc-99m bone scan targeted
d. Arthrography and aspiration hip
e. No ideal imaging exam

Patient with a painful primary total hip arthroplasty. Hardware loosening or wear suspected.

a. *X-ray hip* is the most appropriate (9).
b. CT hip may sometimes be appropriate (5).
c. Tc-99m bone scan targeted may sometimes be appropriate (no consensus).
d. Arthrography and aspiration hip may sometimes be appropriate (5).

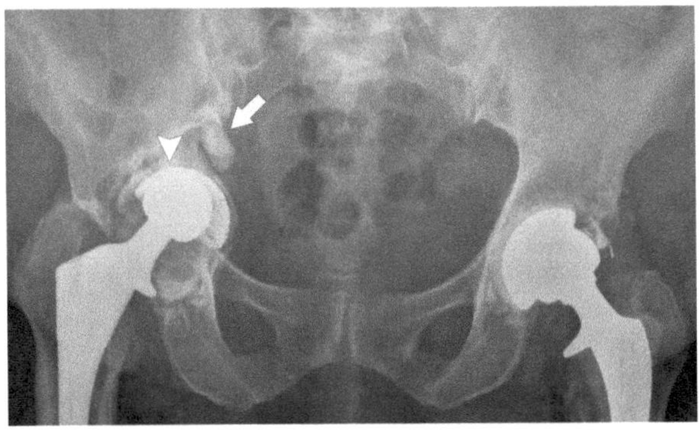

Fig. 5.44 Hardware loosening and wear. Hip X-ray anteroposterior view reveals protrusio displacement of the right hip prosthesis and acetabular disruption with extruded cement (*arrow*). The femoral ball is displaced superolaterally (*arrowhead*), indicating liner wear

A 42-year-old woman with painful primary total hip replacement. Infection is suspected.

a. Tc-99m bone scan targeted
b. Tc-99m bone scan and Ga-67 scan
c. Indium-111 white blood cell scan
d. Arthrography and aspiration hip
e. No ideal imaging exam

Patient with a painful primary total hip arthroplasty. Infection is suspected.

a. Tc-99m bone scan targeted is usually not appropriate. Exam is sensitive but not specific enough to be used as the sole procedure (3).
b. Tc-99m bone scan and Ga-67 scan are usually not appropriate. If bone scan is abnormal, Ga-67 scan can be used to detect inflammation (3).
c. Indium-111 white blood cell scan is usually not appropriate. This can be done without a bone scan to diagnose infection or can follow an abnormal bone scan to confirm infection (3).
d. *Arthrography and aspiration hip* is the most appropriate. This should be the first exam following radiographs. Other studies may be helpful but not indicated routinely (9).

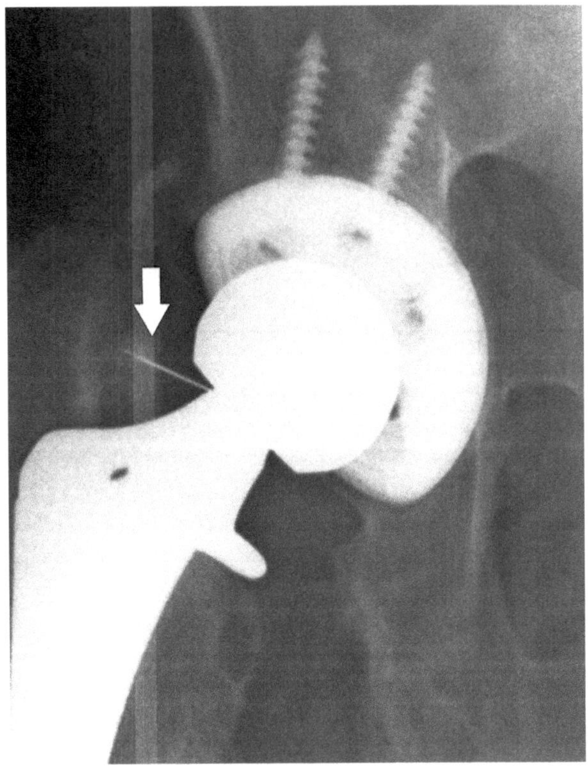

Fig. 5.45 Hip aspiration. Hip aspiration under fluoroscopy demonstrates a 22-G needle (*arrow*) in the hip joint

5.9 Imaging After Total Knee Arthroplasty

A 63-year-old woman with total knee replacement now with pain.

a. X-ray knee
b. CT knee
c. Tc-99m bone scan targeted
d. FDG-PET knee
e. No ideal imaging exam

Pain after total knee arthroplasty. Initial evaluation.

a. *X-ray knee* is the most appropriate. Standing views of both legs can be used to assess the mechanical axis of both lower extremities (9).
b. CT knee is usually not appropriate (1).
c. Tc-99m bone scan targeted is usually not appropriate (1).
d. FDG-PET knee is usually not appropriate (1).

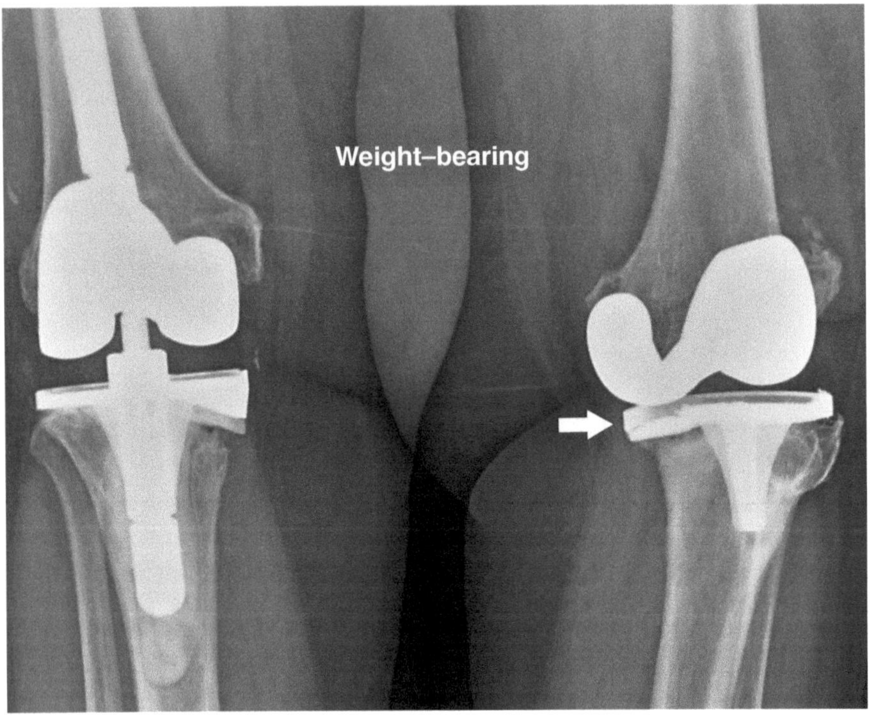

Fig. 5.46 Hardware malposition. Knee X-ray anteroposterior standing view reveals left tibia varus, indicating failure of the medial tibial tray (*arrow*)

A 55-year-old man with total knee replacement and aspirate positive for infection.

a. CT knee
b. Ga-67 scan lower extremity
c. Tc-99m bone scan and In-111 white blood cell scan
d. In-111 white blood cell and Tc-99m sulfur colloid scan
e. No ideal imaging exam

Pain after total knee arthroplasty with positive aspiration for infection.

a. CT knee is usually not appropriate (1).
b. Ga-67 scan lower extremity is usually not appropriate (1).
c. Tc-99m bone scan and In-111 white blood cell scan are usually not appropriate (1).
d. In-111 white blood cell and Tc-99m sulfur colloid scan are usually not appropriate (1).
e. *No ideal imaging exam* is the correct answer.

A 55-year-old man with total knee replacement. Radiograph reveals hardware loosening, but aspirate is negative for infection.

a. X-ray arthrography knee
b. CT knee
c. Tc-99m bone scan targeted
d. FDG-PET knee
e. No ideal imaging exam

Pain after total knee arthroplasty: positive radiograph for loosening. Negative aspiration for infection.

a. X-ray arthrography knee is usually not appropriate (1).
b. CT knee is usually not appropriate (1).
c. Tc-99m bone scan targeted is usually not appropriate (1).
d. FDG-PET knee is usually not appropriate (1).
e. *No ideal imaging exam* is the correct answer.

A 75-year-old woman with total knee replacement. Radiograph demonstrates no hardware loosening, and aspirate is negative for infection.

a. CT knee
b. Tc-99m bone scan targeted
c. In-111 white blood cell and Tc-99m sulfur colloid scan
d. FDG-PET knee
e. No ideal imaging exam

Pain after total knee arthroplasty: negative radiograph for loosening. Negative aspiration for infection.

a. *CT knee* is the most appropriate. Detects osteolysis or component malposition (7).
b. Tc-99m bone scan targeted may sometimes be appropriate. This can be used as a screening test (6).
c. In-111 white blood cell and Tc-99m sulfur colloid scan may sometimes be appropriate. Use if there is persistent high clinical suspicion of infection (6).
d. FDG-PET knee is usually not appropriate (1).

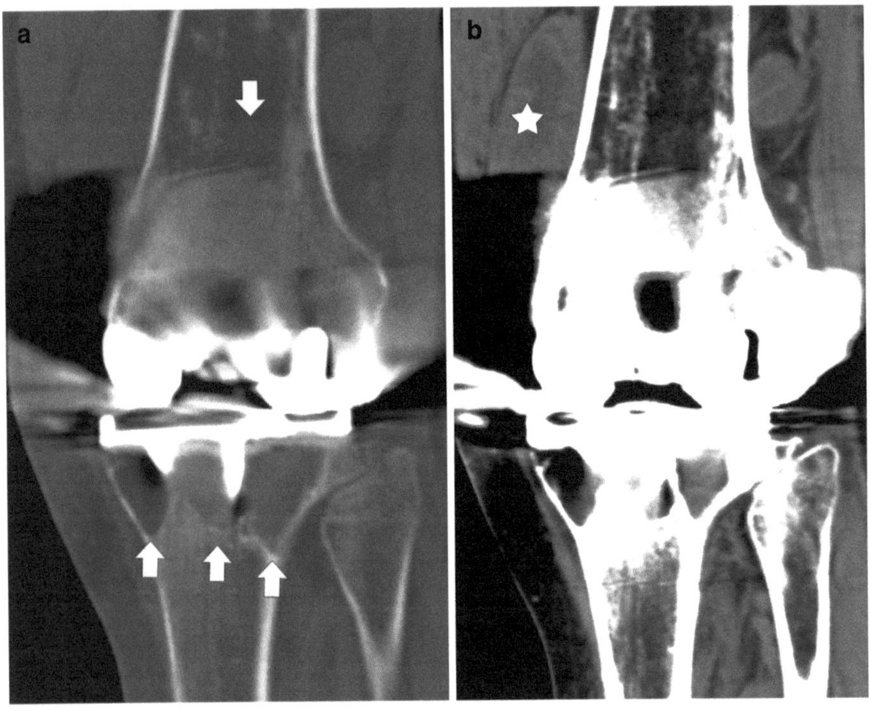

Fig. 5.47 Osteolysis after knee arthroplasty. Knee CT coronal reconstruction images in bone (**a**) and soft tissue (**b**) windows reveal lucency in bone adjacent to hardware (*arrows*) and a complex joint effusion (*star*) suggesting severe synovitis

A 66-year-old man total knee replacement presenting for routine follow-up. He is asymptomatic.

a. X-ray knee
b. Fluoroscopy knee
c. CT knee
d. MRI knee
e. No ideal imaging exam

Routine follow-up of asymptomatic patient with total knee arthroplasty.

a. *X-ray knee* is the most appropriate. Exams should include anteroposterior, lateral standing, and tangential patellar views (9).
b. Fluoroscopy knee is usually not appropriate (1).
c. CT knee is usually not appropriate (1).
d. MRI knee is usually not appropriate (1).

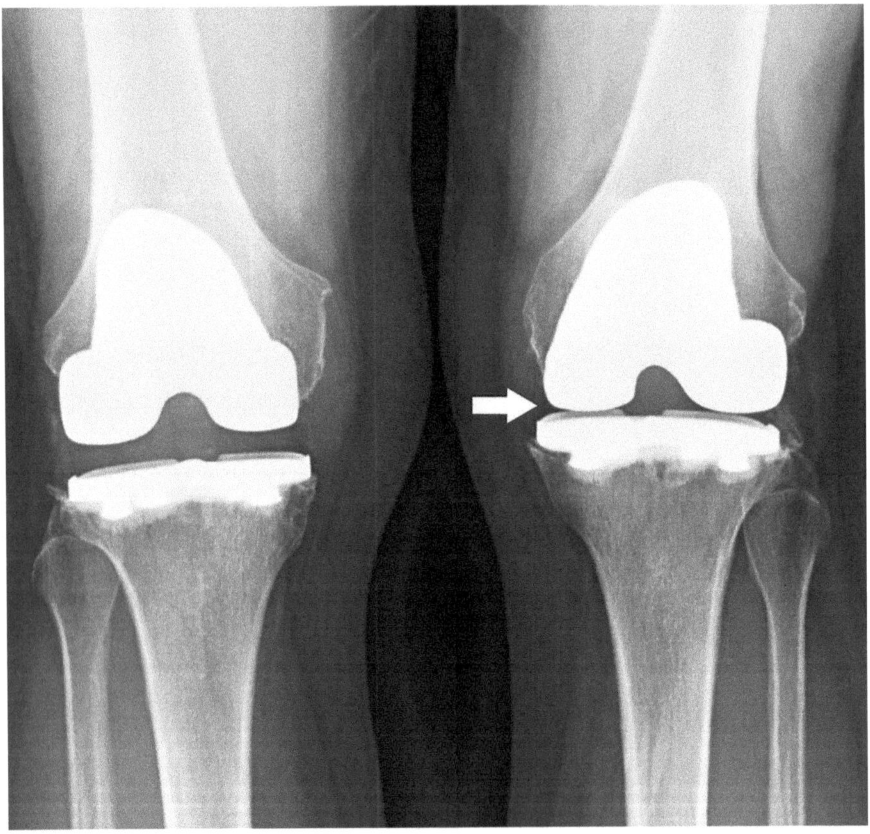

Fig. 5.48 Hardware wear. Knee X-ray anteroposterior standing view reveals thinning of the left polyethylene spacer (*arrow*)

5.10 Suspected Osteomyelitis in Patients with Diabetes Mellitus

A 63-year-old diabetic man with suspected foot osteomyelitis. He has no ulcer or neuroarthropathy.

a. CT foot without contrast
b. MRI foot with contrast
c. Tc-99m 3-phase bone scan and In-111 white blood cell scan foot
d. In-111 white blood cell scan and Tc-99m sulfur colloid marrow scan foot
e. No ideal imaging exam

Soft tissue edema without ulcer or neuroarthropathy.

a. CT foot without contrast is usually not appropriate (1).
b. *MRI foot with contrast* is the most appropriate. Radiographs and MRI are complementary. Both are indicated (9).
c. Tc-99m 3-phase bone scan and In-111 white blood cell scan foot may sometimes be appropriate. Use if MRI is contraindicated (4).
d. In-111 white blood cell scan and Tc-99m sulfur colloid marrow scan foot are usually not appropriate (1).

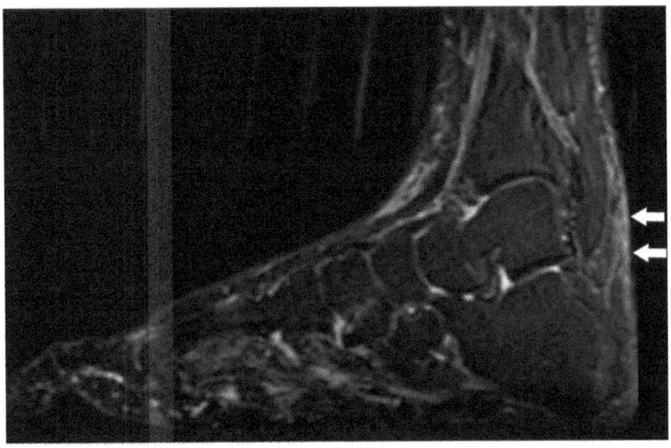

Fig. 5.49 Diabetic foot. Foot MR sagittal T2-weighted image reveals abnormal signal in the posterior soft tissues (*arrows*) but not in the underlying bone

A 22-year-old diabetic man with suspected foot osteomyelitis. He has an ulcer but no exposed bone and no neuroarthropathy.

a. X-ray foot
b. CT foot without contrast
c. Tc-99m 3-phase bone scan and In-111 white blood cell scan foot
d. Tc-99m 3-phase bone scan foot
e. No ideal imaging exam

Ulcer with no exposed bone. No neuroarthropathy.

a. *X-ray foot* is the most appropriate. Radiographs and MRI are complementary. Both are indicated (9).
b. CT foot without contrast is usually not appropriate (1).
c. Tc-99m 3-phase bone scan and In-111 white blood cell scan foot may sometimes be appropriate. Use if MRI is contraindicated (4).
d. Tc-99m 3-phase bone scan foot is usually not appropriate (1).

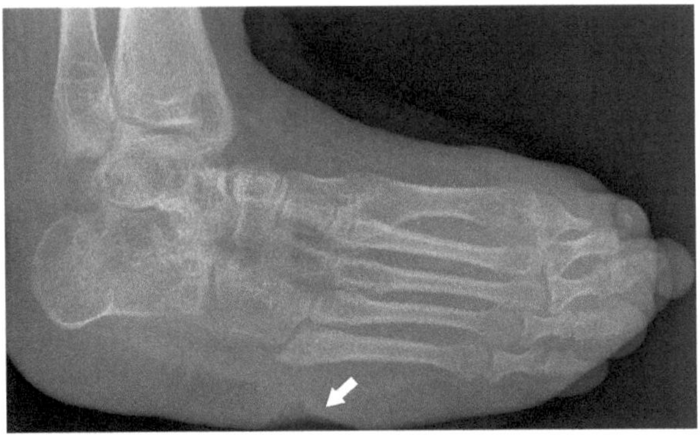

Fig. 5.50 Foot ulcer. Foot X-ray lateral view demonstrates a deep soft tissue ulcer (*arrow*) on the plantar surface with no evidence for underlying osteomyelitis. A clubfoot deformity is also noted

A 79-year-old diabetic man with suspected foot osteomyelitis. He has an ulcer but no exposed bone and no neuroarthropathy.

a. X-ray foot
b. CT foot without contrast
c. Tc-99m 3-phase bone scan and In-111 white blood cell scan foot
d. Tc-99m 3-phase bone scan foot
e. No ideal imaging exam

Ulcer with exposed bone. No neuroarthropathy.

a. *X-ray foot* is the most appropriate. Radiographs and MRI are complementary. Both are indicated (9).
b. CT foot without contrast is usually not appropriate (1).
c. Tc-99m 3-phase bone scan and In-111 white blood cell scan foot may sometimes be appropriate. Use if MRI is contraindicated (4).
d. Tc-99m 3-phase bone scan foot is usually not appropriate (1).

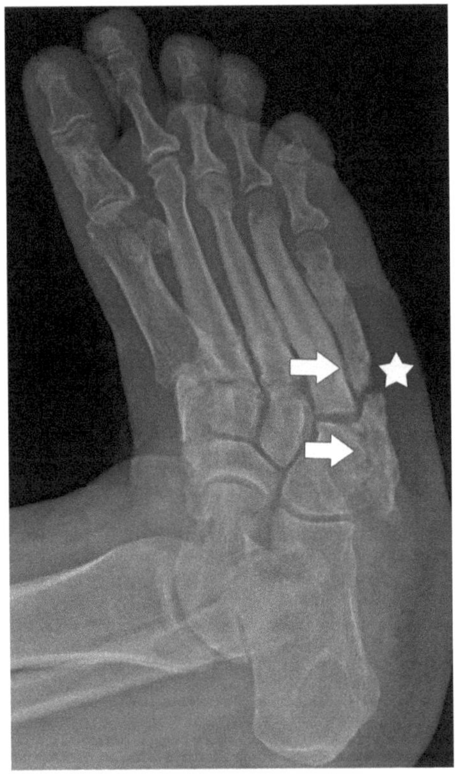

Fig. 5.51 Osteomyelitis. Foot X-ray anteroposterior view reveals bone fragmentation and sclerosis of the proximal fifth metatarsal (*arrows*) and lucency in the adjacent soft tissue (*star*), indicating an ulcer. A clubfoot deformity is also noted

A 60-year-old diabetic man with suspected foot osteomyelitis. He has neuroarthropathy but no ulcer.

a. CT foot without contrast
b. MRI foot
c. Tc-99m 3-phase bone scan
d. Tc-99m 3-phase bone scan and In-111 white blood cell scan of foot
e. No ideal imaging exam

Neuropathy without ulcer.

a. CT foot without contrast may sometimes be appropriate. Use for patients with neuropathy or contraindications to MRI (5).
b. *MRI foot* is the most appropriate. Radiographs and MRI are complementary. Both are indicated (9).
c. Tc-99m 3-phase bone scan may sometimes be appropriate. Use for patients with neuropathy or contraindications to MRI (5).
d. Tc-99m 3-phase bone scan and In-111 white blood cell scan foot are usually not appropriate (2).

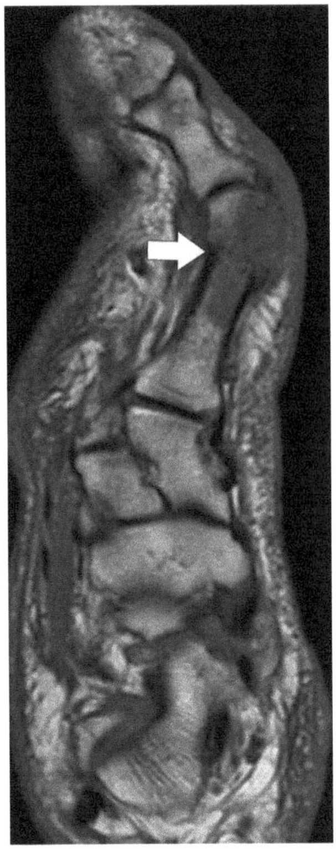

Fig. 5.52 Osteomyelitis. Foot MR axial T1-weighted image reveals abnormal signal (*arrow*) involving the first metatarsal. Also seen is marked edema of the overlying soft tissue

A 66-year-old diabetic man with suspected foot osteomyelitis. He has neuroarthropathy and an ulcer without exposed bone.

a. CT foot without contrast
b. MRI foot
c. In-111 white blood cell scan and Tc-99m sulfur colloid marrow scan foot
d. Tc-99m 3-phase bone scan and In-111 white blood cell scan foot
e. No ideal imaging exam

Neuroarthropathy with ulcer without exposed bone.

a. CT foot without contrast is usually not appropriate (1).
b. *MRI foot* is the most appropriate. Radiographs and MRI are complementary. Both are indicated (9).
c. In-111 white blood cell scan and Tc-99m sulfur colloid marrow scan foot may sometimes be appropriate. Use if MRI is contraindicated (4).
d. Tc-99m 3-phase bone scan and In-111 white blood cell scan foot are usually not appropriate (1).

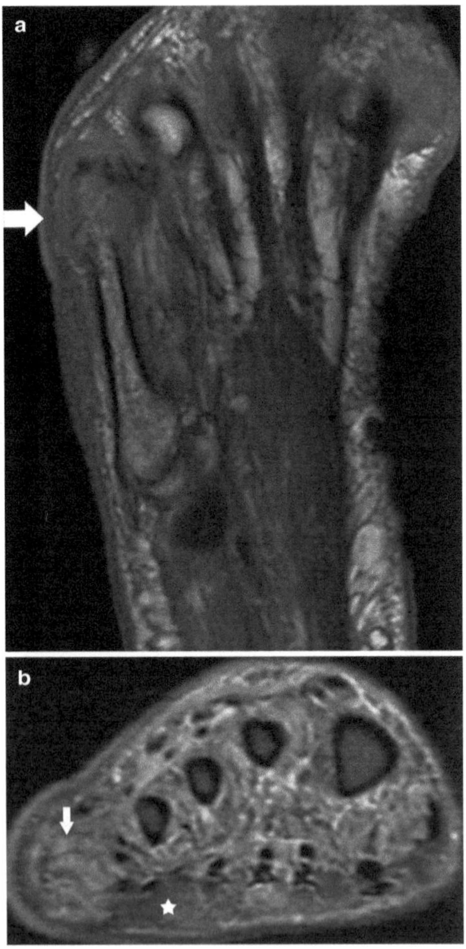

Fig. 5.53 Osteomyelitis. Foot MR axial T1-weighted (**a**) and coronal T2-weighted (**b**) images reveal bone destruction of the distal fifth metatarsal (*arrows*). Also seen is a deep soft tissue ulcer (*star*) on the plantar surface

5.11 Chronic Neck Pain

A 56-year-old man with chronic neck pain.

a. X-ray cervical spine
b. CT cervical spine without contrast
c. MRI cervical spine without contrast
d. Tc-99m bone scan neck
e. No ideal imaging exam

Patient of any age, without or with a history of previous trauma. Initial exam.

a. *X-ray cervical spine* is the most appropriate (9).
b. CT cervical spine without contrast is usually not appropriate (2).
c. MRI cervical spine without contrast is usually not appropriate (2).
d. Tc-99m bone scan neck is usually not appropriate (2).

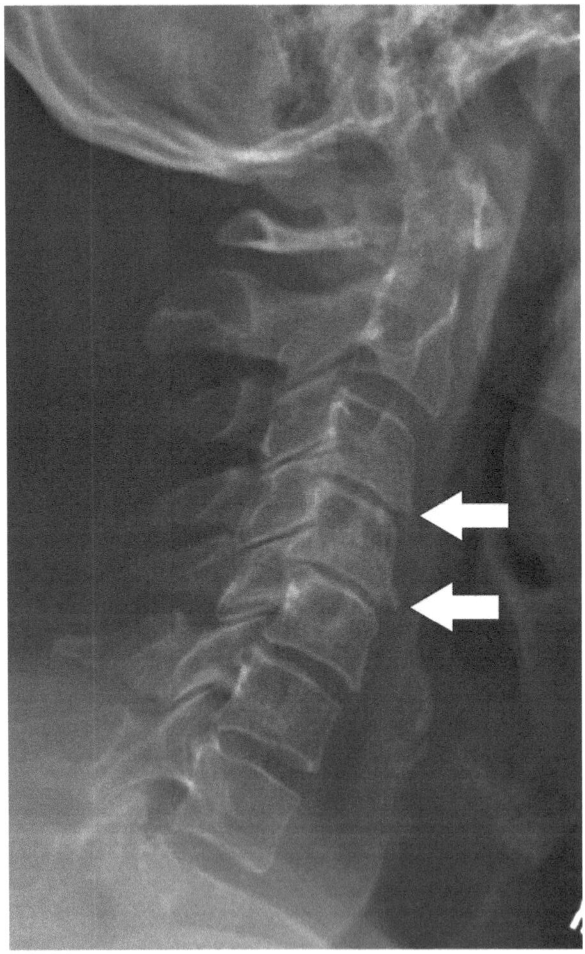

Fig. 5.54 Osteoarthritis. Cervical spine X-ray lateral view reveals disc space narrowing and osteophytes at C3–4 and C4–5 (*arrows*) levels

A 70-year-old man with history of prostate cancer presenting with chronic neck pain.

a. X-ray cervical spine
b. CT cervical spine without contrast
c. MRI cervical spine without contrast
d. Tc-99m bone scan neck
e. No ideal imaging exam

Patient of any age with history of previous malignancy. First study.

a. *X-ray cervical spine* is the most appropriate. Include anteroposterior, lateral, open mouth views (9).
b. CT cervical spine without contrast is usually not appropriate (2).
c. MRI cervical spine without contrast is usually not appropriate (2).
d. Tc-99m bone scan neck is usually not appropriate (2).

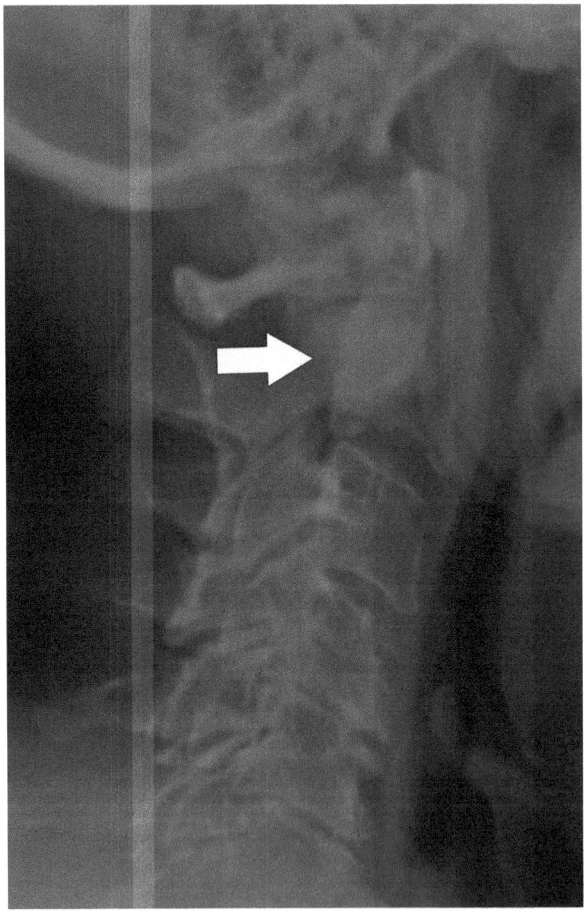

Fig. 5.55 Metastasis. Cervical spine X-ray lateral view in a patient with history of metastatic prostate cancer reveals a sclerotic lesion in C2 (*arrow*)

A 43-year-old woman with history of previous neck surgery now with chronic neck pain.

a. X-ray cervical spine
b. CT cervical spine without contrast
c. MRI cervical spine without contrast
d. Tc-99m bone scan neck
e. No ideal imaging exam

Patient of any age with history of previous neck surgery. First study.

a. *X-ray cervical spine* is the most appropriate. Include anteroposterior, lateral, open mouth, and both oblique views (9).
b. CT cervical spine without contrast is usually not appropriate (2).
c. MRI cervical spine without contrast is usually not appropriate (2).
d. Tc-99m bone scan neck is usually not appropriate (2).

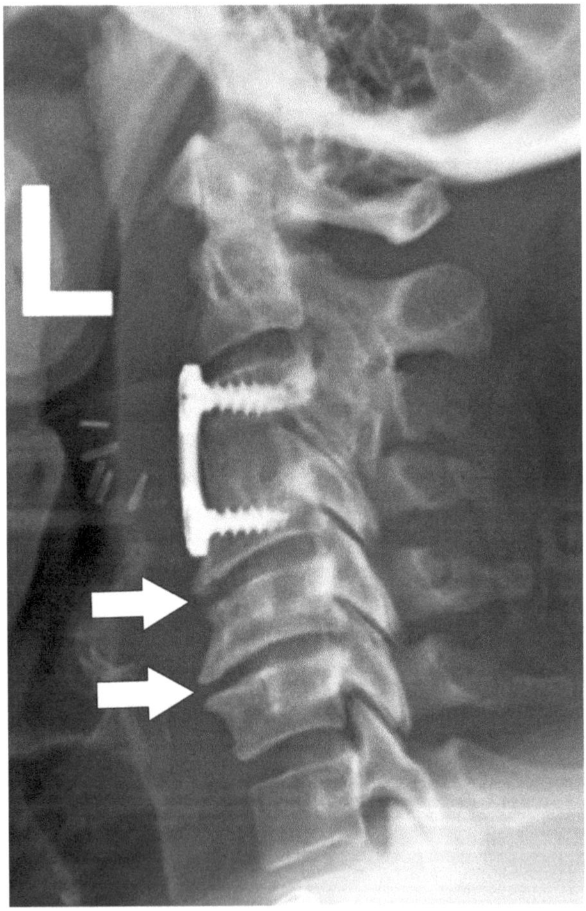

Fig. 5.56 Osteoarthritis. Cervical spine X-ray lateral view in a patient status post C3–4 anterior fusion reveals disc space narrowing and osteophytes at the C4–5 and C5–6 levels (*arrows*)

A 55-year-old man with chronic neck pain and a normal neurologic exam. Radiographs are normal.

a. X-ray myelography cervical spine
b. CT cervical spine without contrast
c. Myelography and postmyelography CT cervical spine
d. MRI cervical spine without contrast
e. No ideal imaging exam

Radiographs are normal. No neurologic findings.

a. X-ray myelography cervical spine is usually not appropriate (2).
b. CT cervical spine without contrast is usually not appropriate (2).
c. Myelography and postmyelography CT cervical spine is usually not appropriate (2).
d. MRI cervical spine without contrast is usually not appropriate (2).
e. *No ideal imaging exam* is the correct answer.

A 33-year-old woman with chronic neck pain and abnormal neurologic exam. Radiographs show spondylosis.

a. X-ray myelography cervical spine
b. Myelography and postmyelography CT cervical spine
c. MRI cervical spine without contrast
d. Facet injection and arthrography cervical spine with selective nerve root block
e. No ideal imaging exam

Radiographs show spondylosis. Neurologic signs or symptoms are present.

a. X-ray myelography cervical spine is usually not appropriate (2).
b. Myelography and postmyelography CT cervical spine may sometimes be appropriate. Use if MRI is contraindicated (5).
c. *MRI cervical spine without contrast* is the most appropriate (9).
d. Facet injection and arthrography cervical spine with selective nerve root block is usually not appropriate (2).

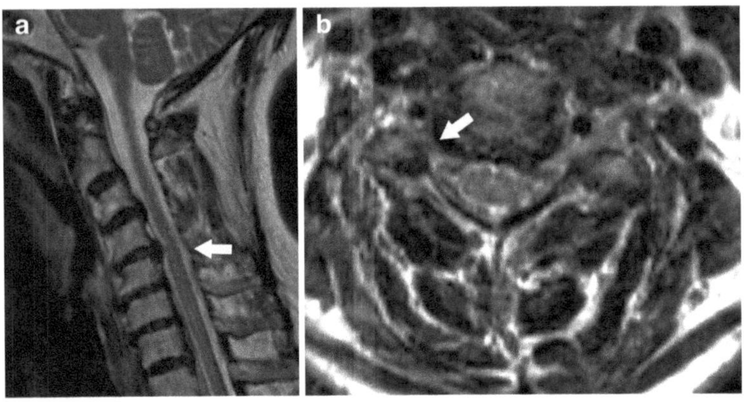

Fig. 5.57 Osteoarthritis. Cervical spine MR sagittal T2-weighted image (**a**) reveals disc bulge at the C4–5 indenting the ventral aspect of the cord. Axial T1-weighted image (**b**) reveals foraminal narrowing of the right C4 nerve root (*arrow*)

A 55-year-old man with chronic neck pain and normal neurologic exam. Radiographs show old trauma.

a. X-ray myelography cervical spine
b. CT cervical spine without contrast
c. Myelography and postmyelography CT cervical spine
d. MRI cervical spine without contrast
e. No ideal imaging exam

Radiographs show old trauma. No neurologic findings.

a. X-ray myelography cervical spine is usually not appropriate (2).
b. CT cervical spine without contrast is usually not appropriate (2).
c. Myelography and postmyelography CT cervical spine is usually not appropriate (2).
d. MRI cervical spine without contrast is usually not appropriate (2).
e. *No ideal imaging exam* is the correct answer.

A 41-year-old man with chronic neck pain and abnormal neurologic exam. Radiographs show old trauma.

a. X-ray myelography cervical spine
b. Myelography and postmyelography CT cervical spine
c. MRI cervical spine without contrast
d. Facet injection and arthrography cervical spine with selective nerve root block
e. No ideal imaging exam

Radiographs show old trauma. Neurologic signs or symptoms are present.

a. X-ray myelography cervical spine is usually not appropriate (2).
b. Myelography and postmyelography CT cervical spine may sometimes be appropriate. Use if MRI contraindicated (5).
c. *MRI cervical spine without contrast* is the most appropriate (9).
d. Facet injection and arthrography cervical spine with selective nerve root block is usually not appropriate (2).

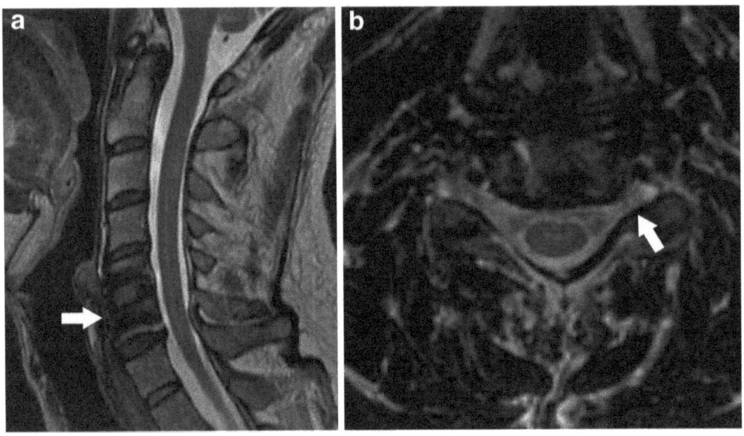

Fig. 5.58 Osteoarthritis. Cervical spine MR sagittal T2-weighted image (**a**) reveals anterior fusion hardware (*arrow*) at the C5–6 level. Axial T2-weighted image (**b**) reveals left C5 nerve root foraminal narrowing (*arrow*)

A 49-year-old man with chronic neck pain. Radiographs show bone and disc margin destruction, suggesting osteomyelitis and discitis.

a. CT cervical spine without contrast
b. Myelography and postmyelography CT cervical spine
c. MRI cervical spine without contrast
d. Tc-99-m bone scan neck
e. No ideal imaging exam

Radiographs show bone or disc margin destruction.

a. CT cervical spine without contrast is usually not appropriate (2).
b. Myelography and postmyelography CT cervical spine is usually not appropriate (2).
c. *MRI cervical spine without contrast* is the most appropriate (9).
d. Tc-99m bone scan neck is usually not appropriate (2).

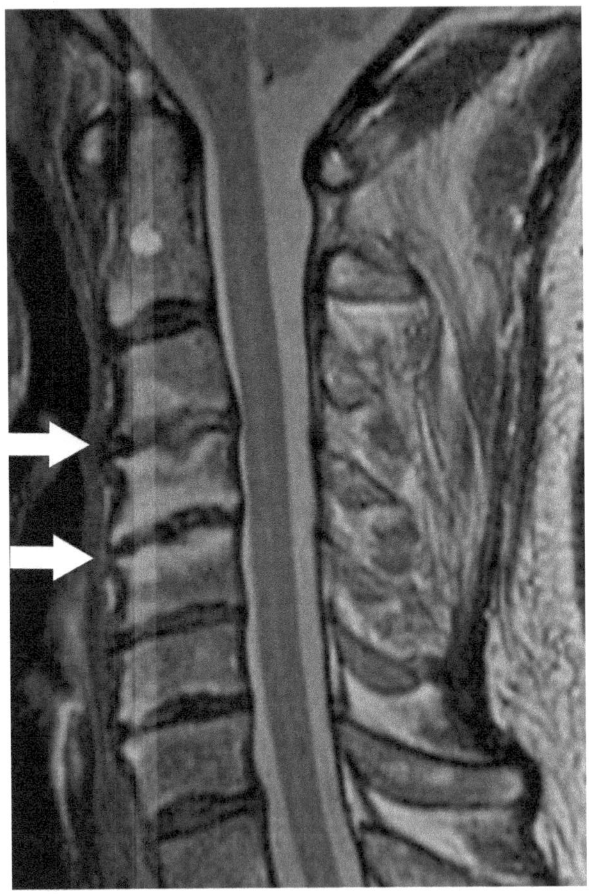

Fig. 5.59 Osteomyelitis and discitis. Cervical spine MR sagittal T2-weighted image reveals abnormal hyperintense signal in the vertebral body marrow adjacent to the C3–4 and C4–5 disc space (*arrows*). Note that the C3–4 disc also demonstrates abnormal signal

Further Reading

Suspected Spine Trauma

Hoffman JR, Mower WR, Wolfson AB, Todd KH, Zucker MI. Validity of a set of clinical criteria to rule out injury to the cervical spine in patients with blunt trauma. National Emergency X-Radiography Utilization Study Group. N Engl J Med. 2000; 343: 94–99.
Stiell IG, Wells GA, Vandemheen KL, Clement CM, Lesiuk H, De Maio VJ, Laupacis A, Schull M, McKnight RD, Verbeek R, Brison R, Cass D, Dreyer J, Eisenhauer MA, Greenberg GH, MacPhail I, Morrison L, Reardon M, Worthington J. The Canadian C-spine rule for radiography in alert and stable trauma patients. JAMA. 2001; 286: 1841–1848.

Suspected Ankle Fracture

Stiell IG, McKnight RD, Greenberg GH, McDowell I, Nair RC, Wells GA, Johns C, Worthington JR. Implementation of the Ottawa ankle rulesJAMA. 1994;271:827–3.

Neurologic Imaging

6

6.1 Head Trauma

Glasgow Coma Scale
Eye-opening response

- Spontaneous (open with blinking at baseline) – 4 points
- To verbal stimuli, command, and speech – 3 points
- To pain only (not applied to face) – 2 points
- No response – 1 point

Verbal response

- Oriented – 5 points
- Confused conversation but able to answer questions – 4 points
- Inappropriate words – 3 points
- Incomprehensible speech – 2 points
- No response – 1 point

Motor response

- Obeys commands for movement – 6 points
- Purposeful movement to painful stimulus – 5 points
- Withdraws in response to pain – 4 points
- Flexion in response to pain (decorticate posturing) – 3 points

S.I. Lee, J.H. Thrall, *Choosing the Correct Radiologic Test*,
DOI 10.1007/978-3-642-15772-1_6, © Springer-Verlag Berlin Heidelberg 2013

- Extension response in response to pain (decerebrate posturing) – 2 points
- No response – 1 point

Head Injury Classification

Severe head injury – score of ≤8 or less

Moderate head injury – score of 9–12

Mild head injury – score of 13–15

A 30-year-old man with minor closed head injury. Exam reveals Glasgow Coma Scale of 14 and no neurologic deficit.

a. X-ray and/or CT cervical spine without contrast
b. CT head without contrast
c. MRI head without contrast
d. MRA head and neck
e. No ideal imaging exam

Minor or mild acute closed head injury (Glasgow Coma Scale ≥13), without risk factors or neurologic deficit.

a. X-ray and/or CT cervical spine without contrast may sometimes be appropriate (5).
b. *CT head without contrast* is the most appropriate. This is known to be low yield (7).
c. MRI head without contrast may sometimes be appropriate (4).
d. MRA head and neck is usually not appropriate. This is rarely indicated in mild trauma (3).

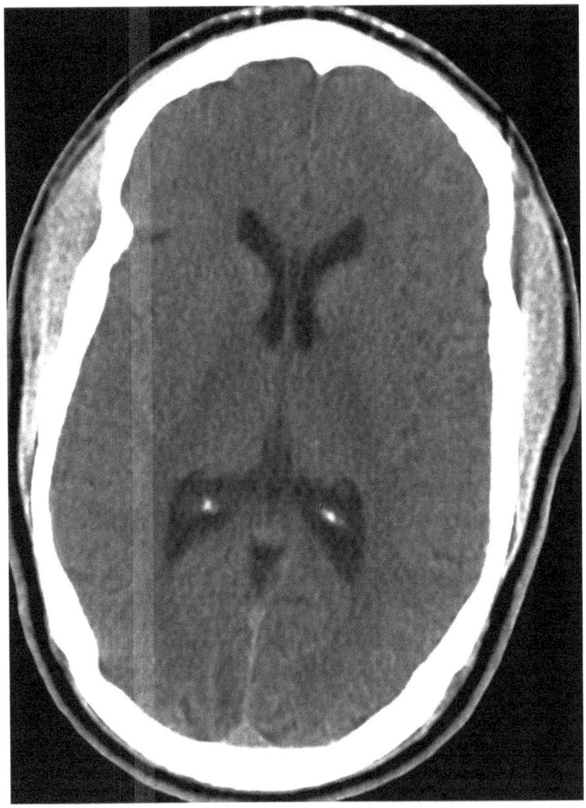

Fig. 6.1 Normal head. Head CT without contrast reveals no abnormalities

A 73-year-old woman with minor closed head injury. Exam reveals a focal neurologic deficit.

a. X-ray and/or CT cervical spine without contrast
b. CT head without contrast
c. MRI head without contrast
d. MRA head and neck
e. No ideal imaging exam

Head trauma – minor or mild acute closed head injury, focal neurologic deficit, and/or risk factors.

a. X-ray and/or CT cervical spine without contrast may sometimes be appropriate (6).
b. *CT head without contrast* is the most appropriate (9).
c. MRI head without contrast may sometimes be appropriate. Use for problem solving (6).
d. MRA head and neck may sometimes be appropriate. Use if vascular injury is suspected (5).

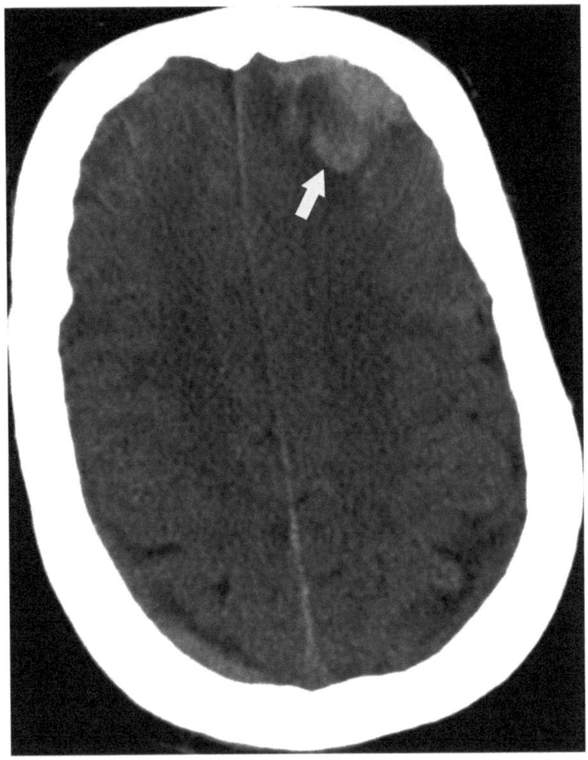

Fig. 6.2 Hemorrhagic contusion. Head CT without contrast shows intraparenchymal blood in the left frontal lobe (*arrow*)

A 19-year-old man with severe acute closed head injury.

a. X-ray and/or CT cervical spine without contrast
b. CT head without contrast
c. MRI head without contrast
d. MRA head and neck
e. No ideal imaging exam

Moderate or severe acute closed head injury.

a. X-ray and/or CT cervical spine without contrast is usually appropriate, but there is a better choice here (8).
b. *CT head without contrast* is the most appropriate (9).
c. MRI head without contrast may sometimes be appropriate (6).
d. MRA head and neck may sometimes be appropriate (5).

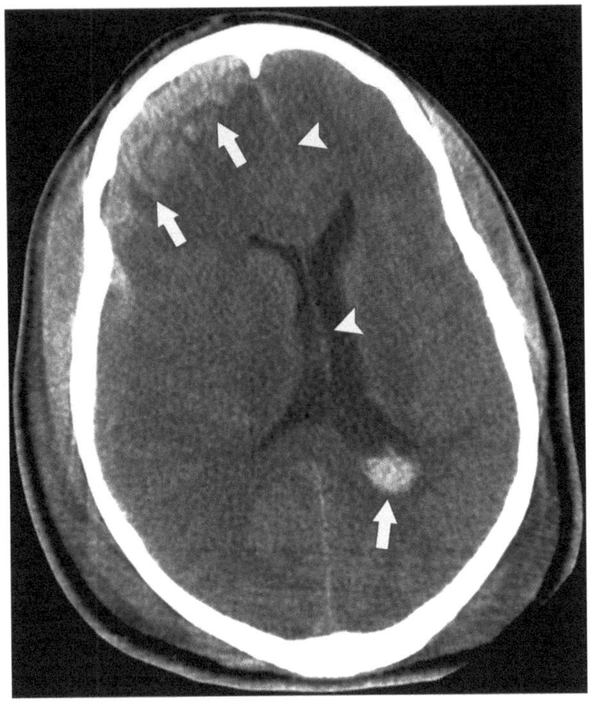

Fig. 6.3 Intracranial hemorrhage with mass effect. Head CT without contrast shows subarachnoid and intraparenchymal blood (*arrows*) and leftward midline shift (*arrowheads*)

A 64-year-old man with subacute closed head injury. Exam reveals neurologic deficits.

a. X-ray and/or CT cervical spine without contrast
b. CT head without contrast
c. MRI head without contrast
d. MRA head and neck
e. No ideal imaging exam

Subacute or chronic closed head injury with cognitive and/or neurologic deficit(s).

a. X-ray and/or CT cervical spine without contrast is usually not appropriate. This assumes that there are no spinal neurologic deficits (2).
b. CT head without contrast may sometimes be appropriate (6).
c. *MRI head without contrast* is the most appropriate (8).
d. MRA head and neck may sometimes be appropriate (4).

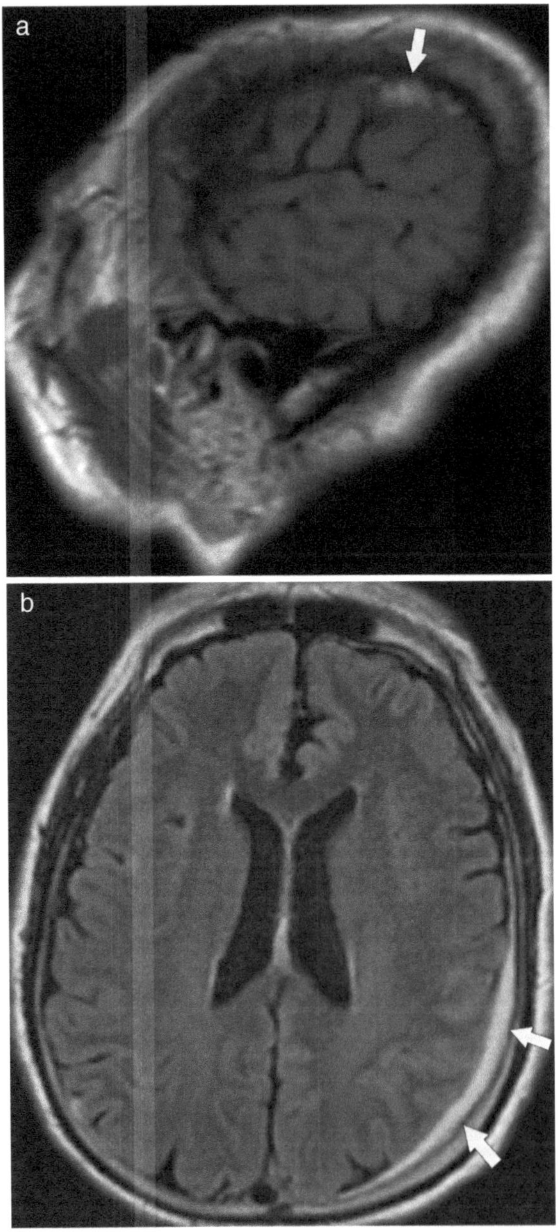

Fig. 6.4 Chronic subdural hemorrhage. Head MR sagittal T1-weighted (**a**) and axial FLAIR (**b**) images reveal a left subdural collection (*arrows*) with signal intensity consistent with old blood

A 59-year-old woman with closed head injury. Vertebral artery dissection is suspected.

a. X-ray and/or CT cervical spine without contrast
b. CT head without and with contrast
c. MRA head and neck
d. Cervicocerebral arteriogram
e. No ideal imaging exam

Closed head injury; rule out carotid or vertebral artery dissection.

a. X-ray and/or CT cervical spine without contrast may sometimes be appropriate (5).
b. CT head without and with contrast may sometimes be appropriate (6).
c. *MRA head and neck* is the most appropriate (8).
d. Cervicocerebral arteriogram may sometimes be appropriate. Use for problem solving (6).

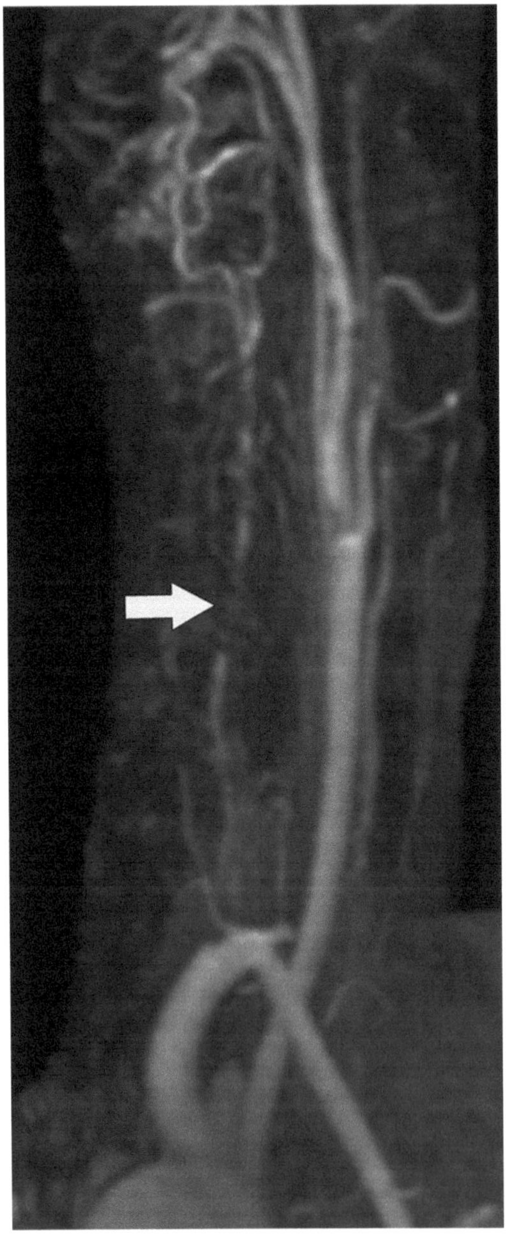

Fig. 6.5 Left vertebral artery dissection. Neck MRA 3-D reconstruction images show signal dropout (*arrow*) in the left midvertebral artery

A 7-year-old boy with penetrating head injury. He is clinically stable and neurologically intact.

a. X-ray head
b. CT head without contrast
c. MRI head without contrast
d. MRA head and neck
e. No ideal imaging exam

Penetrating injury, stable and neurologically intact.

a. X-ray head is usually appropriate, but there is a better choice here. Use if calvarium is site of injury (8).
b. *CT head without contrast* is the most appropriate (9).
c. MRI head without contrast may sometimes be appropriate (5).
d. MRA head and neck may sometimes be appropriate (6).

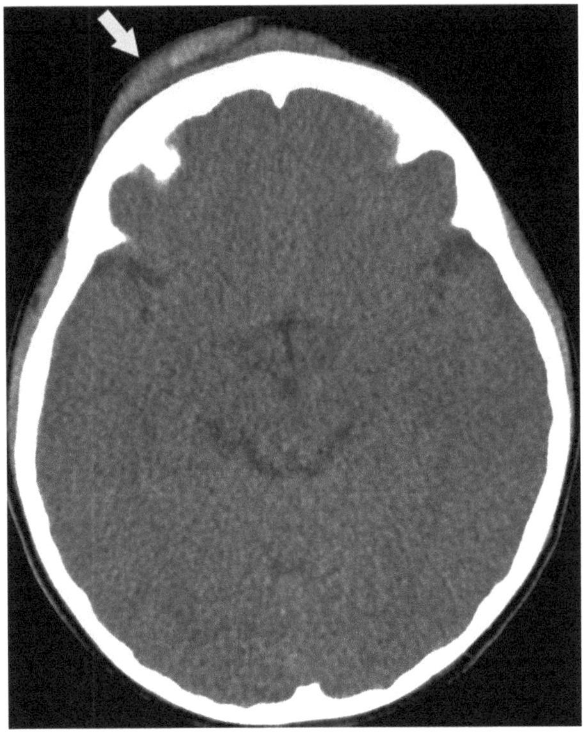

Fig. 6.6 Scalp hematoma. Head CT without contrast shows a subcutaneous blood (*arrow*). No intracranial injury is seen

An 80-year-old woman with head trauma. A skull fracture is suspected.

a. X-ray head
b. X-ray and/or CT cervical spine without contrast
c. CT head without contrast
d. MRI head without contrast
e. No ideal imaging exam

Skull fracture.

a. X-ray head may sometimes be appropriate (5).
b. X-ray and/or CT cervical spine without contrast may sometimes be appropriate (6).
c. *CT head without contrast* is the most appropriate (9).
d. MRI head without contrast may sometimes be appropriate (6).

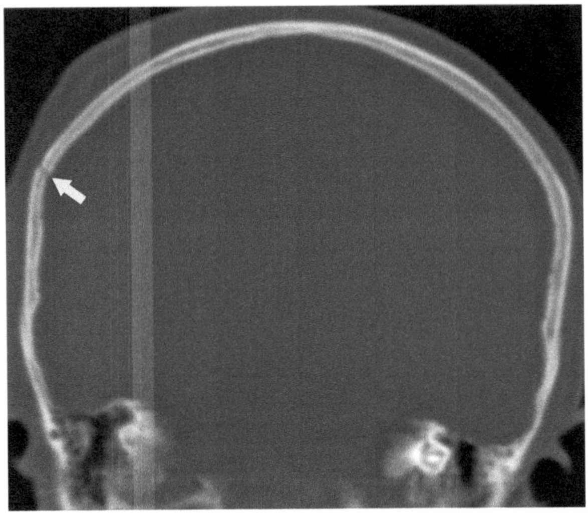

Fig. 6.7 Skull fracture. Head CT coronal reconstruction image shows a parietal skull fracture (*arrow*)

6.2 Cerebrovascular Disease

An 87-year-old woman with suspected cerebrovascular disease and a cervical bruit.

a. US carotid with Doppler
b. CT head without and with contrast
c. MRI head without and with contrast
d. Cervicocerebral arteriogram
e. No ideal imaging exam

Asymptomatic; structural lesion on physical exam (cervical bruit) and/or risk factors.

a. *US carotid with Doppler* is the most appropriate. Results may need to be confirmed with a second noninvasive study (8).
b. CT head without and with contrast may sometimes be appropriate (5).
c. MRI head without and with contrast may sometimes be appropriate (5).
d. Cervicocerebral arteriogram is usually not appropriate (2).

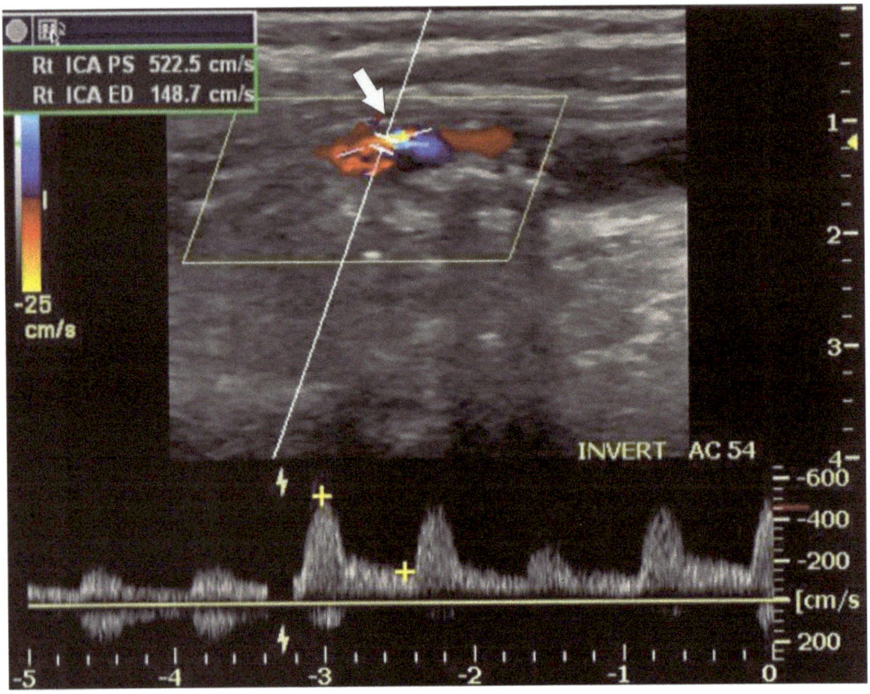

Fig. 6.8 Carotid artery stenosis. Carotid artery US with Doppler shows turbulent flow (*arrow*) with high velocity (*calipers*) indicating narrowing

A 56-year-old man with suspected cerebrovascular disease and a recent transient ischemic attack.

a. US transcranial with Doppler
b. US carotid with Doppler
c. MRI head and MRA of head and neck
d. Cervicocerebral arteriogram
e. No ideal imaging exam

Carotid territory or vertebrobasilar transient ischemic attack, initial screening survey.

a. US transcranial with Doppler is usually not appropriate (3).
b. US carotid with Doppler may sometimes be appropriate (6).
c. *MRI head and MRA of head and neck* are the most appropriate. Combined vascular and cerebral evaluation should be considered. MR is preferred over CT if treatment is not unreasonably delayed (8).
d. Cervicocerebral arteriogram is usually not appropriate (3).

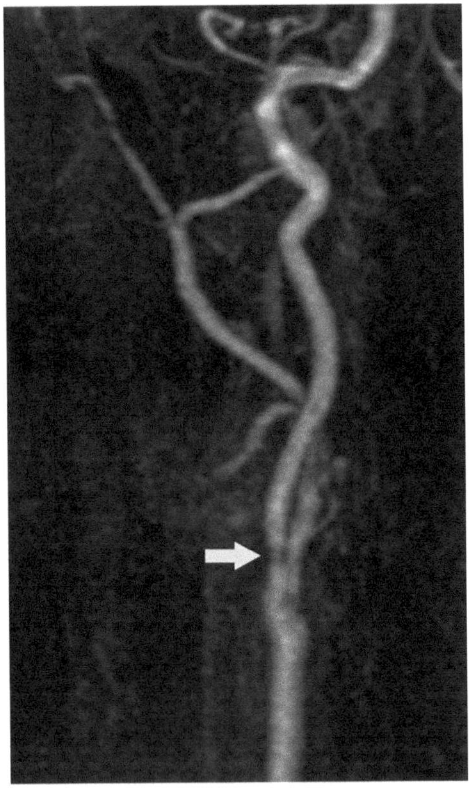

Fig. 6.9 Internal carotid artery stenosis. Neck MRA 3-D reconstruction images show narrowing (*arrow*) at the origin of the internal carotid artery

A 92-year-old woman with suspected cerebrovascular disease and a new focal-fixed neurologic deficit starting 2 hours ago.

a. US transcranial with Doppler
b. US carotid with Doppler
c. MRI head and MRA of head and neck
d. Cervicocerebral arteriogram
e. No ideal imaging exam

New focal neurologic defect, fixed or worsening for less than 3 hours.

a. US transcranial with Doppler is usually not appropriate (2).
b. US carotid with Doppler is usually not appropriate (2).
c. *MRI head and MRA of head and neck* are the most appropriate. Combined vascular and cerebral evaluation should be considered. MR is preferred over CT if treatment is not unreasonably delayed (8).
d. Cervicocerebral arteriogram may sometimes be appropriate. Use if intra-arterial therapy is being considered (5).

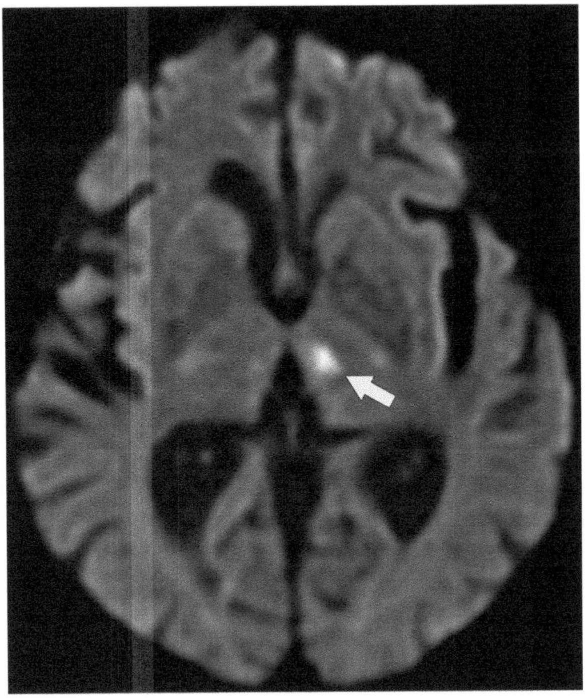

Fig. 6.10 Early stroke. Head MR axial diffusion-weighted image shows a focus of restricted diffusion in the left thalamus (*arrow*)

A 77-year-old woman with suspected cerebrovascular disease and new focal-fixed neurologic deficit starting 10 hours ago.

a. US transcranial with Doppler
b. US carotid with Doppler
c. MRI head and MRA of head and neck
d. Cervicocerebral arteriogram
e. No ideal imaging exam

New focal neurologic defect, fixed or worsening for 3–24 hours.

a. US transcranial with Doppler is usually not appropriate (2).
b. US carotid with Doppler is usually not appropriate (2).
c. *MRI head and MRA of head and neck* are the most appropriate. Combined vascular and cerebral evaluation should be considered. MR is preferred over CT if treatment is not unreasonably delayed (8).
d. Cervicocerebral arteriogram may sometimes be appropriate. Use if intra-arterial therapy is considered (6).

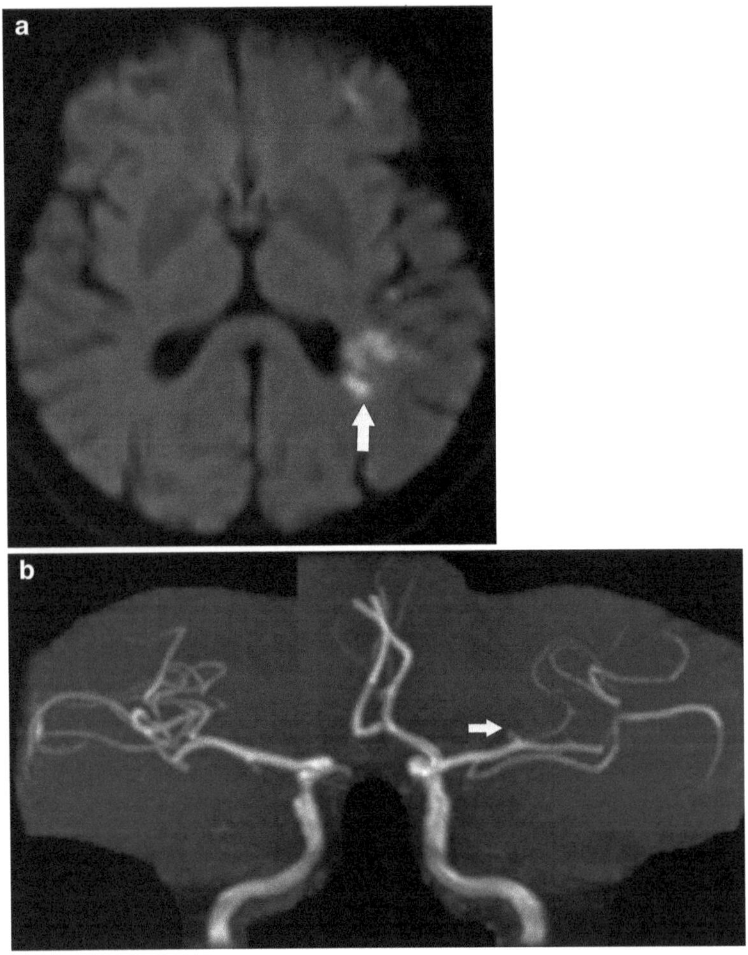

Fig. 6.11 Left hemispheric stroke. Head MR axial diffusion-weighted image (**a**) shows a focus of restricted diffusion in the left parietal lobe (*arrow*). Concurrent head MRA 3-D reconstruction image (**b**) shows thrombus of one of the left middle cerebral artery branches (*arrow*)

An 84-year-old woman with suspected unruptured intracranial aneurysm and a positive family history.

a. US transcranial with Doppler
b. MRI head
c. MRA head
d. Cervicocerebral arteriogram
e. No ideal imaging exam

Risk for unruptured aneurysm and positive family history.

a. US transcranial with Doppler is usually not appropriate (1).
b. MRI head may sometimes be appropriate (6).
c. *MRA head* is the most appropriate. MR is preferred over CT if treatment is not unreasonably delayed (8).
d. Cervicocerebral arteriogram is usually not appropriate (1).

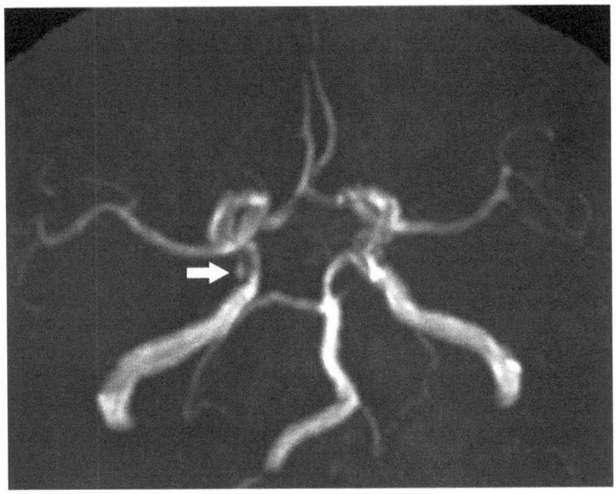

Fig. 6.12 Intracranial aneurysm. Head MRA 3-D reconstruction image shows a small aneurysm (*arrow*) arising from the right circle of Willis

A 53-year-old woman with clinically suspected subarachnoid hemorrhage.

a. CT head without contrast
b. CTA head
c. MRI head
d. MRA head
e. No ideal imaging exam

Clinically suspected subarachnoid hemorrhage (SAH), not yet confirmed.

a. *CT head without contrast* is the most appropriate (9).
b. CTA head is usually not appropriate (2).
c. MRI head may sometimes be appropriate (4).
d. MRA head may sometimes be appropriate (4).

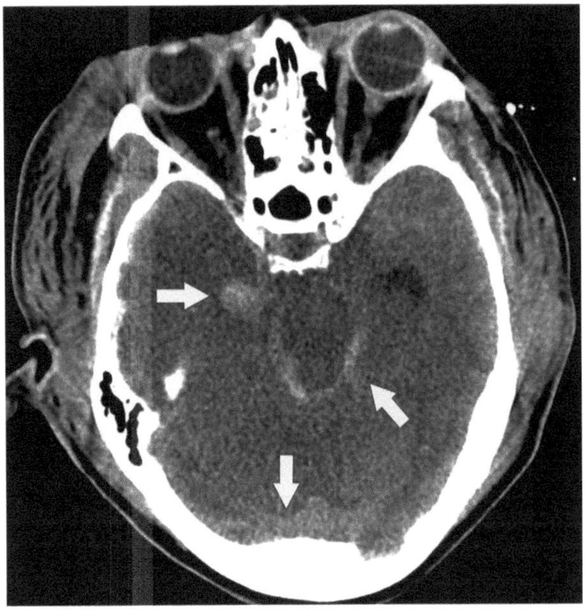

Fig. 6.13 Subarachnoid hemorrhage. Head CT without contrast reveals high-density blood in the ventricles, sulci, and cisterns (*arrows*)

A 43-year-old woman with subarachnoid hemorrhage confirmed by lumbar puncture.

a. US transcranial with Doppler
b. MRI head
c. MRA head
d. Cervicocerebral arteriogram
e. No ideal imaging exam

Proven SAH by lumbar puncture or imaging.

a. US transcranial with Doppler may sometimes be appropriate. Use for vasospasm (5).
b. MRI head may sometimes be appropriate (6).
c. MRA head may sometimes be appropriate. Use for treatment planning (6).
d. *Cervicocerebral arteriogram* is the most appropriate. Use for treatment planning (8).

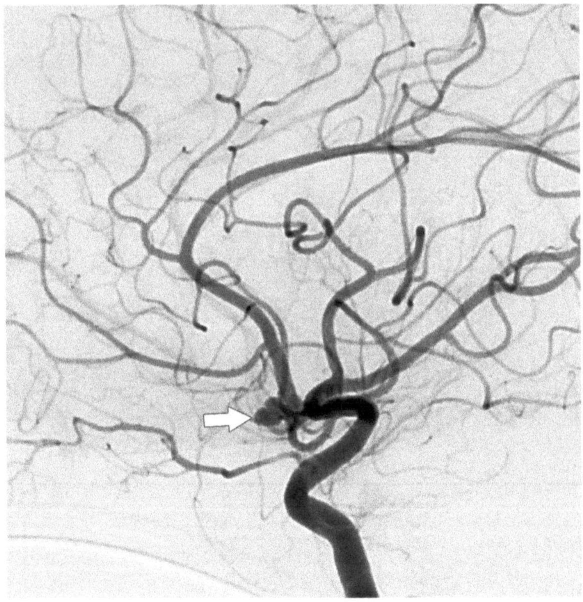

Fig. 6.14 Bleeding intracranial aneurysm. Head angiogram lateral view shows an aneurysm (*arrow*) arising from the anterior communicating artery

A 43-year-old woman with subarachnoid hemorrhage on head CT. Angiogram was negative.

a. US transcranial Doppler
b. CT head without contrast
c. CT head without and with contrast
d. Repeat cervicocerebral arteriogram
e. No ideal imaging exam

Proven SAH, negative angiogram, and follow-up.

a. US transcranial Doppler may sometimes be appropriate (5).
b. CT head without contrast may sometimes be appropriate (5).
c. CT head without and with contrast may sometimes be appropriate (4).
d. *Repeat cervicocerebral arteriogram* is the most appropriate (8).

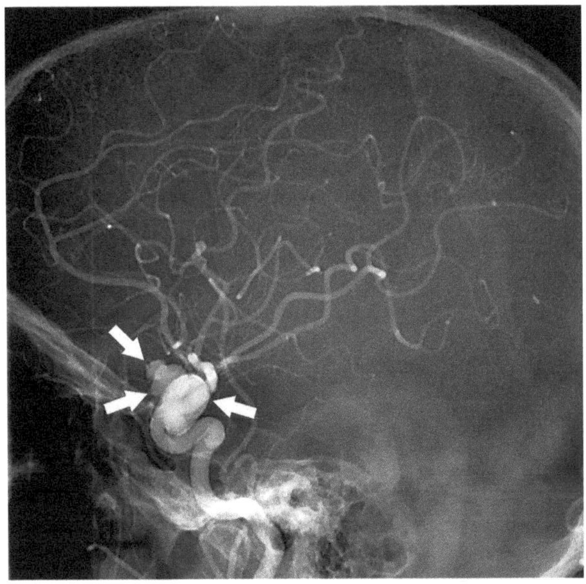

Fig. 6.15 Intracranial aneurysms. Head angiogram lateral view shows aneurysms (*arrows*) in the supraclinoid segment of the internal carotid artery

A 68-year-old woman with suspected parenchymal intracranial hemorrhage.

a. CT head without contrast
b. CT head without and with contrast
c. MRI head
d. Cervicocerebral arteriogram
e. No ideal imaging exam

Clinically suspected parenchymal hemorrhage (hematoma), not yet confirmed.

a. *CT head without contrast* is the most appropriate (8).
b. CT head without and with contrast is usually appropriate, but there is a better choice here (7).
c. MRI head is usually appropriate, but there is a better choice here (7).
d. Cervicocerebral arteriogram is usually not appropriate (3).

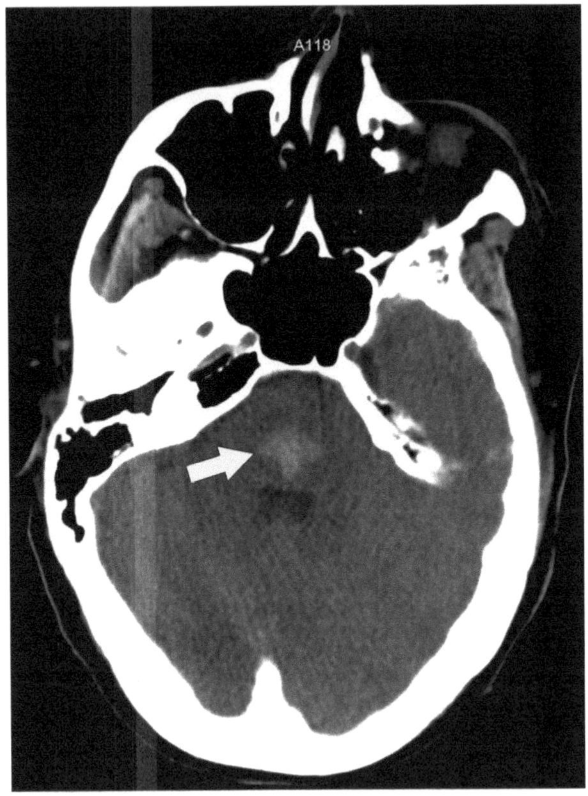

Fig. 6.16 Intraparenchymal hemorrhage. Head CT without contrast shows blood in the brainstem (*arrow*)

An 18-year-old woman with known parenchymal intracranial hemorrhage on head CT.

a. CTA neck
b. MRA neck
c. MRI head and MRA head
d. Cervicocerebral arteriogram
e. No ideal imaging exam

Proven parenchymal hemorrhage (hematoma).

a. CTA neck may sometimes be appropriate (5).
b. MRA neck may sometimes be appropriate (5).
c. *MRI head and MRA head* are the most appropriate. Combined vascular and cerebral evaluation should be considered. MR is preferred over CT if treatment is not unreasonably delayed (8).
d. Cervicocerebral arteriogram is usually appropriate, but there is a better choice here. Use if arteriovenous malformation is suspected (7).

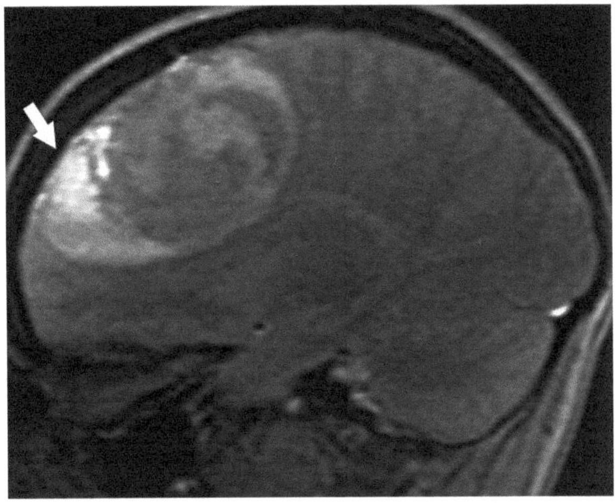

Fig. 6.17 Intraparenchymal hemorrhage. Head MR sagittal T1-weighted image shows hyperintense signal in the frontal lobe (*arrow*) consistent with acute hematoma

6.3 Focal Neurologic Deficit

A 52-year-old woman with multifocal neurologic deficits.

a. CT head without contrast
b. CTA head and neck
c. MRI head
d. MRA head and neck
e. No ideal imaging exam

Multiple focal neurologic deficits.

a. CT head without contrast is usually appropriate, but there is a better choice here. Use as an acute screening exam (7).
b. CTA head and neck is usually appropriate, but there is a better choice here. Use if vascular abnormality is suspected (6).
c. *MRI head* is the most appropriate (8).
d. MRA head and neck may sometimes be appropriate. Use if vascular abnormality is suspected (6).

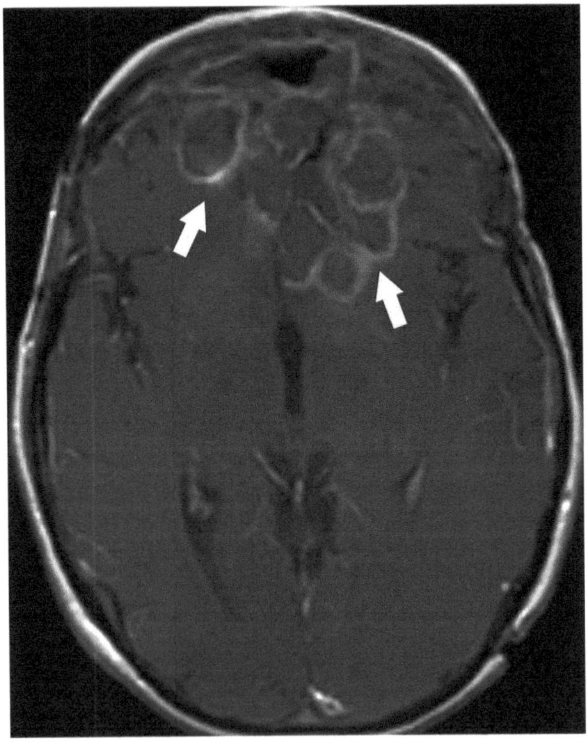

Fig. 6.18 Intracranial abscess. Head MR with axial postcontrast image shows a multiloculated abscess (*arrows*) involving the frontal lobes bilaterally

A 55-year-old man with single sudden-onset focal neurologic deficit. Exam has been stable.

a. CT head without and with contrast
b. MRI head
c. MRA head and neck
d. Cervicocerebral arteriogram
e. No ideal imaging exam

Single focal neurologic deficit, sudden onset, stable, or incompletely resolving.

a. CT head without and with contrast may sometimes be appropriate. Use if MRI is unavailable or contraindicated (5).
b. *MRI head* is the most appropriate. Both CT and MR may be necessary. CT evaluates for suspected hemorrhage in the acute setting and MR for infarction and masses (8).
c. MRA head and neck is usually appropriate, but there is a better choice here (7).
d. Cervicocerebral arteriogram is usually not appropriate. Use for problem solving (3).

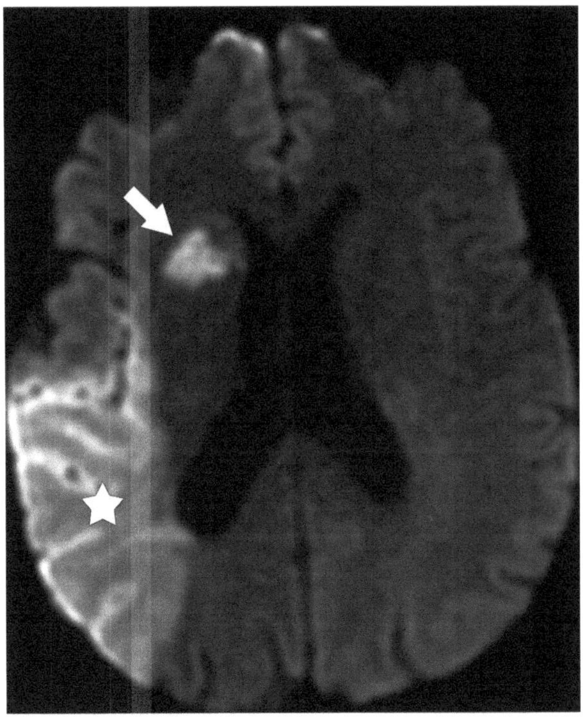

Fig. 6.19 Right hemispheric stroke. Head MR axial diffusion-weighted image shows areas of restricted diffusion in the temporal and parietal lobes (*star*) and the corona radiata (*arrow*) consistent with infarction in the middle cerebral artery territory

A 61-year-old man with single sudden-onset focal neurologic deficit and progressive symptoms.

a. CT head without and with contrast
b. MRI head
c. MRA head and neck
d. Cervicocerebral arteriogram
e. No ideal imaging exam

Single focal neurologic deficit, sudden onset, and progressive.

a. CT head without and with contrast may sometimes be appropriate. Use if MRI is unavailable or contraindicated (6).
b. *MRI head* is the most appropriate. Both CT and MR may be necessary. CT evaluates for suspected hemorrhage in the acute setting and MR for infarction and masses (8).
c. MRA head and neck is usually appropriate, but there is a better choice here (7).
d. Cervicocerebral arteriogram is usually not appropriate. Use for problem solving (3).

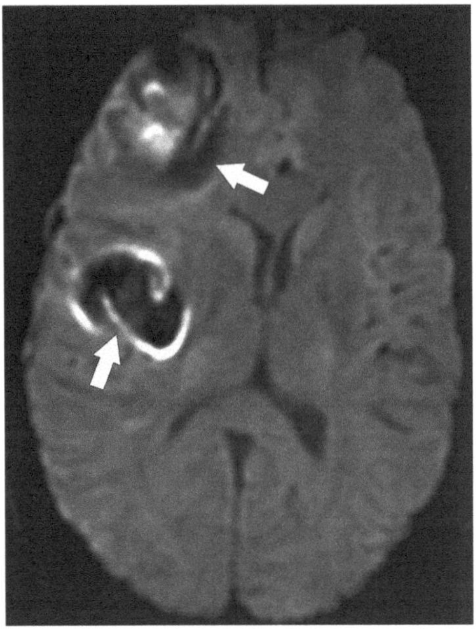

Fig. 6.20 Hemorrhagic stroke. Head MR axial diffusion-weighted image shows areas of increased susceptibility indicating blood in the right frontal and temporal lobes (*arrows*)

An 87-year-old woman initially presented with a single focal neurologic deficit. Symptoms have now completely resolved.

a. CT head without and with contrast
b. MRI head
c. MRA head and neck
d. Cerebral angiogram
e. No ideal imaging exam

Single focal neurologic deficit, completely resolving.

a. CT head without and with contrast may sometimes be appropriate. Use if MRI is unavailable or contraindicated (6).
b. *MRI head* is the most appropriate. Both CT and MR may be necessary. CT evaluates for suspected hemorrhage in the acute setting and MR for infarction and masses (8).
c. MRA head and neck is usually appropriate, but there is a better choice here (7).
d. Cerebral angiogram is usually not appropriate. Use for problem solving (3).

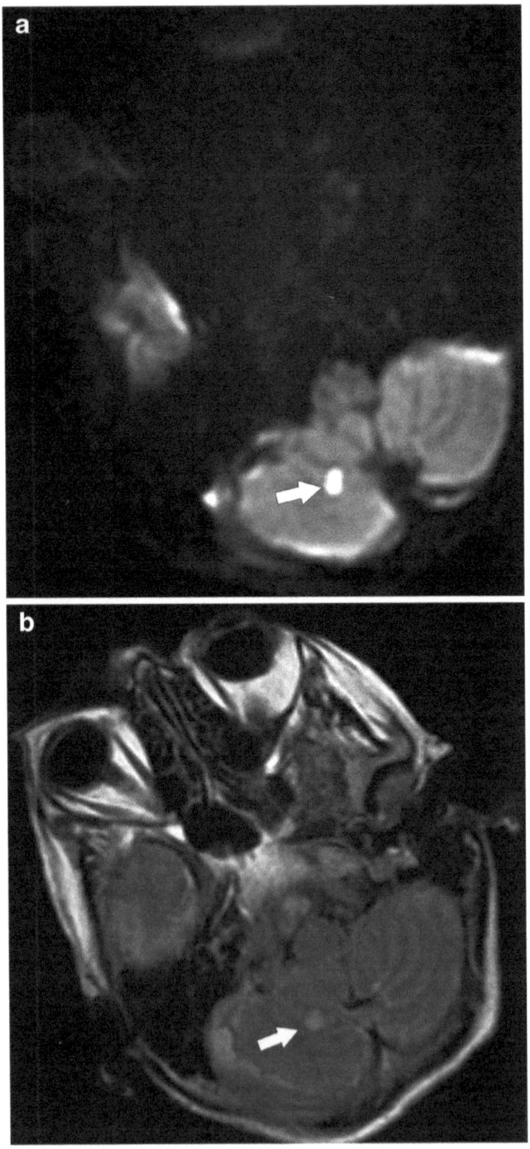

Fig. 6.21 Cerebellar stroke. Head MR axial images show a tiny stroke in the right cerebellum (*arrows*) that is easily detected on the diffusion weighted (**a**) but less well seen on the FLAIR (**b**) sequence

An 84-year-old woman with a focal neurologic deficit and acute unexplained confusion.

a. CT head without and with contrast
b. MRI head
c. MRA head and neck
d. Cervicocerebral arteriogram
e. No ideal imaging exam

Unexplained acute confusion or altered level of consciousness.

a. CT head without and with contrast may sometimes be appropriate. Use if MRI is unavailable or contraindicated (5).
b. *MRI head* is the most appropriate. Both CT and MR may be necessary. CT evaluates for suspected hemorrhage in the acute setting and MR for infarction and masses (8).
c. MRA head and neck may sometimes be appropriate. Use if vascular abnormality is suspected (6).
d. Cervicocerebral arteriogram is usually not appropriate (2).

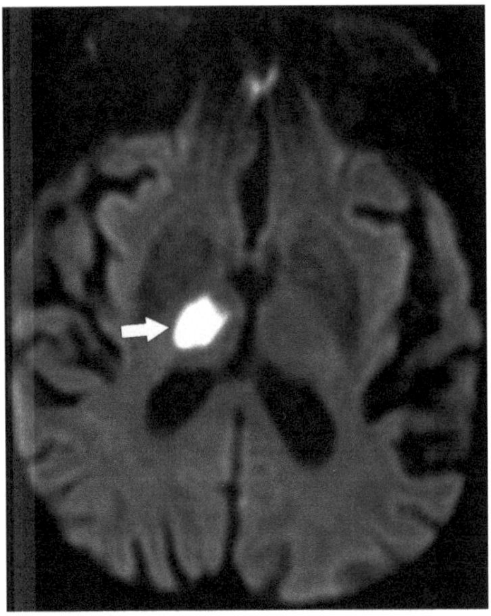

Fig. 6.22 Right thalamic stroke. Head MR axial diffusion-weighted image shows an area of restricted diffusion (*arrow*) in the right thalamus

6.4 Headache

A 40-year-old man with chronic headaches with no new recent features.

a. CT head
b. CTA head
c. MRI head
d. MRA head
e. No ideal imaging exam

Chronic headache with no new features.

a. CT head may sometimes be appropriate (4).
b. CTA head is usually not appropriate (2).
c. MRI head may sometimes be appropriate (4).
d. MRA head is usually not appropriate (2).
e. *No ideal imaging exam* is the correct answer.

A 47-year-old woman with chronic headaches which have recently increased in intensity.

a. CT head without and with contrast
b. CTA head
c. MRI head without and with contrast
d. MRA head
e. No ideal imaging exam

Chronic headache with new features.

a. CT head without and with contrast may sometimes be appropriate. Use if MRI is unavailable or contraindicated (4).
b. CTA head may sometimes be appropriate. It is not generally appropriate for screening or as first imaging exam. It should be used in combination with CT (4).
c. *MRI head without and with contrast* is the most appropriate (8).
d. MRA head may sometimes be appropriate. Use in selected cases when vascular disease suspected (5).

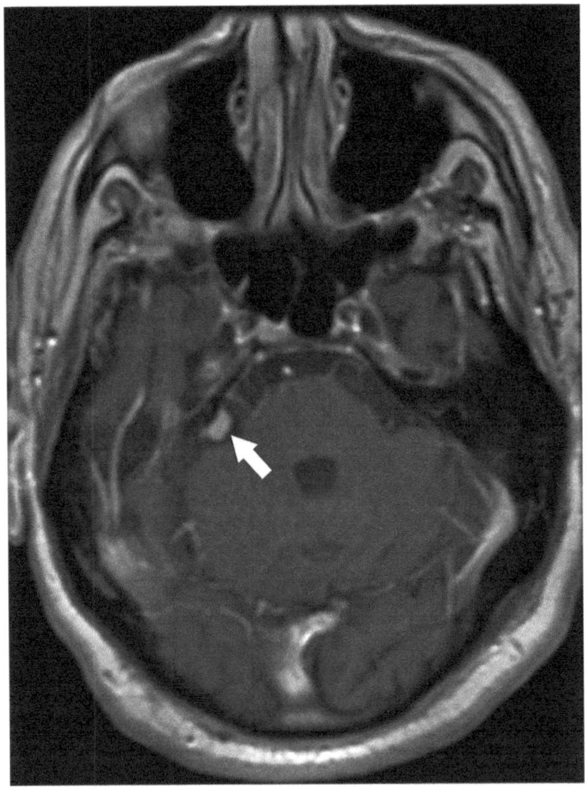

Fig. 6.23 Meningioma. Head MR axial postcontrast image shows a 1-cm enhancing extra-axial mass (*arrow*) at the right cerebellopontine angle

An 82-year-old man with sudden-onset “worst headache of his life”.

a. CT head without contrast
b. CTA head
c. MRA head
d. Cervicocerebral arteriogram
e. No ideal imaging exam

Sudden onset of severe headache ("worst headache of one's life, thunderclap headache").

a. *CT head without contrast* is the most appropriate (9).
b. CTA head is usually appropriate, but there is a better choice here. Selection of CT versus MRI depends on local preference and availability (8).
c. MRA head is usually appropriate, but there is a better choice here. Selection of CT versus MRI depends on local preference and availability (8).
d. Cervicocerebral arteriogram is usually appropriate, but there is a better choice here (7).

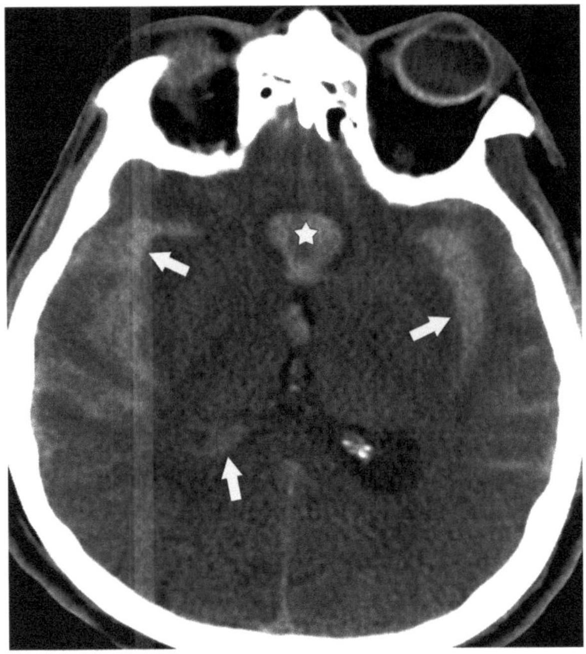

Fig. 6.24 Subarachnoid hemorrhage from aneurysm. Head CT without contrast shows blood bilaterally in the sulci and in the right lateral ventricle (*arrows*). A rounded high-density collection (*star*) is the ruptured basilar artery aneurysm representing the bleeding source

A 40-year-old woman presents with sudden-onset unilateral headache. Vertebral artery dissection is suspected.

a. US carotid with Doppler
b. CT head without contrast
c. CTA head and neck
d. Cervicocerebral arteriogram
e. No ideal imaging exam

Sudden onset of unilateral headache, or suspected carotid or vertebral dissection or ipsilateral Horner's syndrome.

a. US carotid with Doppler is usually not appropriate (3).
b. CT head without contrast is usually appropriate, but there is a better choice here (7).
c. *CTA head and neck* is the most appropriate. Selection of CT versus MRI depends on local preference and availability (8).
d. Cervicocerebral arteriogram is usually appropriate, but there is a better choice here (7).

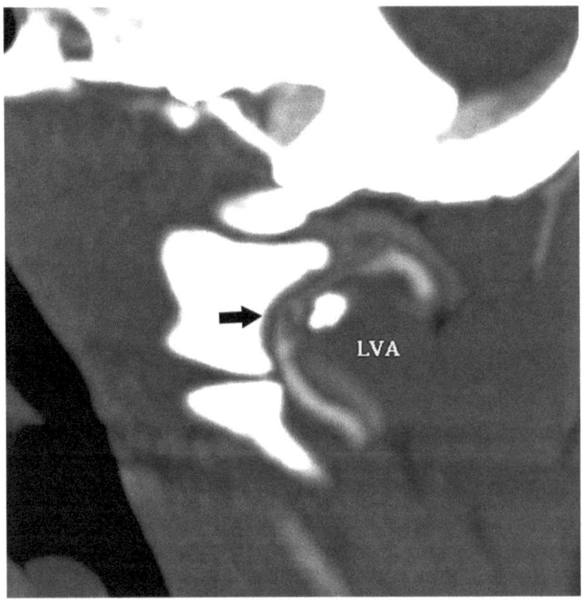

Fig. 6.25 Vertebral artery dissection. Neck CTA sagittal reconstruction image shows a left vertebral artery (*LVA*) dissection at the C1 level (*arrow*)

A 21-year-old man presents with headache suspected to be secondary to sinusitis.

a. X-ray head
b. US transcranial
c. CT head without and with contrast
d. MRI head without and with contrast
e. No ideal imaging exam

Headache, suspected complication of sinusitis and/or mastoiditis.

a. X-ray head is usually not appropriate (NA).
b. US transcranial is usually not appropriate (2).
c. CT head without and with contrast may sometimes be appropriate. Sinus imaging may also be indicated (6).
d. *MRI head without and with contrast* is the most appropriate (8).

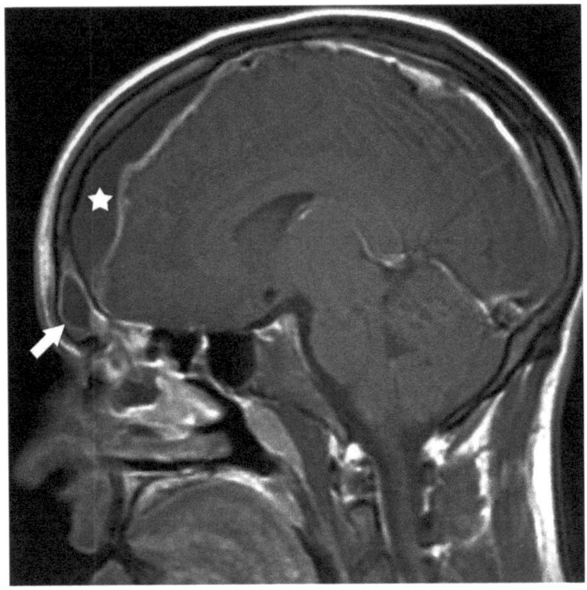

Fig. 6.26 Epidural abscess from sinusitis. Head MR sagittal postcontrast image reveals a rim-enhancing epidural collection (*star*). Fluid is seen in the frontal sinus (*arrow*)

A 65-year-old woman with headache, temporal tenderness, and elevated sedimentation rate. Temporal arteritis is suspected.

a. CT head without contrast
b. CTA head and neck
c. MRI head without contrast
d. MRA head and neck
e. No ideal imaging exam

New headache in patient older than age 60, sedimentation rate higher than 55, temporal tenderness, and suspected temporal arteritis.

a. CT head without contrast may sometimes be appropriate (6).
b. CTA head and neck may sometimes be appropriate (5).
c. *MRI head without contrast* is the most appropriate (8).
d. MRA head and neck may sometimes be appropriate (5).

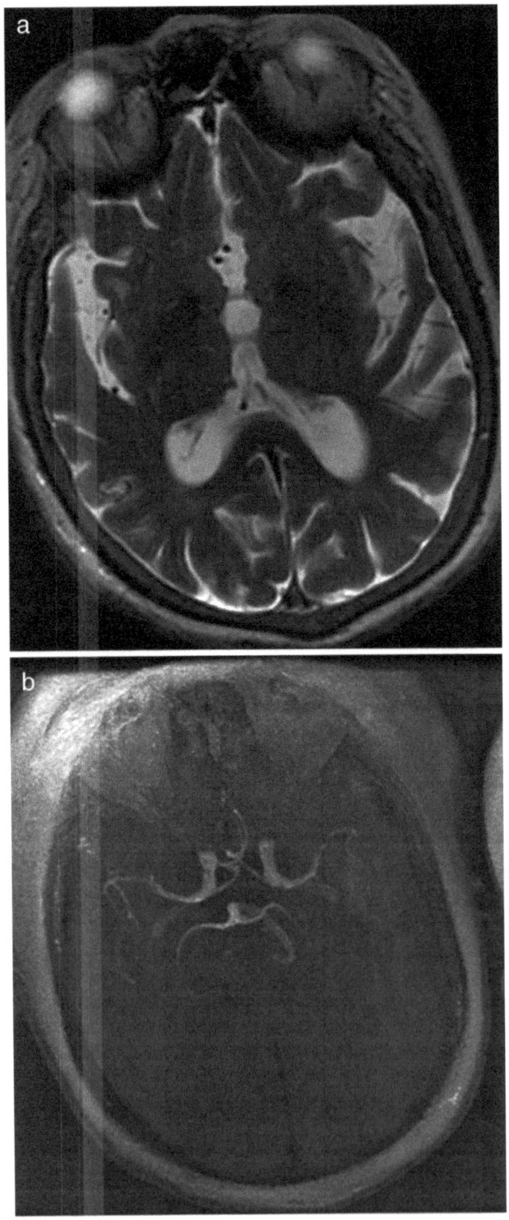

Fig. 6.27 Temporal arteritis. Head MR axial T2 image of the brain (**a**) shows no evidence of ischemia. Concurrent head MRA (**b**) reveals no evidence of arteritis in the intracranial vessels

A 53-year-old woman who is positive for human immunodeficiency virus now with headache.

a. CT head without and with contrast
b. CTA head
c. MRI head without and with contrast
d. MRA head
e. No ideal imaging exam

New headache in human immunodeficiency virus-positive individual.

a. CT head without and with contrast may sometimes be appropriate (5).
b. CTA head may sometimes be appropriate. This is indicated if vascular lesion is suspected (5).
c. *MRI head without and with contrast* is the most appropriate (8).
d. MRA head is usually not appropriate. This is indicated if vascular lesion is suspected (2).

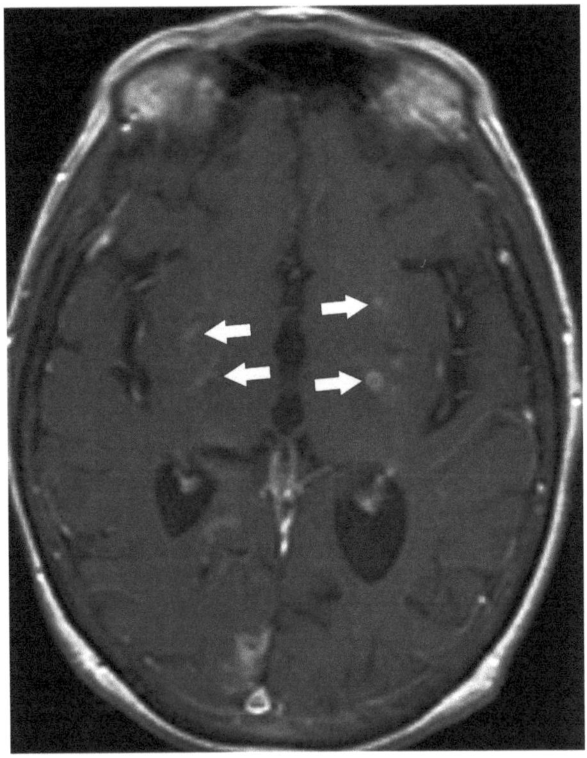

Fig. 6.28 Cryptococcal abscesses. Head MR axial postcontrast image shows enhancing foci bilaterally in the basal ganglia (*arrows*)

A 25-year-old pregnant woman with new-onset headache.

a. CTA head
b. MRI head without contrast
c. MRI head without and with contrast
d. MRA head
e. No ideal imaging exam

New headache in pregnant patient.

a. CTA head is usually not appropriate. Use if MRI not available, contraindicated, or inconclusive. CT venography may also be performed (2).
b. *MRI head without contrast* is the most appropriate. Selection of CT versus MRI depends on local preference and availability (8).
c. MRI head without and with contrast may sometimes be appropriate. Pregnancy is a relative contraindication to gadolinium administration (5).
d. MRA head may sometimes be appropriate. MR venography should also be performed (5).

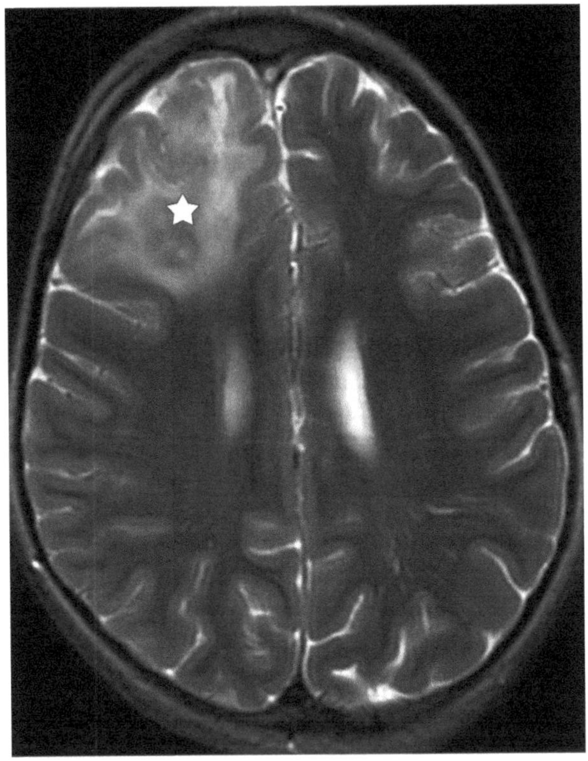

Fig. 6.29 Intracranial edema from venous sinus thrombosis. Head MR axial T2-weighted image shows hyperintensity in the right frontal lobe with mass effect (*star*)

A 59-year-old man with new-onset headache. Meningitis is suspected.

a. CTA head
b. MRI head without contrast
c. MRI head without and with contrast
d. MRA head
e. No ideal imaging exam

New headache; suspected meningitis/encephalitis.

a. CTA head may sometimes be appropriate. Use for problem solving or if there is a strong suspicion of vascular disease (6).
b. MRI head without contrast may sometimes be appropriate (6).
c. *MRI head without and with contrast* is the most appropriate. Selection of CT versus MRI depends on local preference and availability (8).
d. MRA head may sometimes be appropriate. MR venography should also be performed (6).

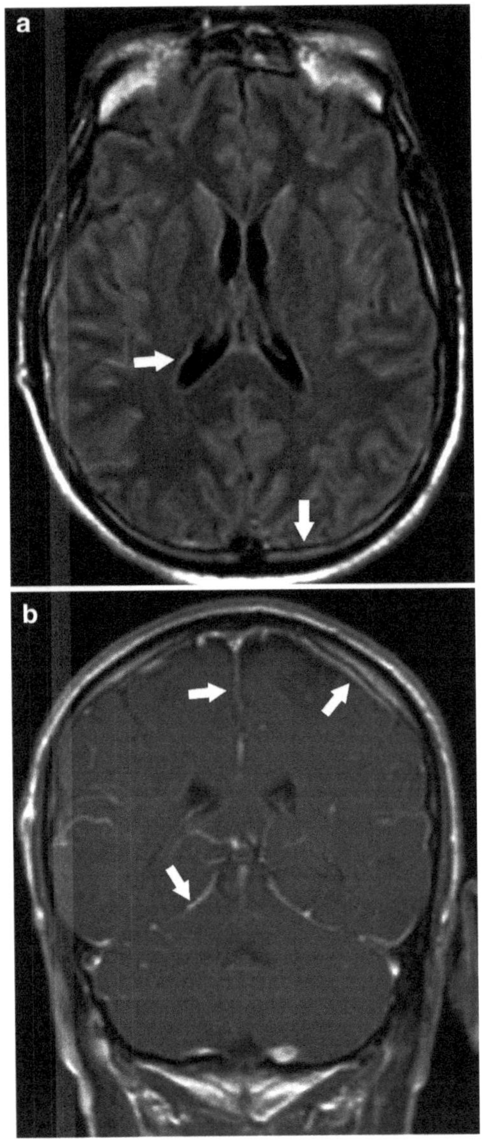

Fig. 6.30 Meningitis. Head MR axial FLAIR (**a**) and coronal postcontrast (**b**) images show abnormal meningeal signal and enhancement (*arrows*)

6.5 Suspected Spine Trauma

NEXUS Criteria

C-spine imaging is recommended in trauma patients unless they meet all of the following criteria.

- No posterior midline cervical spine tenderness
- No evidence of intoxication
- Normal level of alertness
- No focal neurological deficit
- No clinically apparent painful injuries that might distract from pain of a cervical spine injury

Canadian C-Spine Rules (CCR)
No imaging is necessary if the following criteria are met.

Absence of high-risk factors:

- Age >65 years
- Dangerous mechanism – fall from an elevation of 3 ft or 5 stairs, axial load to the head (e.g., diving), motor vehicle collision at high speed or with rollover or ejection, collision involving a motorized recreational vehicle, or bicycle collision
- Paresthesias in the extremities

Low-risk factors that allow safe assessment of range of motion:

- Simple rear-end motor vehicle collision – excludes being pushed into oncoming traffic, being hit by a bus, a large truck, or a high-speed vehicle, or a rollover
- Sitting position
- Ambulatory at any time
- Delayed onset of neck pain
- No midline cervical tenderness
- Able to actively rotate neck 45° left and right

A 23-year-old man with cervical spine trauma. He is alert. Exam reveals no focal neurologic deficits or tenderness over the midline cervical spine.

a. X-ray cervical spine
b. CT cervical spine without contrast
c. MRI cervical spine without contrast
d. Myelography and postmyelography CT cervical spine
e. No ideal imaging exam

Cervical spine imaging not indicated by NEXUS or CCR clinical criteria; patient meets low-risk criteria.

a. X-ray cervical spine is usually not appropriate (1).
b. CT cervical spine without contrast is usually not appropriate. Exam includes sagittal and coronal reformations (1).
c. MRI cervical spine without contrast is usually not appropriate (1).
d. Myelography and postmyelography CT cervical spine is usually not appropriate (1).
e. *No ideal imaging exam* is the correct answer.

A 71-year-old man with cervical spine trauma. On exam, tenderness over the midline cervical spine is noted.

a. X-ray cervical spine
b. CT cervical spine without contrast
c. MRI cervical spine without contrast
d. Myelography and postmyelography CT cervical spine
e. No ideal imaging exam

Suspected acute cervical spine trauma, imaging indicated by clinical criteria (NEXUS or CCR), not otherwise specified.

a. X-ray cervical spine may sometimes be appropriate. This is useful if CT reconstructions are not optimal (6).
b. *CT cervical spine without contrast* is the most appropriate. Exam includes sagittal and coronal reformations (9).
c. MRI cervical spine without contrast is usually not appropriate (1).
d. Myelography and postmyelography CT cervical spine is usually not appropriate (1).

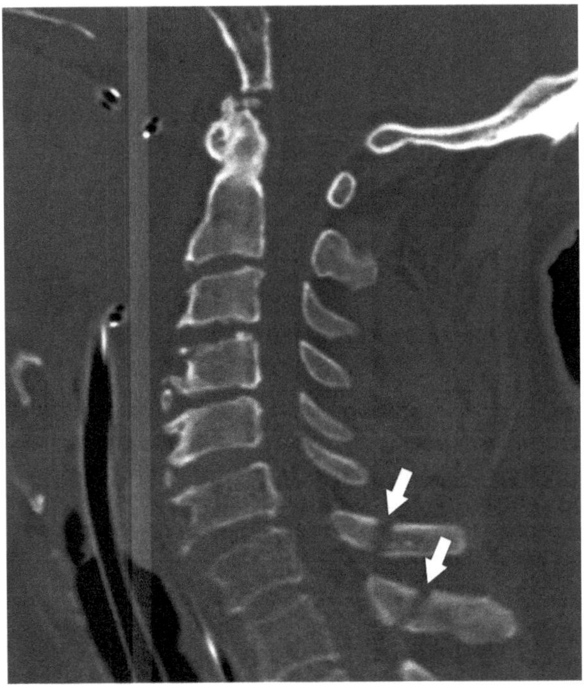

Fig. 6.31 Cervical spine fracture. Cervical spine CT sagittal reconstruction image shows fractures (*arrows*) through the C7 and T1 spinous processes

A 57-year-old man with cervical spine trauma. Cord injury is suspected.

a. X-ray cervical spine
b. MRI cervical spine without contrast
c. MRA neck
d. Myelography and postmyelography CT cervical spine
e. No ideal imaging exam

Suspected acute cervical spine trauma, imaging indicated by clinical criteria (NEXUS or CCR), myelopathy.

a. X-ray cervical spine may sometimes be appropriate. This is useful if CT reconstructions are not optimal (6).
b. *MRI cervical spine without contrast* is the most appropriate. MRI and CT provide complementary information. It is appropriate to perform both exams (9).
c. MRA neck is usually not appropriate (1).
d. Myelography and postmyelography CT cervical spine may sometimes be appropriate. Use if MRI is contraindicated or inconclusive (5).

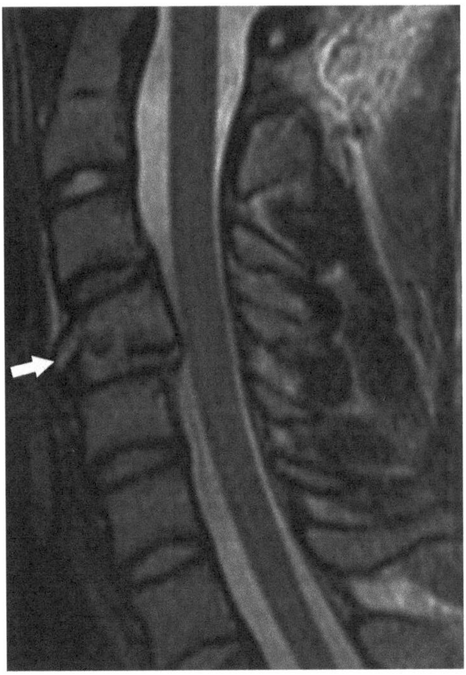

Fig. 6.32 Cervical spine fracture with cord injury. Cervical spine MR sagittal T2-weighted image shows a C3 vertebral body fracture (*arrow*) resulting in cord compression and edema

A 67-year-old man with spine trauma. He is undergoing treatment planning for a mechanically unstable spine.

a. X-ray cervical spine
b. CT cervical spine without contrast
c. MRI cervical spine without contrast
d. Myelography and postmyelography CT cervical spine
e. No ideal imaging exam

Acute cervical spine trauma, imaging indicated by clinical criteria (NEXUS or CCR), treatment planning for mechanically unstable spine.

a. X-ray cervical spine may sometimes be appropriate. Exam should be individualized in consultation with referring physician for surgical planning (6).
b. *CT cervical spine without contrast* is the most appropriate. Exam includes sagittal and coronal reformations (9).
c. MRI cervical spine without contrast is usually appropriate, but there is a better choice here. Use for thorough evaluation of ligamentous injury (8).
d. Myelography and postmyelography CT cervical spine may sometimes be appropriate (4).

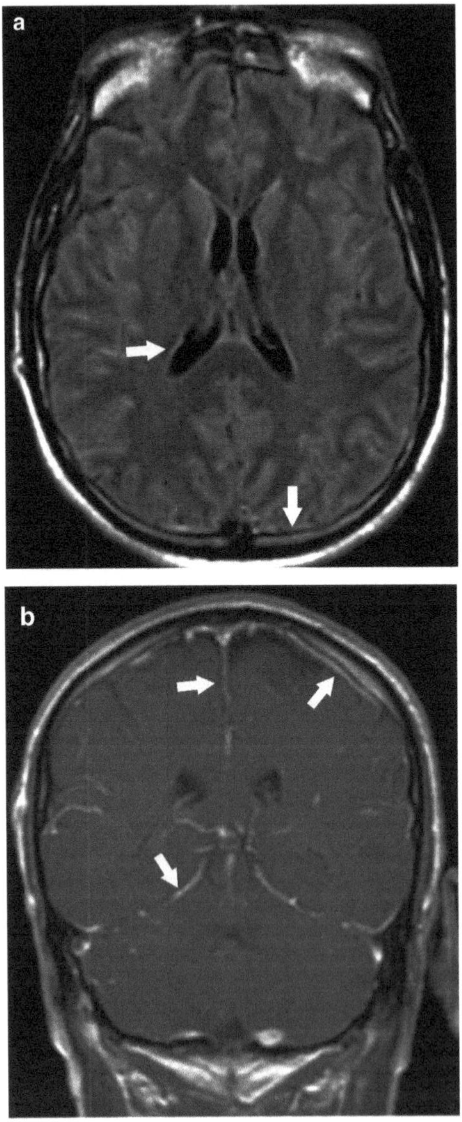

Fig. 6.33 Unstable cervical spine fracture. Cervical spine CT sagittal reconstruction image in bone window (**a**) shows a C3 vertebral body fracture (*arrow*). The same image in soft tissue window (**b**) shows cord compression (*arrow*)

A 27-year-old woman with cervical spine trauma. Arterial injury is suspected.

a. X-ray cervical spine
b. CTA head and neck
c. Myelography and postmyelography CT cervical spine
d. Cervicocerebral arteriogram
e. No ideal imaging exam

Suspected acute cervical spine trauma, imaging indicated by clinical criteria (NEXUS or CCR), clinical or imaging findings suggest arterial injury.

a. X-ray cervical spine is usually not appropriate (1).
b. *CTA head and neck* is the most appropriate. Either CTA or MRA can be performed depending on institutional preference (9).
c. Myelography and postmyelography CT cervical spine is usually not appropriate (1).
d. Cervicocerebral arteriogram may sometimes be appropriate. Use for treatment planning or problem solving (5).

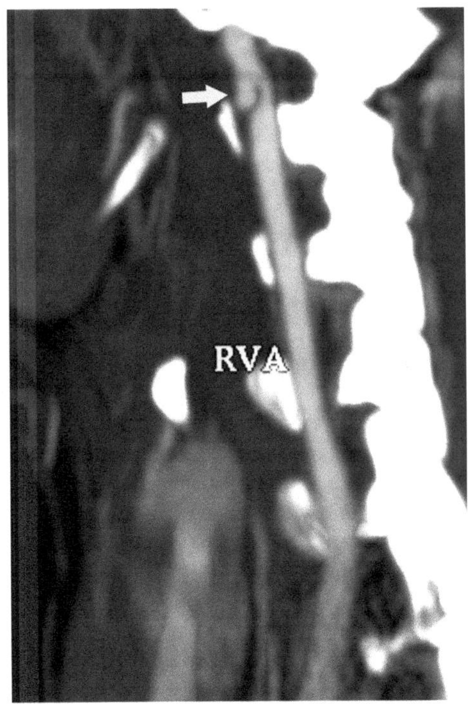

Fig. 6.34 Vertebral artery pseudoaneurysm. Neck CTA sagittal 3-D reconstruction image shows a right vertebral artery (*RVA*) pseudoaneurysm (*arrow*) at the C2–3 level

A 76-year-old woman with cervical spine trauma. Ligamentous injury is suspected.

a. X-ray cervical spine
b. MRI cervical spine without contrast
c. Myelography and postmyelography CT cervical spine
d. Cervicocerebral arteriogram
e. No ideal imaging exam

Suspected acute cervical spine trauma, imaging indicated by clinical criteria (NEXUS or CCR), clinical or imaging findings suggest ligamentous injury.

a. X-ray cervical spine is usually not appropriate. Use if needed for surgical planning (1).
b. *MRI cervical spine without contrast* is the most appropriate. Often both CT and MRI are needed to evaluate for soft tissue and ligamentous damage (8).
c. Myelography and postmyelography CT cervical spine is usually not appropriate (1).
d. Cervicocerebral arteriogram is usually not appropriate (1).

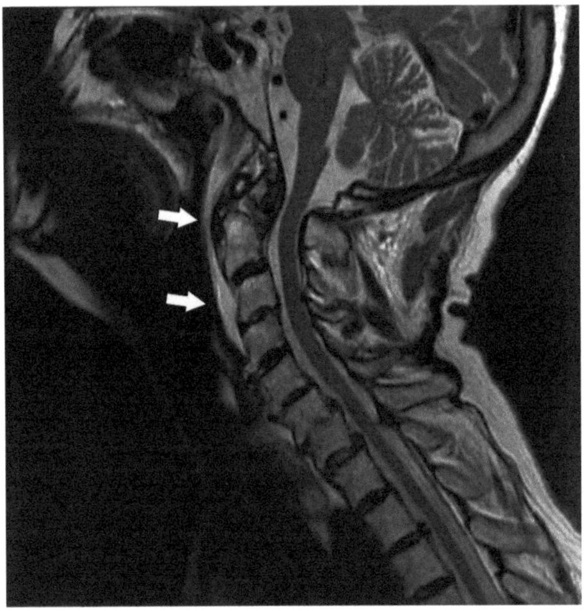

Fig. 6.35 Cervical spine ligamentous injury. Cervical spine MR sagittal T2-weighted image shows prevertebral soft tissue edema (*arrows*) anterior to C1–C4

An 82-year-old man with suspected thoracolumbar spine injury from blunt trauma.

a. X-ray thoracic or lumbar spine
b. CT thoracic or lumbar spine without contrast
c. MRI thoracic or lumbar spine without contrast
d. Myelography and postmyelography CT thoracic or lumbar spine
e. No ideal imaging exam

Blunt trauma meeting criteria for thoracic or lumbar imaging, with or without localizing signs.

a. X-ray thoracic or lumbar spine is usually not appropriate. This is useful for patients with localizing signs (3).
b. *CT thoracic or lumbar spine without contrast* is the most appropriate. Sagittal and coronal reformation from dedicated spine CT or derived from chest, abdomen, and pelvis CT can be used (9).
c. MRI thoracic or lumbar spine without contrast may sometimes be appropriate. Usefulness depends on clinical findings and results of the CT. Use if cord or soft tissue injury is suspected (5).
d. Myelography and postmyelography CT thoracic or lumbar spine is usually not appropriate. Use if MRI is contraindicated (3).

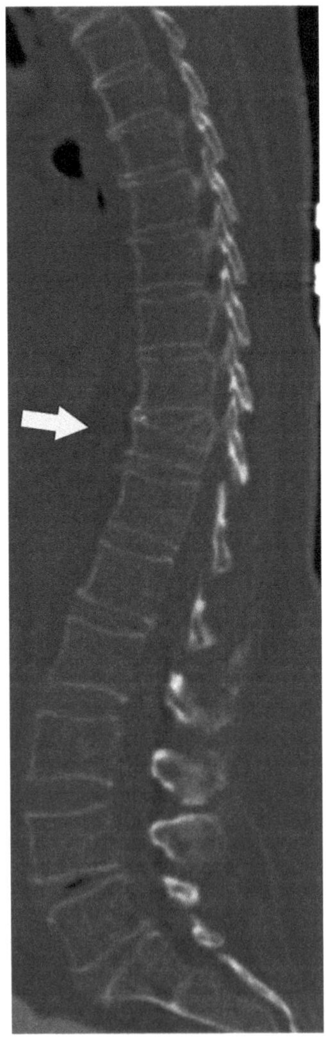

Fig. 6.36 Thoracic spine fracture. Thoracolumbar spine CT sagittal reconstruction image shows a T10 vertebral body fracture (*arrow*)

6.6 Low Back Pain

A 40-year-old presents with low back pain of <6 weeks duration. He is otherwise asymptomatic with no significant medical history.

a. X-ray lumbar spine
b. CT lumbar spine without contrast
c. MRI lumbar spine without contrast
d. Myelography and postmyelography CT lumbar spine
e. No ideal imaging exam

Uncomplicated acute low back pain and/or radiculopathy, nonsurgical presentation, and no red flags.

a. X-ray lumbar spine is usually not appropriate (2).
b. CT lumbar spine without contrast is usually not appropriate (2).
c. MRI lumbar spine without contrast is usually not appropriate (2).
d. Myelography and postmyelography CT lumbar spine is usually not appropriate (2).
e. *No ideal imaging exam* is the correct answer.

An 89-year-old woman with known osteoporosis now with low back pain.

a. X-ray lumbar spine
b. CT lumbar spine without contrast
c. MRI lumbar spine without contrast
d. Myelography and postmyelography CT lumbar spine
e. No ideal imaging exam

Low-velocity trauma, osteoporosis, and/or age >70 years.

a. X-ray lumbar spine may sometimes be appropriate (6).
b. CT lumbar spine without contrast may sometimes be appropriate. MRI is preferred. CT is useful if MRI is contraindicated or unavailable and/or for problem solving (6).
c. *MRI lumbar spine without contrast* is the most appropriate (8).
d. Myelography and postmyelography CT lumbar spine is usually not appropriate (1).

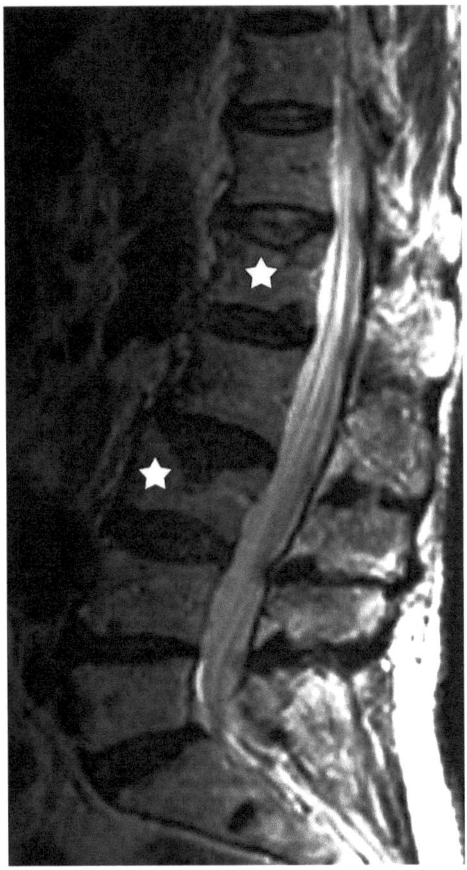

Fig. 6.37 Lumbar spine fractures from osteoporosis. Lumbar spine MR sagittal T2-weighted image shows compression fractures of the L1 and L3 vertebrae (*stars*)

A 75-year-old man, chronically immunosuppressed, now with low back pain.

a. X-ray lumbar spine
b. CT lumbar spine without contrast
c. MRI lumbar spine without and with contrast
d. Myelography and postmyelography CT lumbar spine
e. No ideal imaging exam

Suspicion of cancer, infection, or immunosuppression.

a. X-ray lumbar spine may sometimes be appropriate (5).
b. CT lumbar spine without contrast may sometimes be appropriate. MRI is preferred. CT is useful if MRI is contraindicated or unavailable and/or for problem solving (6).
c. *MRI lumbar spine without and with contrast* is the most appropriate (8).
d. Myelography and postmyelography CT lumbar spine is usually not appropriate (2).

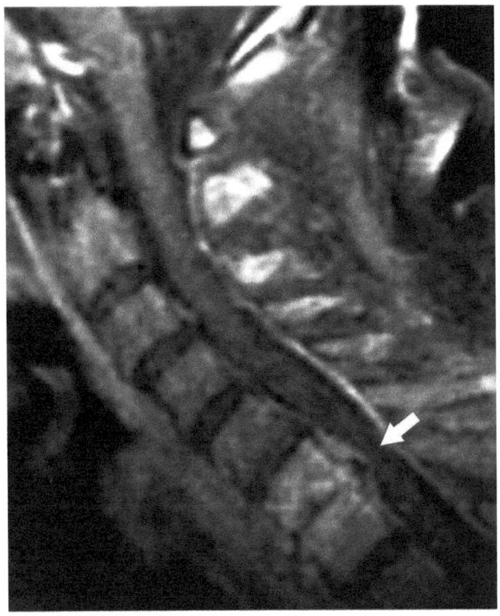

Fig. 6.38 Cervical spine osteomyelitis. Cervical spine MR sagittal postcontrast image shows abnormal enhancement of the C6–7 vertebrae and disc collapse (*arrow*)

A 49-year-old man with low back pain and radiculopathy who is undergoing evaluation for surgical treatment.

a. X-ray lumbar spine
b. CT lumbar spine without contrast
c. MRI lumbar spine without contrast
d. Myelography and postmyelography CT lumbar spine
e. No ideal imaging exam

Low back pain and/or radiculopathy, surgery or intervention candidate.

a. X-ray lumbar spine may sometimes be appropriate. This is usually not sufficient for decision making without MR and/or CT imaging (4).
b. CT lumbar spine without contrast may sometimes be appropriate. MRI is preferred. CT is useful if MRI is contraindicated or unavailable and/or for problem solving (5).
c. *MRI lumbar spine without contrast* is the most appropriate (8).
d. Myelography and postmyelography CT lumbar spine may sometimes be appropriate. This may be indicated if MRI is contraindicated or nondiagnostic (5).

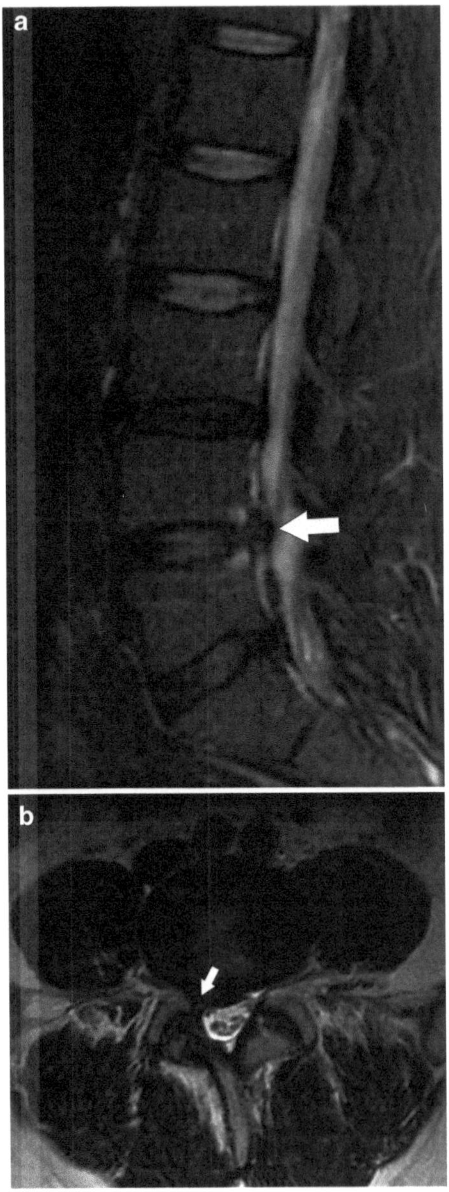

Fig. 6.39 Disc herniation with nerve root compression. Lumbar spine MR sagittal T2-weighted image (**a**) shows L4–5 disc herniation (*arrow*) which on axial T2-weighted image (**b**) is seen to compress the right L5 nerve root (*arrow*)

A 50-year-old man with prior lumbar spine surgery now with low back pain.

a. X-ray lumbar spine
b. CT lumbar spine without contrast
c. MRI lumbar spine without and with contrast
d. Myelography and postmyelography CT lumbar spine
e. No ideal imaging exam

Prior lumbar surgery.

a. X-ray lumbar spine may sometimes be appropriate. Flexion and extension views may be useful (5).
b. CT lumbar spine without contrast may sometimes be appropriate. This is most useful in postfusion patients or when MRI is contraindicated or inconclusive (6).
c. *MRI lumbar spine without and with contrast* is the most appropriate. Use to differentiate disc versus scar (8).
d. Myelography and postmyelography CT lumbar spine may sometimes be appropriate (6).

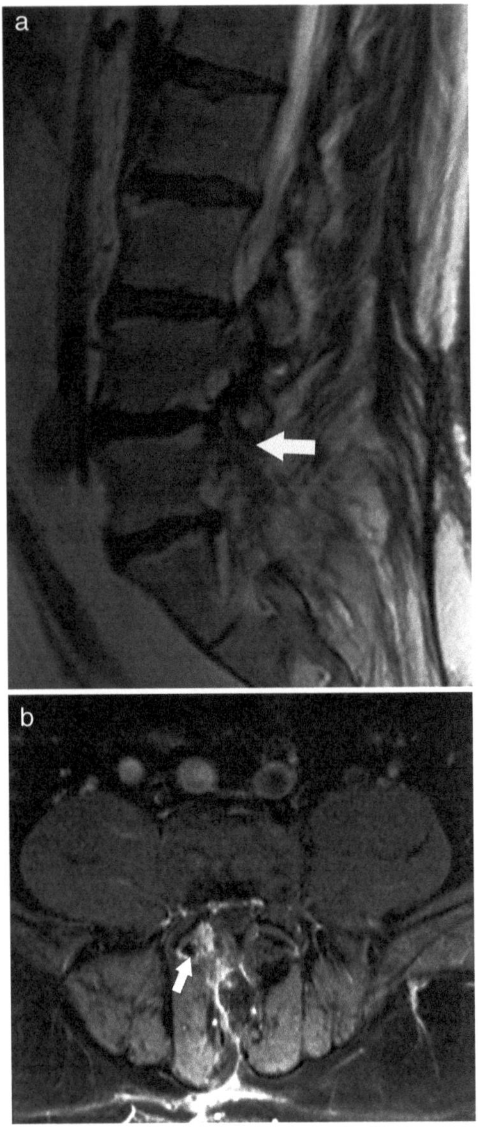

Fig. 6.40 Postspine surgery scar with nerve root impingement. Lumbar spine MR sagittal T2-weighted (**a**) and axial postcontrast (**b**) images show soft tissue (*arrows*) encasing the right S1 nerve root

A 93-year-old woman presents with low back pain and cauda equina syndrome.

a. X-ray lumbar spine
b. CT lumbar spine
c. MRI lumbar spine without contrast
d. Myelography and postmyelography CT lumbar spine
e. No ideal imaging exam

Cauda equina syndrome.

a. X-ray lumbar spine may sometimes be appropriate (4).
b. CT lumbar spine may sometimes be appropriate. It may be indicated if MRI is inconclusive or contraindicated and myelography is not feasible. Use of contrast depends on clinical circumstances (6).
c. *MRI lumbar spine without contrast* is the most appropriate. Use of contrast depends on clinical circumstances (9).
d. Myelography and postmyelography CT lumbar spine may sometimes be appropriate. Use if MRI is nondiagnostic or contraindicated (6).

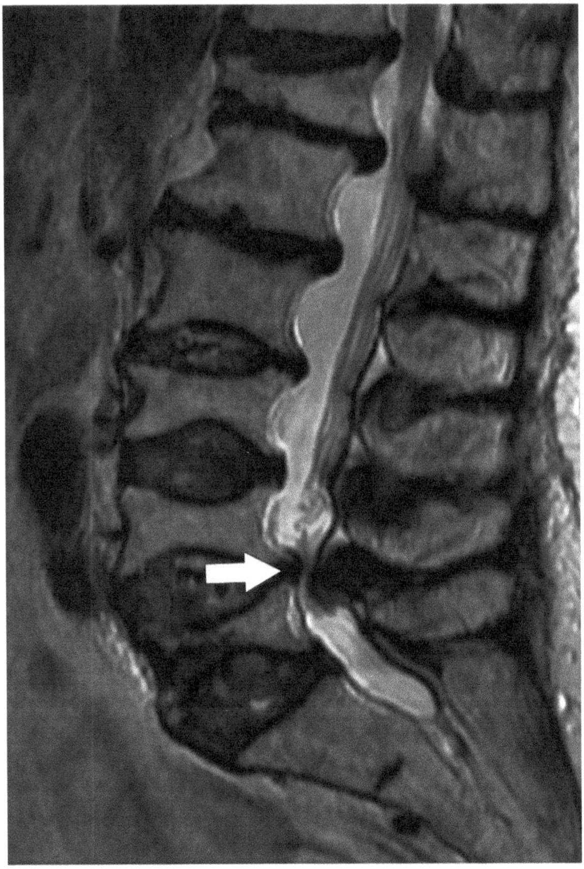

Fig. 6.41 Spinal stenosis. Lumbar spine MR sagittal T2-weighted image shows a posterior L3–4 disc herniation (*arrow*) compressing the cauda equina

Further Reading

Head Trauma

Teasdale G, Jennett B. Assessment of coma and impaired consciousness. Lancet 1974; 81–84.

Suspected Spine Trauma

Hoffman JR, Mower WR, Wolfson AB, Todd KH, Zucker MI. Validity of a set of clinical criteria to rule out injury to the cervical spine in patients with blunt trauma. National Emergency X-Radiography Utilization Study Group. N Engl J Med. 2000; 343: 94–99.

Stiell IG, Wells GA, Vandemheen KL, Clement CM, Lesiuk H, De Maio VJ, Laupacis A, Schull M, McKnight RD, Verbeek R, Brison R, Cass D, Dreyer J, Eisenhauer MA, Greenberg GH, MacPhail I, Morrison L, Reardon M, Worthington J. The Canadian C-spine rule for radiography in alert and stable trauma patients. JAMA. 2001; 286: 1841–1848.

7 Pediatric Imaging

7.1 Headache

A 12-year-old boy with isolated episode of headache with no associated neurological signs or symptoms.

a. CT head without contrast
b. CT head with contrast
c. MRI head without contrast
d. MRI head with contrast
e. No ideal imaging exam

S.I. Lee, J.H. Thrall, *Choosing the Correct Radiologic Test*,
DOI 10.1007/978-3-642-15772-1_7,

Isolated headache unaccompanied by neurologic signs and symptoms or historical data.

a. CT head without contrast is usually not appropriate (2).
b. CT head with contrast is usually not appropriate (2).
c. MRI head without contrast is usually not appropriate (2).
d. MRI head with contrast is usually not appropriate (2).
e. *No ideal imaging exam* is the correct answer.

A 7-year-old boy with headaches with positive neurological signs or symptoms.

a. CT head with contrast
b. MRI head without contrast
c. MRA head
d. Arteriography cerebral
e. No ideal imaging exam

Headaches with positive neurologic signs or symptoms.

a. CT head with contrast is usually not appropriate (3).
b. *MRI head without contrast* is the most appropriate (8).
c. MRA head may sometimes be appropriate (5).
d. Arteriography cerebral is usually not appropriate (2).

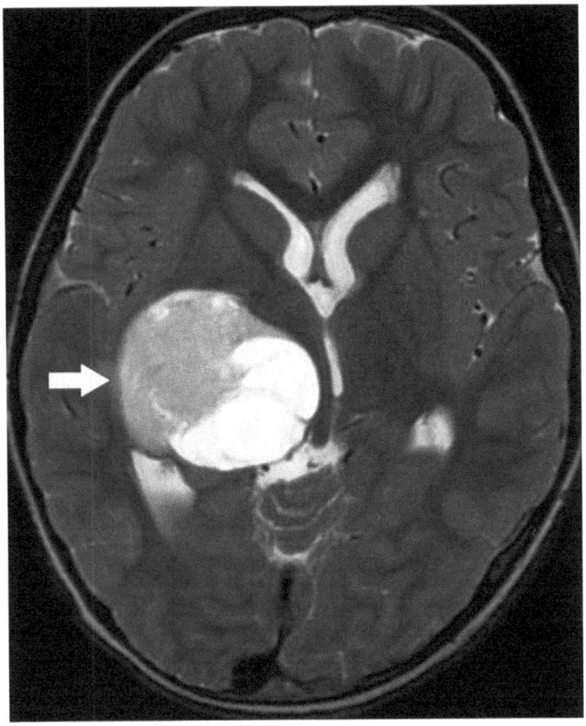

Fig. 7.1 Pilocytic astrocytoma. Brain MR axial T2-weighted image shows a mass in the right midbrain (*arrow*)

A 9-year-old girl with "thunderclap" headache and no family history of migraine headaches.

a. CT head without contrast
b. CTA head
c. MRI head without contrast
d. MRA head
e. No ideal imaging exam

Acute severe "thunderclap" headache and absence of family history of migraine.

a. *CT head without contrast* is the most appropriate (9).
b. CTA head is usually appropriate, but there is a better choice here (7).
c. MRI head without contrast is usually appropriate, but there is a better choice here (8).
d. MRA head is usually appropriate, but there is a better choice here (7).

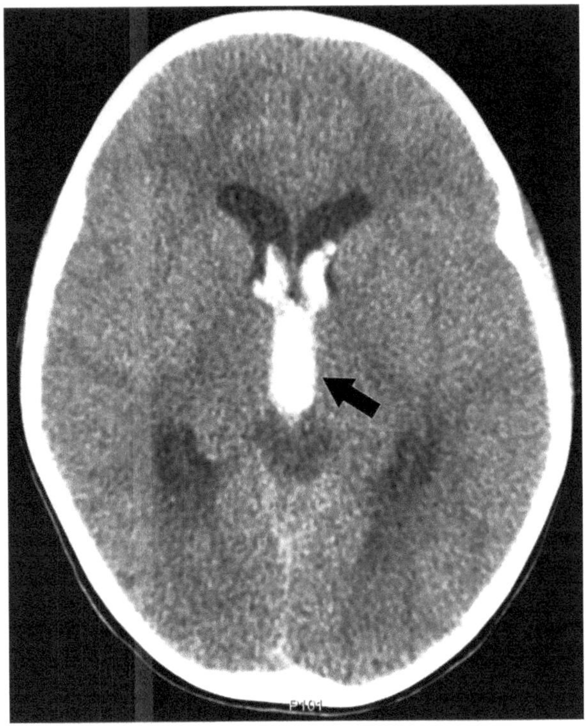

Fig. 7.2 Intracranial hemorrhage. Head CT without contrast demonstrates blood in the ventricle (*arrow*)

A 11-year-old boy with migraine headache without neurological signs or symptoms.

a. CT head without contrast
b. CT head with contrast
c. MRI head without contrast
d. MRI head with contrast
e. No ideal imaging exam

Migraine with or without aura and without neurologic findings.

a. CT head without contrast is usually not appropriate (2).
b. CT head with contrast is usually not appropriate (2).
c. MRI head without contrast is usually not appropriate (2).
d. MRI head with contrast is usually not appropriate (2).
e. *No ideal imaging exam* is the correct answer.

7.2 Sinusitis

A 4-year-old girl with acute sinusitis.

a. X-ray paranasal sinuses
b. CT paranasal sinuses without contrast
c. CT paranasal sinuses with contrast
d. MRI paranasal sinuses without contrast
e. No ideal imaging exam

Child with uncomplicated acute sinusitis.

a. X-ray paranasal sinuses is usually not appropriate. One to four projections are acquired (1).
b. CT paranasal sinuses without contrast is usually not appropriate (1).
c. CT paranasal sinuses with contrast is usually not appropriate (NA).
d. MRI paranasal sinuses without contrast is usually not appropriate (1).
e. *No ideal imaging exam* is the correct answer.

A 13-year-old boy with acute sinusitis unresponsive to therapy.

a. X-ray paranasal sinuses
b. CT paranasal sinuses without contrast
c. CT paranasal sinuses with contrast
d. MRI paranasal sinuses without contrast
e. No ideal imaging exam

Child with persistent acute (unresponsive to therapy), recurrent, or chronic sinusitis.

a. X-ray paranasal sinuses is usually not appropriate. One to four projections are acquired (1).
b. *CT paranasal sinuses without contrast* is the most appropriate (9).
c. CT paranasal sinuses with contrast is usually not appropriate (NA).
d. MRI paranasal sinuses without contrast is usually not appropriate (3).

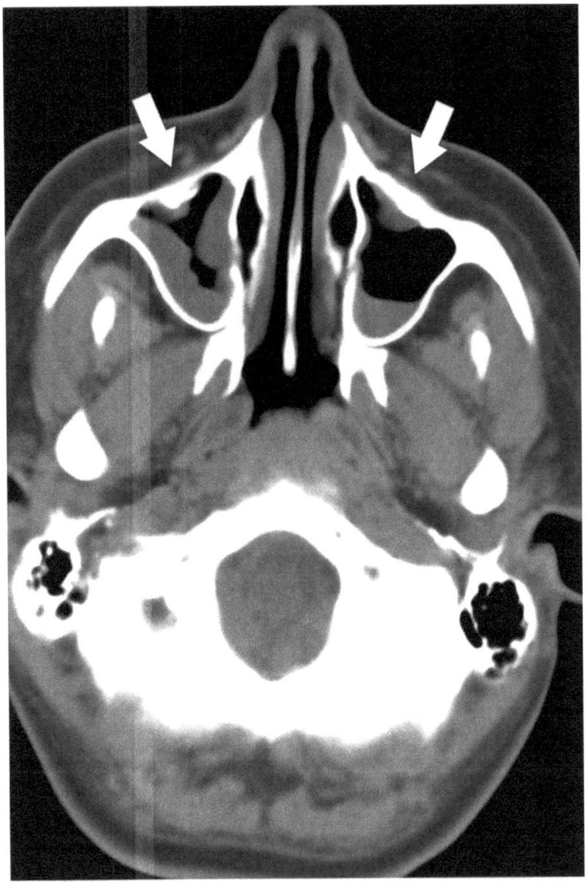

Fig. 7.3 Sinusitis. Sinus CT shows bilateral mucosal thickening of the maxillary sinuses (*arrows*) consistent with chronic sinusitis. Air-fluid level in the left maxillary sinus indicates acute sinusitis

7.3 Seizures

A 3-month-old boy with seizures.

a. US head
b. CT head without contrast
c. MRI head without contrast
d. FDG-PET head
e. No ideal imaging exam

Neonatal seizures.

a. *US head* is the most appropriate (9).
b. CT head without contrast is usually not appropriate (3).
c. MRI head without contrast may sometimes be appropriate. It is useful in detecting for hypoxic ischemic encephalopathy and congenital malformations (5).
d. FDG-PET head is usually not appropriate (1).

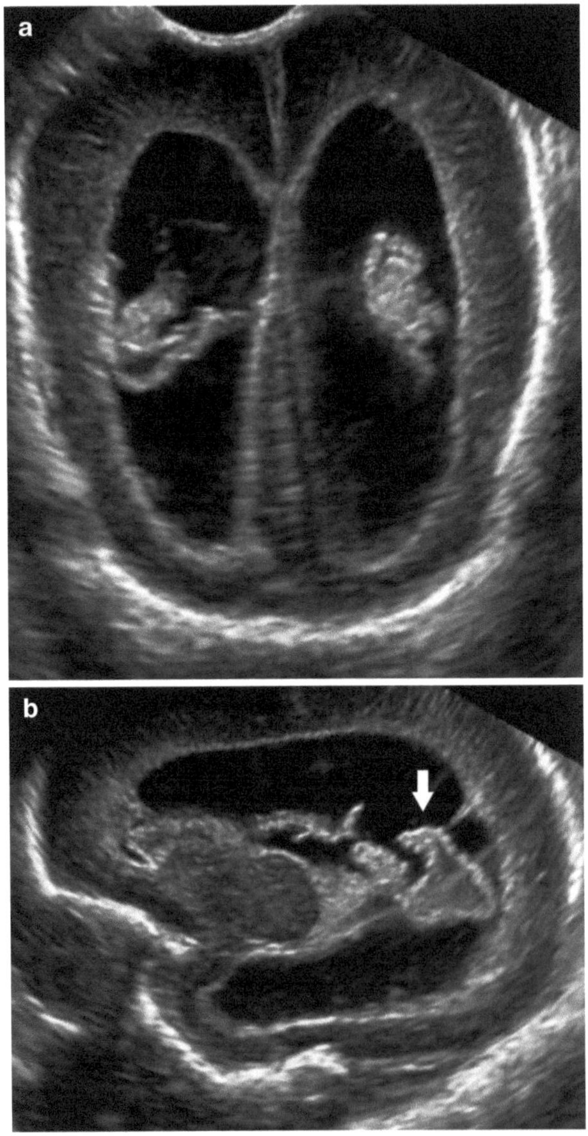

Fig. 7.4 Intracranial hemorrhage. Head US coronal (**a**) and parasagittal (**b**) views reveal bilaterally enlarged ventricles containing hematoma (*arrow*)

A 9-month-old girl with febrile seizures.

a. US head
b. CT head without contrast
c. MRI head without contrast
d. FDG-PET head
e. No ideal imaging exam

Febrile seizures.

a. US head is usually not appropriate (1).
b. CT head without contrast is usually not appropriate. It is used in child with complex febrile seizure (2).
c. MRI head without contrast is usually not appropriate. It is used in child with complex febrile seizure (2).
d. FDG-PET head is usually not appropriate (1).
e. *No ideal imaging exam* is the correct answer.

A 8-year-old girl with posttraumatic seizures.

a. US head
b. CT head without contrast
c. MRI head without contrast
d. FDG-PET head
e. No ideal imaging exam

Posttraumatic seizures.

a. US head is usually not appropriate (1).
b. *CT head without contrast* is the most appropriate (9).
c. MRI head without contrast may sometimes be appropriate. Exam is more sensitive than CT in detecting blood products and gliosis in the chronic posttraumatic setting (5).
d. FDG-PET head is usually not appropriate (1).

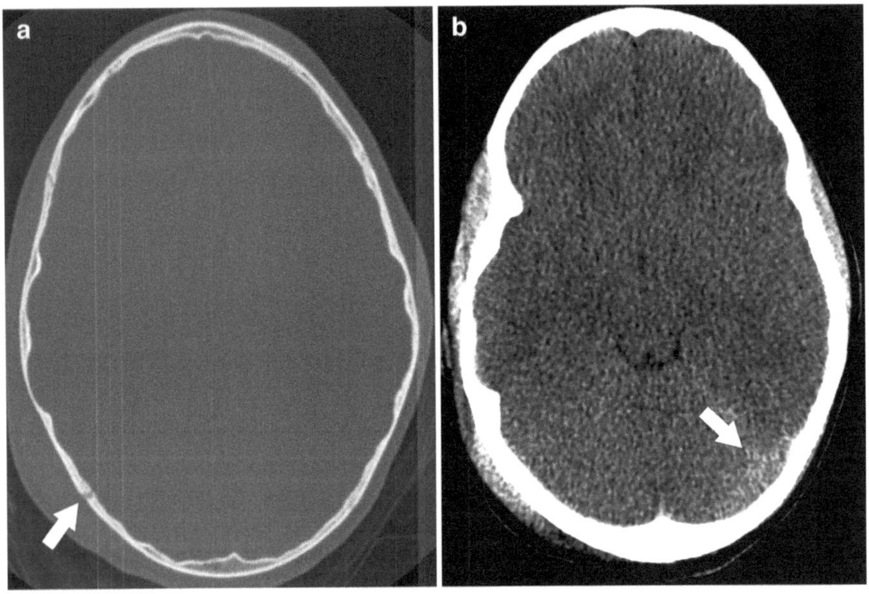

Fig. 7.5 Intracranial hemorrhage with skull fracture. Head CT bone window (**a**) shows a right parietal skull fracture (*arrow*). Soft tissue window (**b**) shows left subdural blood (*arrow*)

A 15-year-old boy with partial seizures.

a. US head
b. CT head without contrast
c. MRI head without contrast
d. FDG-PET head
e. No ideal imaging exam

Partial seizures.

a. US head is usually not appropriate (1).
b. CT head without contrast may sometimes be appropriate. Use if MRI unavailable or contraindicated (5).
c. *MRI head without contrast* is the most appropriate (9).
d. FDG-PET head may sometimes be appropriate. Use in children with recurrent seizures. (5)

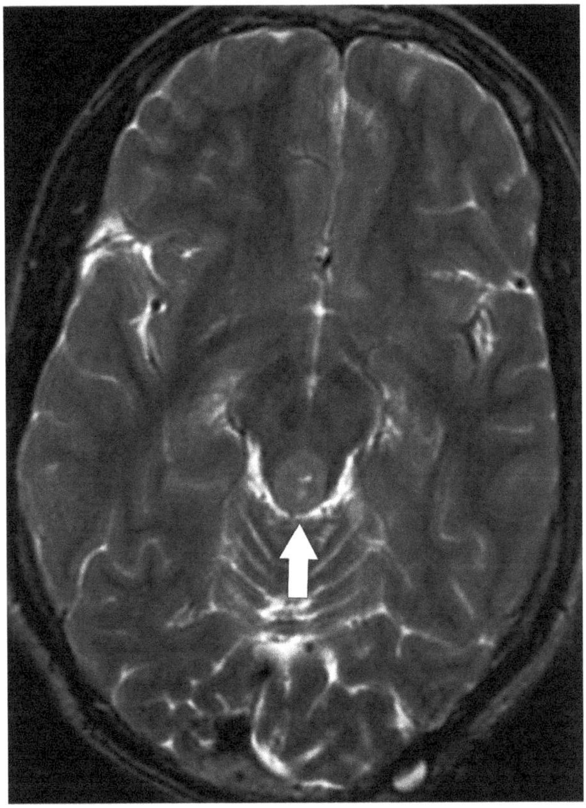

Fig. 7.6 Pilocytic astrocytoma. Brain MR axial T2-weighted image shows a 2.5-cm mass (*arrow*) in the dorsal midbrain

A 4-year-old girl with first episode of generalized seizure. She is otherwise normal neurologically.

a. US head
b. CT head without contrast
c. MRI head without contrast
d. FDG-PET head
e. No ideal imaging exam

First generalized seizure in a child that is otherwise neurologically normal.

a. US head is usually not appropriate (1).
b. CT head without contrast may sometimes be appropriate (4).
c. MRI head without contrast may sometimes be appropriate (5).
d. FDG-PET head is usually not appropriate (1).
e. *No ideal imaging exam* is the correct answer.

A 15-year-old girl with first episode of generalized seizure and history of developmental delay.

a. US head
b. CT head without contrast
c. MRI head without contrast
d. FDG-PET head
e. No ideal imaging exam

Generalized seizure in a child with a history of neurologic abnormality.

a. US head is usually not appropriate (1).
b. CT head without contrast may sometimes be appropriate (6).
c. *MRI head without contrast* is the most appropriate (9).
d. FDG-PET head is usually not appropriate (2).

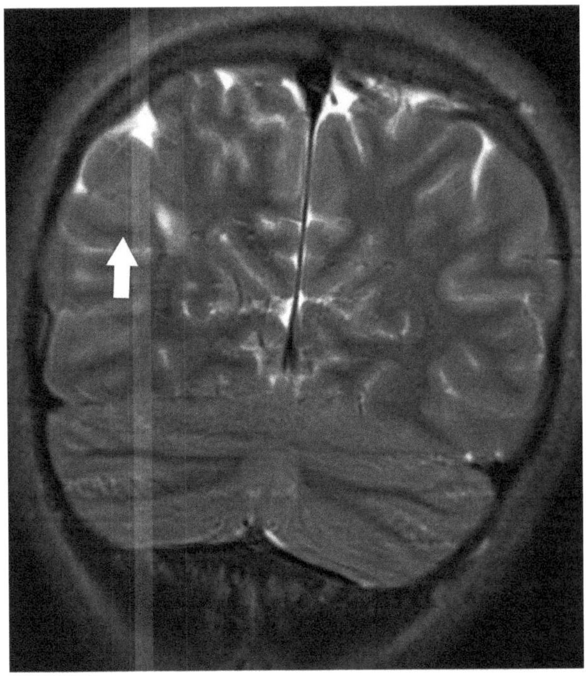

Fig. 7.7 Cortical dysplasia. Brain MR coronal T2-weighted image shows a focal area of cortical thickening and abnormal gyral fold (*arrow*) in the right parietal lobe

A 12-year-old boy with intractable seizures.

a. US head
b. CT head without contrast
c. MRI head without contrast
d. FDG-PET head
e. No ideal imaging exam

Intractable or refractory seizures.

a. US head is usually not appropriate (1).
b. CT head without contrast may sometimes be appropriate (5).
c. *MRI head without contrast* is the most appropriate (9).
d. FDG-PET head may sometimes be appropriate (6).

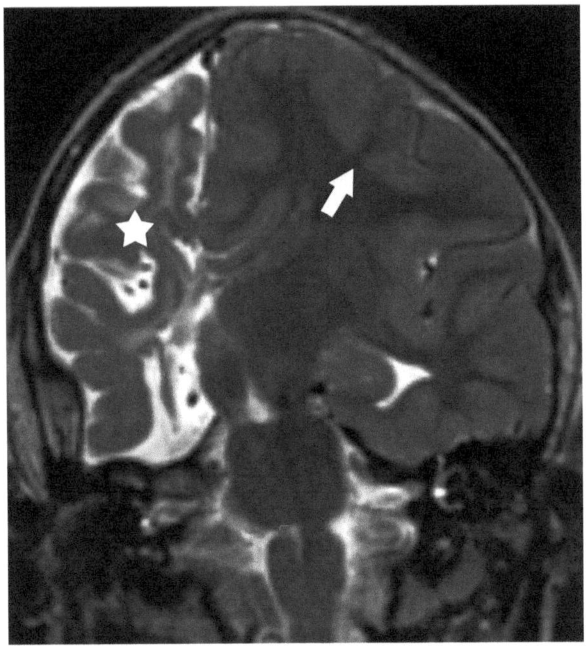

Fig. 7.8 Cortical dysplasia. Brain MR coronal T2-weighted images reveal right cerebral atrophy (*star*) and polymicrogyria (*arrow*) of the left parietal lobe

7.4 Head Trauma

A 1-year-old with mild acute closed head injury from trauma.

a. US head with Doppler
b. CT head without contrast
c. MRI head without contrast
d. FDG-PET head
e. No ideal imaging exam

Mild or moderate acute closed head injury in a child <2 years old.

a. US head with Doppler is usually not appropriate (1).
b. *CT head without contrast* is the most appropriate (9).
c. MRI head without contrast is usually appropriate, but there is a better choice here (7).
d. FDG-PET head is usually not appropriate (1).

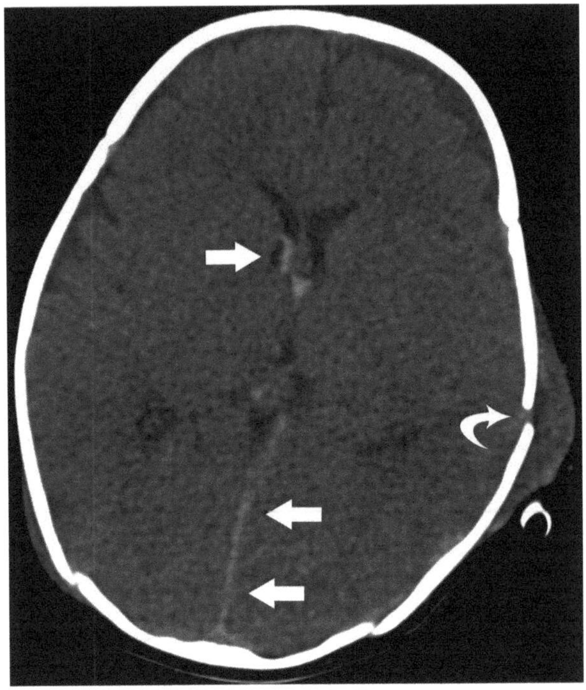

Fig. 7.9 Head trauma. Head CT shows subdural blood (*arrows*) and a skull fracture (*curved arrow*)

7.5 Suspected Spine Trauma

A 6-year-old boy with suspected spine trauma. He is alert, with no neck or back pain. Exam reveals a supple neck.

a. X-ray cervical spine
b. CT cervical spine without contrast
c. CT thoracic and lumbar spine without contrast
d. MRI cervical spine without contrast
e. No ideal imaging exam

Child who is alert, with a supple neck and without neck or back pain or history of distracting injury.

a. X-ray cervical spine is usually not appropriate (1).
b. CT cervical spine without contrast is usually not appropriate. Sagittal and coronal reformations should be performed (1).
c. CT thoracic and lumbar spine without contrast is usually not appropriate. Images can be acquired as a dedicated spine scan with sagittal and coronal reformations or be derived from a body CT scan (1).
d. MRI cervical spine without contrast is usually not appropriate (NA).
e. *No ideal imaging exam* is the correct answer.

A 8-year-old girl with a known cervical spine fracture.

a. X-ray thoracic and lumbar spine
b. CT thoracic and lumbar spine without contrast
c. CT thoracic and lumbar spine post myelography
d. MRI thoracic or lumbar spine without contrast
e. No ideal imaging exam

Child with a known cervical spine fracture.

a. X-ray thoracic and lumbar spine is usually appropriate, but there is a better choice here (8).
b. *CT thoracic and lumbar spine without contrast* is the most appropriate. Images can be acquired as a dedicated spine scan with sagittal and coronal reformations or be derived from a body CT scan (9).
c. CT thoracic and lumbar spine post myelography is usually not appropriate (NA).
d. MRI thoracic or lumbar spine without contrast is usually not appropriate (NA).

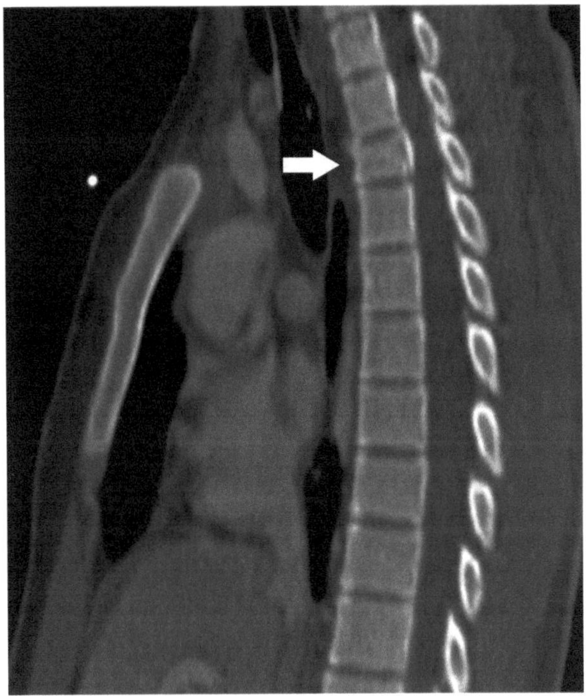

Fig. 7.10 Thoracic spine fracture. Sagittal reformation from a thoracoabdominal CT reveals a burst fracture of the T3 vertebral body (*arrow*)

7.6 Vomiting in Infants

A 3-day-old boy with bilious vomiting.

a. X-ray abdomen
b. X-ray fluoroscopy upper GI series
c. US abdomen
d. Radionuclide gastric motility scan
e. No ideal imaging exam

Bilious vomiting in neonate up to 1 week old.

a. *X-ray abdomen* is the most appropriate. Initial X-ray will help determine further workup strategy (9).
b. X-ray fluoroscopy upper GI series is usually appropriate, but there is a better choice here (8).
c. US abdomen is usually not appropriate (NA).
d. Radionuclide gastric motility scan is usually not appropriate (NA).

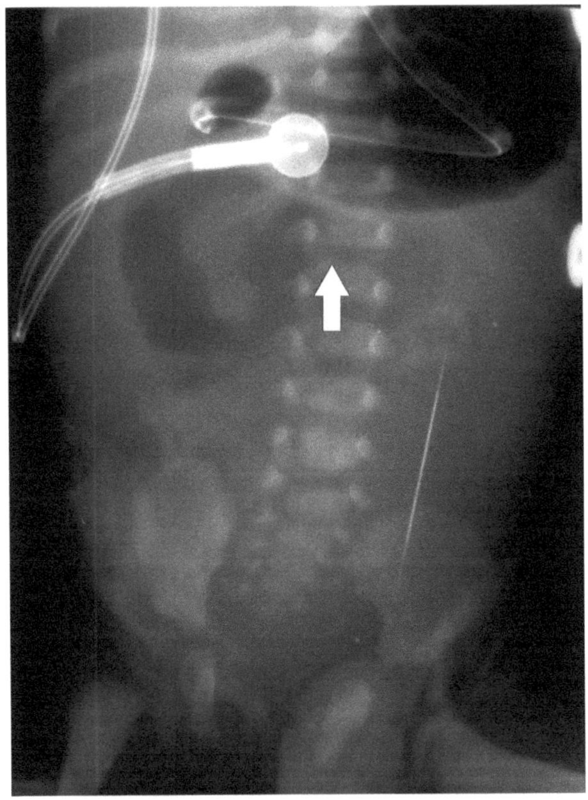

Fig. 7.11 Midgut volvulus. Abdominal X-ray shows a distended stomach and proximal duodenum with an abrupt transition (*arrow*) to collapsed bowel in the distal duodenum

A 4-week-old boy with bilious vomiting.

a. X-ray abdomen
b. X-ray fluoroscopy upper GI series
c. US abdomen
d. Radionuclide gastric motility scan
e. No ideal imaging exam

Bilious vomiting in infant 1 week to 3 months old.

a. X-ray abdomen may sometimes be appropriate (5).
b. *X-ray fluoroscopy upper GI series* is the most appropriate (9).
c. US abdomen is usually not appropriate (2).
d. Radionuclide gastric motility scan is usually not appropriate (1).

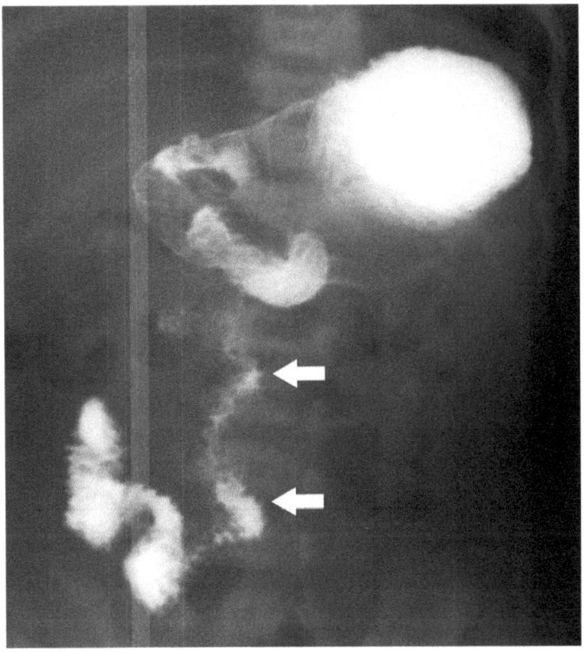

Fig. 7.12 Midgut volvulus. Abdominal X-ray from upper GI shows small bowel that fails to cross the midline and spirals caudally (*arrows*)

A 6-week-old girl with intermittent nonbilious vomiting since birth.

a. X-ray abdomen
b. X-ray fluoroscopy upper GI series
c. US abdomen
d. Radionuclide gastric motility scan
e. No ideal imaging exam

Intermittent nonbilious vomiting since birth.

a. X-ray abdomen is usually not appropriate (1).
b. X-ray fluoroscopy upper GI series may sometimes be appropriate (6).
c. US abdomen is usually not appropriate (3).
d. Radionuclide gastric motility scan is usually not appropriate (2).
e. *No ideal imaging exam* is the correct answer.

A 4-week-old boy with intermittent nonbilious vomiting since birth.

a. X-ray abdomen
b. X-ray fluoroscopy upper GI series
c. US abdomen
d. Radionuclide gastric motility scan
e. No ideal imaging exam

A 4-week-old boy with new-onset projectile nonbilious vomiting.

a. X-ray abdomen is usually not appropriate (2).
b. X-ray fluoroscopy upper GI series may sometimes be appropriate (6).
c. *US abdomen* is the most appropriate (8).
d. Radionuclide gastric motility scan is usually not appropriate (1).

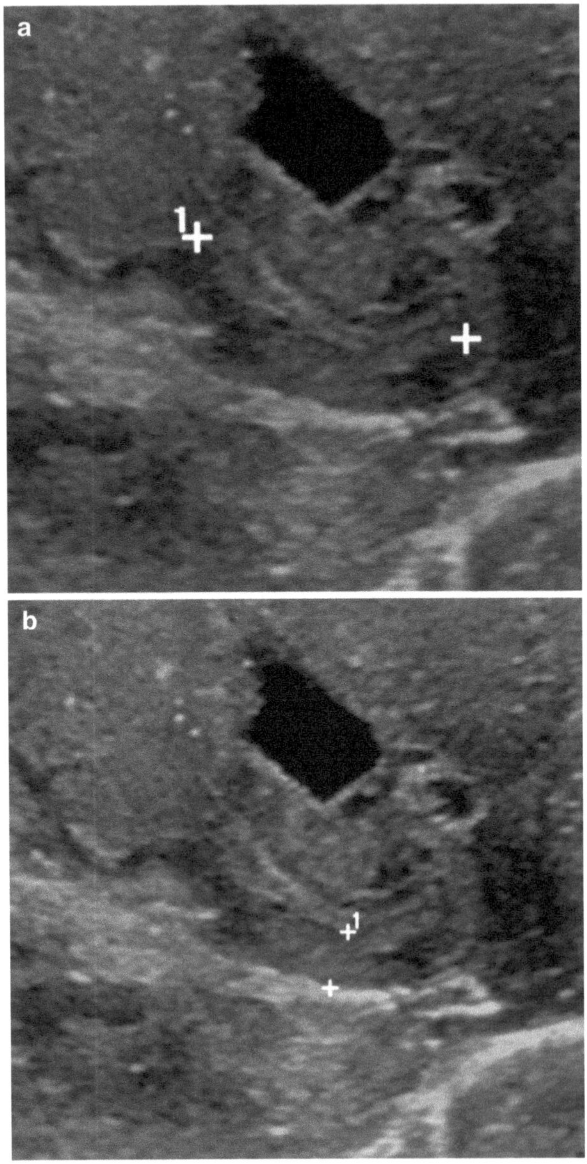

Fig. 7.13 Hypertrophic pyloric stenosis. Abdomen ultrasound measures (*calipers*) the length (**a**) and wall thickness (**b**) of the pylorus which is >2 cm and >4 mm, respectively

7.7 Right Lower Quadrant Abdominal Pain

A 12-year-old boy with right lower quadrant pain, fever, and leukocytosis.

a. X-ray abdomen
b. US abdomen
c. CT abdomen and pelvis
d. MRI abdomen and pelvis
e. No ideal imaging exam

Fever, leukocytosis, with possible appendicitis in a child <14 years old.

a. X-ray abdomen may sometimes be appropriate (6).
b. *US abdomen* is the most appropriate (8).
c. CT abdomen and pelvis is usually appropriate, but there is a better choice here (7).
d. MRI abdomen and pelvis may sometimes be appropriate (5).

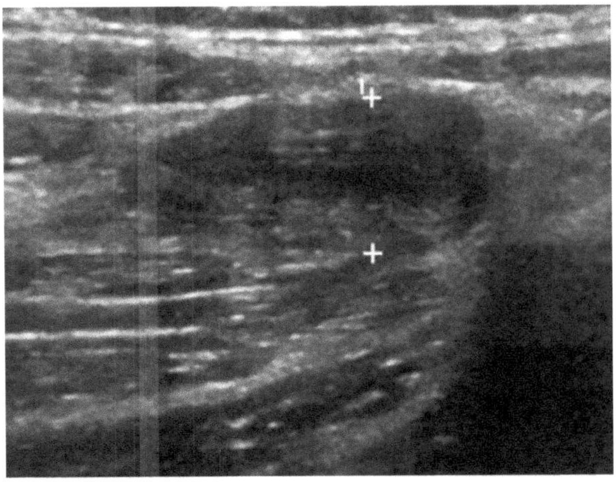

Fig. 7.14 Appendicitis. Abdomen ultrasound reveals an abnormally thickened appendix (*calipers*) measuring 9 mm that does not deform with compression

7.8 Urinary Tract Infection

A 1-year-old girl with urinary tract infection and maximum temperature <38.5 °C.

a. US kidneys and bladder
b. X-ray fluoroscopy voiding cystourethrography
c. Radionuclide cystography
d. Radionuclide renal cortical scintigraphy
e. No ideal imaging exam

Child aged 0–2 years with maximum temperature <38.5 °C.

a. *US kidneys and bladder* is the most appropriate (9).
b. X-ray fluoroscopy voiding cystourethrography is usually appropriate, but there is a better choice here. Exam is accurate in evaluation of reflux. It confers higher radiation dose but provides better anatomic differentiation than radionuclide cystography. In girls, exam should be used only when significant anatomic abnormality is suspected (7).
c. Radionuclide cystography is usually appropriate, but there is a better choice here. Exam is accurate in evaluation of reflux. It confers lower radiation dose but provides poorer anatomic differentiation than X-ray fluoroscopy voiding cystourethrography. In girls, exams should be used when no anatomic abnormality is suspected (8).
d. Radionuclide renal cortical scintigraphy may sometimes be appropriate (6).

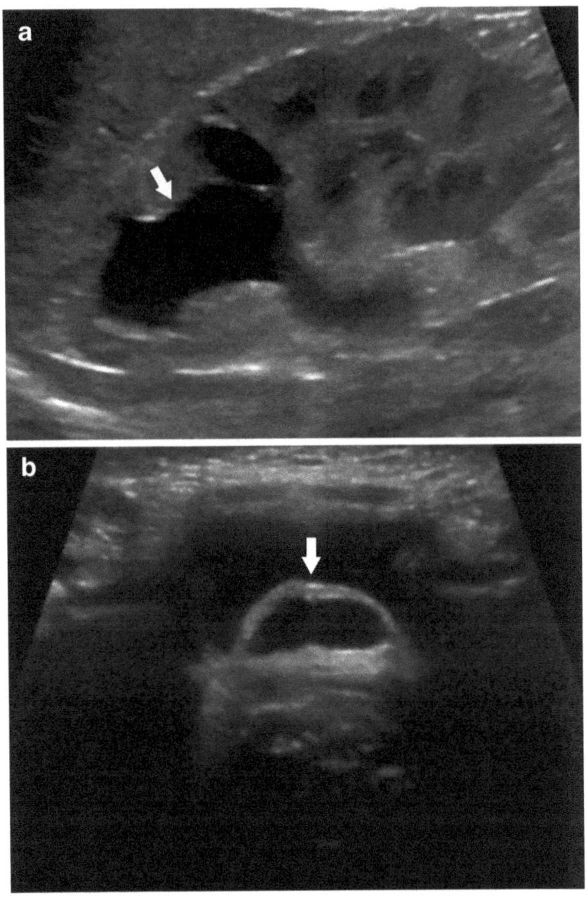

Fig. 7.15 Duplex collecting system, hydronephrosis, and ureterocele. Renal ultrasound (**a**) shows a duplex right renal collecting system with dilatation of the upper pole (*arrow*). A bladder image (**b**) from the same exam shows a ureterocele (*arrow*)

A 1-year-old boy with urinary tract infection and maximum temperature >38.5 °C.

a. US kidneys and bladder
b. X-ray fluoroscopy voiding cystourethrography
c. Radionuclide cystography
d. Radionuclide renal cortical scintigraphy
e. No ideal imaging exam

Child aged 0–2 years with maximum temperature ≥38.5 °C.

a. *US kidneys and bladder* is the most appropriate (9).
b. X-ray fluoroscopy voiding cystourethrography is usually appropriate, but there is a better choice here. Exam is accurate in evaluation of reflux. It confers higher radiation dose but provides better anatomic differentiation than radionuclide cystography (8).
c. Radionuclide cystography is usually not appropriate. Exam is accurate in evaluation of reflux. It confers lower radiation dose but provides poorer anatomic differentiation than X-ray fluoroscopy voiding cystourethrography (2).
d. Radionuclide renal cortical scintigraphy is usually appropriate, but there is a better choice here. Pinhole and/or SPECT acquisition should be performed (7).

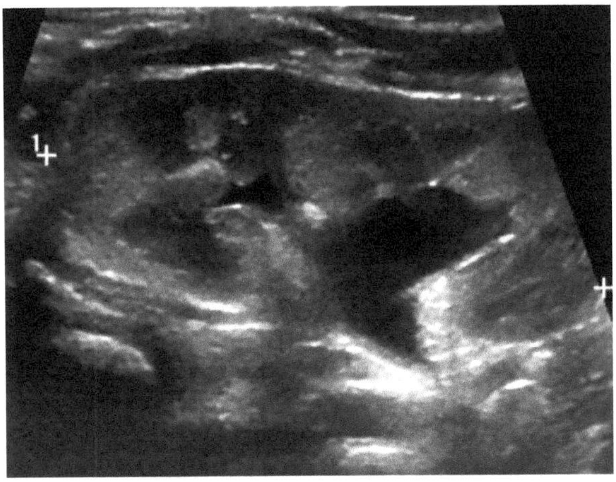

Fig. 7.16 Hydronephrosis. Renal ultrasound shows a dilated collecting system within the left kidney (*calipers*)

A 3-year-old boy with urinary tract infection and maximum temperature <38.5 °C.

a. X-ray fluoroscopy voiding cystourethrography
b. MRI abdomen and pelvis
c. Radionuclide cystography
d. Radionuclide renal cortical scintigraphy
e. No ideal imaging exam

Child aged 2–7 years with maximum temperature <38.5 °C.

a. *X-ray fluoroscopy voiding cystourethrography* is the most appropriate. Exam is accurate in evaluation of reflux. It confers higher radiation dose but provides better anatomic differentiation than radionuclide cystography (8).
b. MRI abdomen and pelvis may sometimes be appropriate. It is an acceptable method of cortical imaging. Child needs to be sedated (4).
c. Radionuclide cystography is usually not appropriate. Exam is accurate in evaluation of reflux. It confers lower radiation dose but provides poorer anatomic differentiation than X-ray fluoroscopy voiding cystourethrography (2).
d. Radionuclide renal cortical scintigraphy may sometimes be appropriate. Pinhole and/or SPECT acquisition should be performed (4).

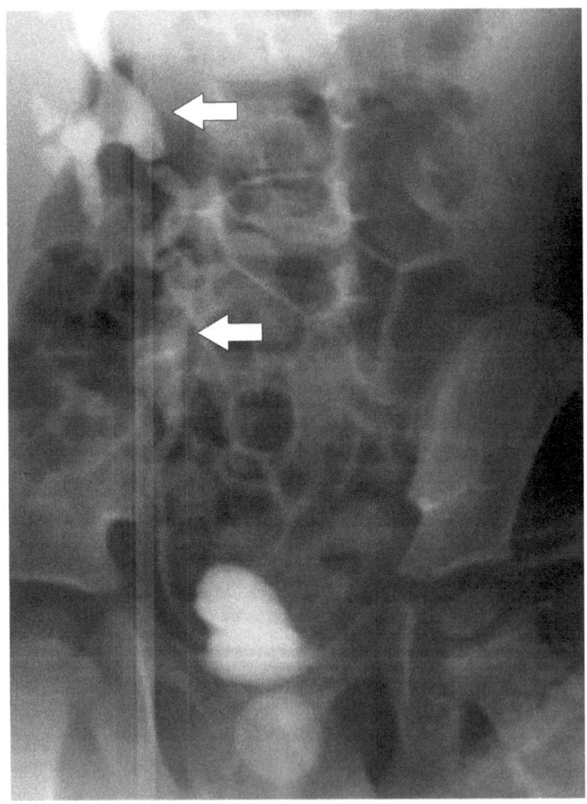

Fig. 7.17 Vesicoureteral reflux. Abdominal X-ray AP view from a voiding cystourethrogram demonstrates contrast reflux into the right renal collecting system and ureter (*arrows*)

A 5-year-old girl with urinary tract infection and maximum temperature >38.5 °C.

a. X-ray fluoroscopy voiding cystourethrography
b. MRI abdomen and pelvis
c. Radionuclide cystography
d. Radionuclide renal cortical scintigraphy
e. No ideal imaging exam

Child aged 2–7 years with maximum temperature ≥38.5 °C.

a. X-ray fluoroscopy voiding cystourethrography is usually appropriate, but there is a better choice here. Exam is accurate in evaluation of reflux. It confers higher radiation dose but better anatomic differentiation than radionuclide cystography. In girls, exam should be used only when significant anatomic abnormality is suspected (7).
b. MRI abdomen and pelvis may sometimes be appropriate. It is an acceptable method of cortical imaging. Child needs to be sedated (4).
c. *Radionuclide cystography* is the most appropriate. Exam is accurate in evaluation of reflux. It confers lower radiation dose but provides poorer anatomic differentiation than X-ray fluoroscopy voiding cystourethrography. In girls, exams should be used when no anatomic abnormality is suspected (8).
d. Radionuclide renal cortical scintigraphy may sometimes be appropriate. Pinhole and/or SPECT acquisition should be performed (4).

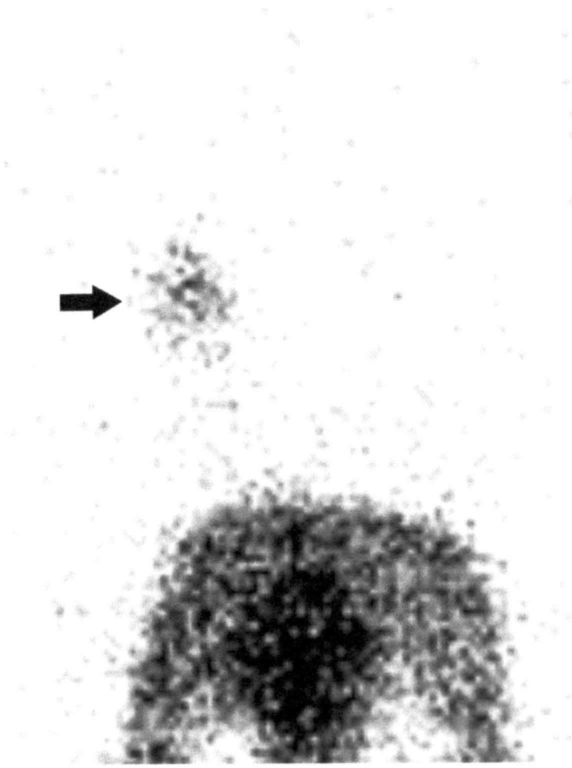

Fig. 7.18 Vesicoureteral reflux. Radionucleotide cystogram posterior planar view shows tracer reflux into the left renal collecting system (*arrow*)

A 9-year-old boy with urinary tract infection.

a. US kidneys and bladder
b. X-ray fluoroscopy voiding cystourethrography
c. Radionuclide cystography
d. CT abdomen with contrast
e. No ideal imaging exam

Child or adolescent older than 8 years.

a. *US kidneys and bladder* is the most appropriate (9).
b. X-ray fluoroscopy voiding cystourethrography is sometimes appropriate (5).
c. Radionuclide cystography is sometimes appropriate (5).
d. CT abdomen with contrast is sometimes appropriate (4).

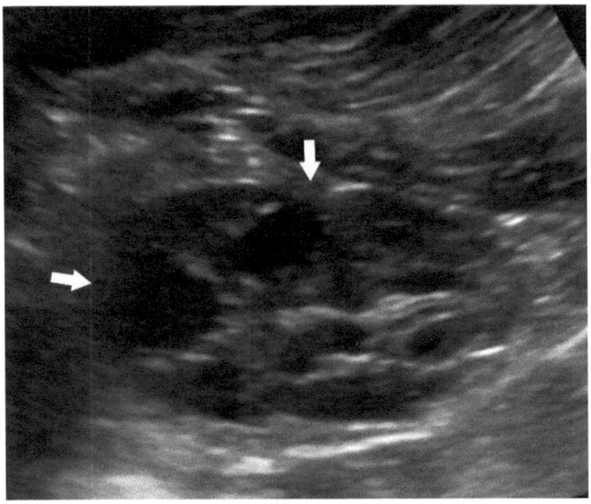

Fig. 7.19 Hydronephrosis and renal cortical scarring. Renal ultrasound of left kidney shows hydronephrosis and focal areas of cortical thinning (*arrows*)

7.9 Hematuria

A 5-year-old girl with isolated episode of hematuria.

a. US kidneys and bladder
b. X-ray fluoroscopy voiding cystourethrography
c. Radionuclide cystography
d. Radionuclide renal cortical scintigraphy
e. No ideal imaging exam

Child aged >8 years with maximum temperature ≥38.5 °C.

a. *US kidneys and bladder* is the most appropriate (8).
b. X-ray fluoroscopy voiding cystourethrography may sometimes be appropriate (5).
c. Radionuclide cystography may sometimes be appropriate (5).
d. Radionuclide renal cortical scintigraphy is usually not appropriate (2).

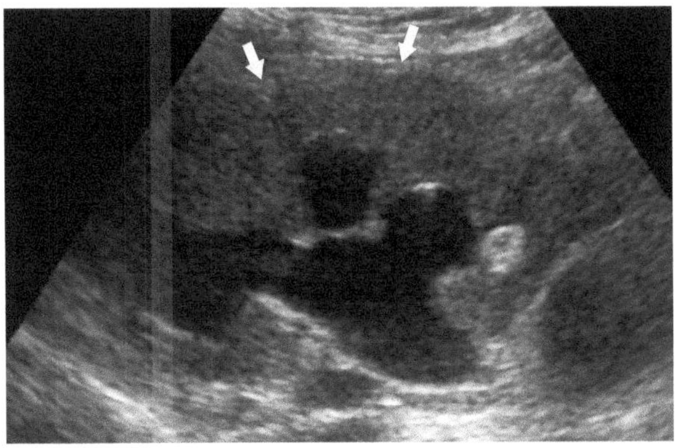

Fig. 7.20 Hydronephrosis and renal cortical scarring. Renal ultrasound of left kidney shows hydronephrosis and focal areas of cortical thinning (*arrows*)

A 5-year-old girl with isolated episode of hematuria.

a. X-ray abdomen and pelvis
b. X-ray fluoroscopy voiding cystourethrography
c. US kidneys and bladder
d. CT abdomen and pelvis
e. No ideal imaging exam

Isolated hematuria.

a. X-ray abdomen and pelvis is usually not appropriate (2).
b. X-ray fluoroscopy voiding cystourethrography is usually not appropriate. Exam may be useful if abnormality is found on US (3).
c. *US kidneys and bladder* is the most appropriate (7).
d. CT abdomen and pelvis is usually not appropriate. Exam may be useful if abnormality is found on US (3).

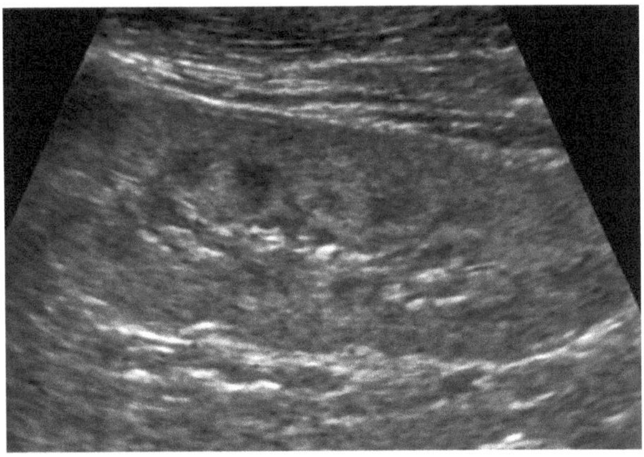

Fig. 7.21 Glomerulonephritis. Renal ultrasound shows a normal-sized left kidney with an echogenic cortex. Right kidney (not shown) appeared similar

A 11-year-old girl with painful hematuria and no history of trauma.

a. X-ray abdomen and pelvis
b. X-ray fluoroscopy voiding cystourethrography
c. US kidneys and bladder
d. CT abdomen and pelvis
e. No ideal imaging exam

Nontraumatic painful hematuria.

a. X-ray abdomen and pelvis may sometimes be appropriate (6).
b. X-ray fluoroscopy voiding cystourethrography is usually not appropriate (2).
c. US kidneys and bladder is usually appropriate, but there is a better choice here (7).
d. *CT abdomen and pelvis* is the most appropriate. Use to evaluate for stones (8).

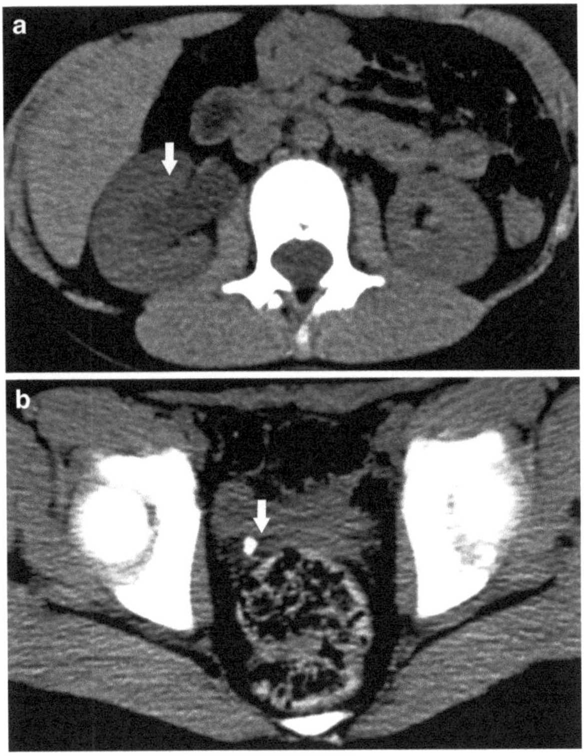

Fig. 7.22 Obstructive urolithiasis. Abdominopelvic CT without intravenous contrast image of the kidneys (**a**) shows right hydronephrosis (*arrow*). Image of the bladder (**b**) shows a stone (*arrow*) at the right ureterovesical junction (*arrow*)

A 15-year-old boy with macroscopic hematuria and history of trauma.

a. X-ray abdomen and pelvis
b. X-ray intravenous urography
c. US kidneys and bladder
d. CT abdomen and pelvis
e. No ideal imaging exam

Traumatic macroscopic hematuria.

a. X-ray abdomen and pelvis is usually not appropriate (2).
b. X-ray intravenous urography is usually not appropriate (2).
c. US kidneys and bladder is usually not appropriate (2).
d. *CT abdomen and pelvis* is the most appropriate (9).

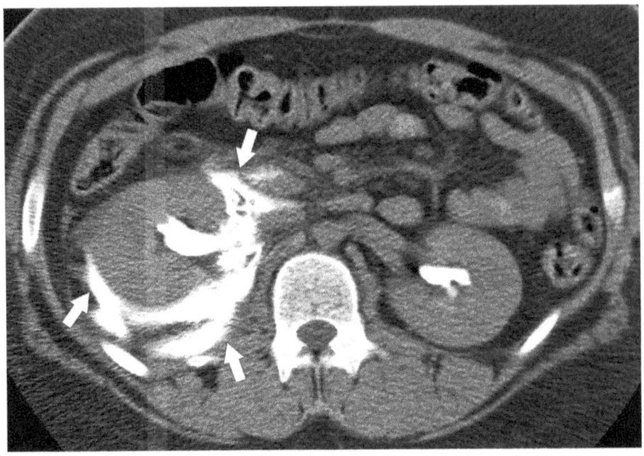

Fig. 7.23 Ureteral injury. Abdominopelvic CT with contrast during the excretory phase demonstrates urine leak (*arrows*) outside the kidney

A 15-year-old boy with microscopic hematuria and history of trauma.

a. X-ray abdomen and pelvis
b. X-ray intravenous urography
c. US kidneys and bladder
d. CT abdomen and pelvis
e. No ideal imaging exam

Traumatic microscopic hematuria.

a. X-ray abdomen and pelvis is usually not appropriate (2).
b. X-ray intravenous urography is usually not appropriate (2).
c. US kidneys and bladder may sometimes be appropriate. Use to evaluate for mass or developmental anomaly (4).
d. *CT abdomen and pelvis* is the most appropriate. Use in the presence of risk factors such as pelvic fractures, flank pain and tenderness, hypotension, or other signs of injury (7).

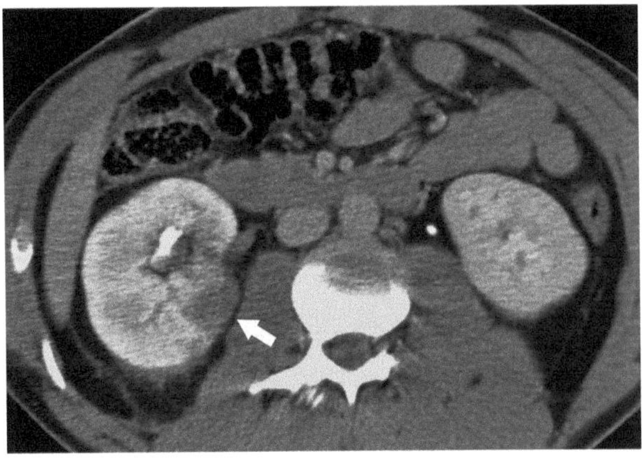

Fig. 7.24 Renal fracture. Abdominopelvic CT with contrast demonstrates a hematoma in the right renal cortex (*arrow*)

7.10 Developmental Dysplasia of the Hip

A 2-month-old boy with suspected developmental dysplasia of the hip. Physical exam (Ortolani or Barlow maneuvers) is positive or equivocal.

a. X-ray hips
b. US hips
c. CT pelvis
d. Tc-99m bone scan lower extremity
e. No ideal imaging exam

Child younger than 4 months of age with positive or equivocal physical findings.

a. X-ray hips AP view is usually not appropriate (2).
b. *US hips* is the most appropriate. Wait until the patient is at least 2 weeks of age to perform the US (7).
c. CT pelvis is usually not appropriate (NA).
d. Tc-99m bone scan lower extremity is usually not appropriate (NA).

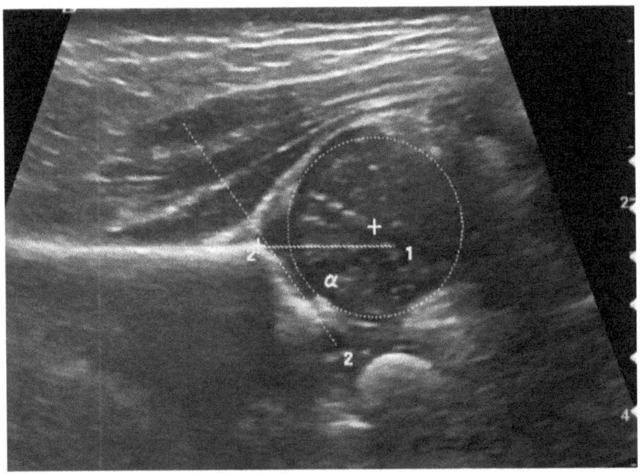

Fig. 7.25 Developmental hip dysplasia. Hip ultrasound shows an alpha (acetabular roof) angle of <60° at the left hip

A 2-month-old boy with suspected developmental dysplasia of the hip and history of breech presentation. Physical exam (Ortolani or Barlow maneuvers) is negative.

a. X-ray hips
b. US hips
c. CT pelvis
d. Tc-99m bone scan lower extremity
e. No ideal imaging exam

Child younger than 4 months of age with breech presentation or positive family history but without physical findings.

a. X-ray hips AP view is usually not appropriate (2).
b. US hips may sometimes be appropriate. Wait until the patient is at least 2 weeks of age to perform the exam (6).
c. CT pelvis is usually not appropriate (NA).
d. Tc-99m bone scan lower extremity is usually not appropriate (NA).
e. *No ideal imaging exam* is the correct answer.

A 6-month-old girl with suspected developmental dysplasia of the hip with limited abduction.

a. X-ray hips
b. US hips
c. CT pelvis
d. Tc-99m bone scan lower extremity
e. No ideal imaging exam

Child 4 months of age or older with limited abduction or abnormal gait.

a. *X-ray hips* is the most appropriate (8).
b. US hips is usually not appropriate. Wait until the patient is at least 2 weeks of age to perform the exam (3).
c. CT pelvis is usually not appropriate (NA).
d. Tc-99m bone scan lower extremity is usually not appropriate (NA).

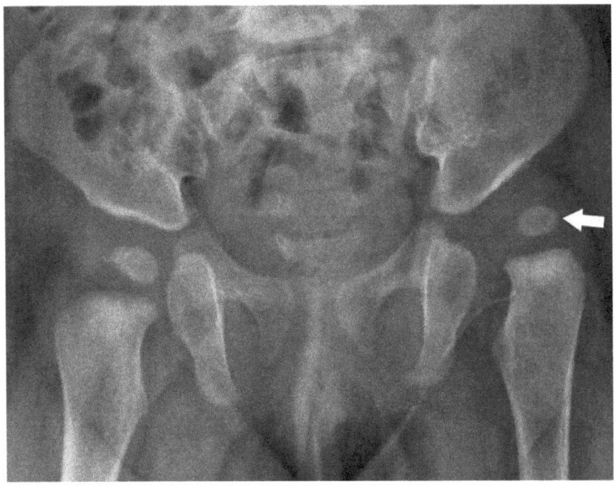

Fig. 7.26 Developmental dysplasia of the hip. Hip X-ray AP view shows abnormal left acetabular shape and superior and lateral displacement of the left femoral head (*arrow*)

7.11 Limping Child

A 5-year-old girl with limp and a nonfocal clinical exam.

a. X-ray pelvis and lower extremity
b. US hips
c. MRI pelvis and lower extremity
d. Tc-99m 3-phase bone scan lower extremity
e. No ideal imaging exam

Nonfocal clinical exam.

a. *X-ray pelvis and lower extremity* is the most appropriate. Pelvis, femur (including knee), lower leg, and foot are all imaged (8).
b. US hips may sometimes be appropriate. Use as follow-up study as needed (5).
c. MRI pelvis and lower extremity may sometimes be appropriate. Use as follow-up study as needed (6).
d. Tc-99m 3-phase bone scan lower extremity may sometimes be appropriate. Use if limping persists and radiographs are negative (6).

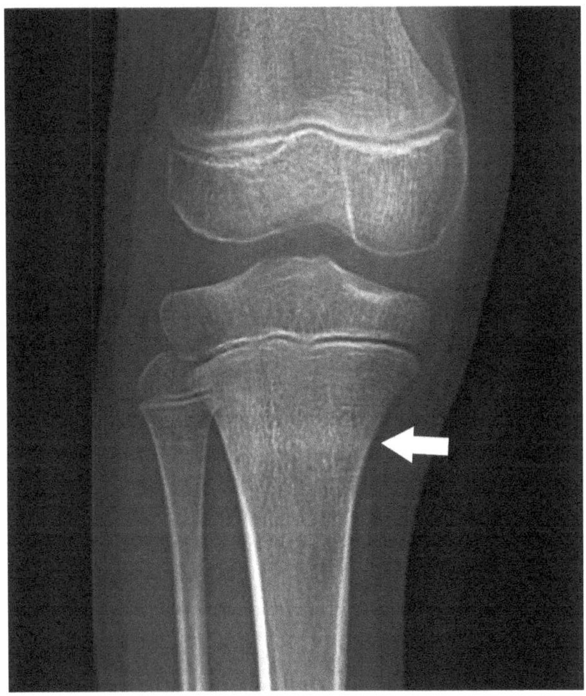

Fig. 7.27 Stress fracture. Lower leg X-ray AP view shows a faint line of sclerosis in the proximal tibia (*arrow*)

A 8-year-old boy with limp and a focal finding on exam. Septic arthritis is not suspected.

a. X-ray area of interest
b. US area of interest
c. MRI area of interest
d. Tc-99m 3-phase bone scan lower extremity
e. No ideal imaging exam

Focal clinical exam but nonsuspicious for septic arthritis.

a. *X-ray area of interest* is the most appropriate. Consider imaging region above and below area of concern (9).
b. US area of interest is usually not appropriate (3).
c. MRI area of interest is usually appropriate, but there is a better choice here. Use as follow-up study as needed (7).
d. Tc-99m 3-phase bone scan lower extremity is usually appropriate, but there is a better choice here. Use as follow-up study as needed (7).

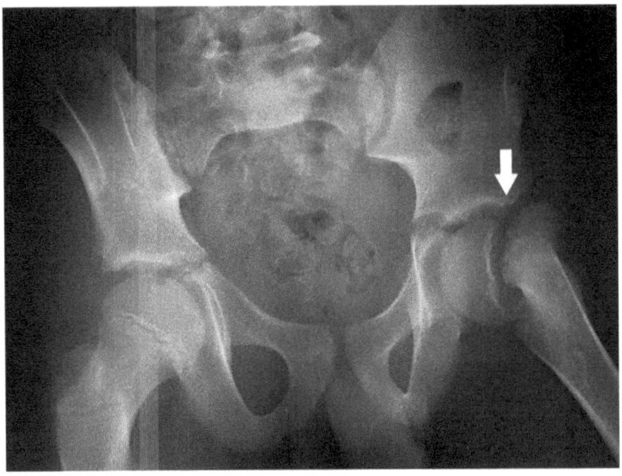

Fig. 7.28 Slipped capital femoral epiphysis. Pelvis X-ray AP view shows a left femoral epiphysis dislocated from the femoral neck (*arrow*)

A 5-year-old girl with limp. Septic arthritis is suspected.

a. X-ray area of interest
b. US area of interest
c. MRI area of interest
d. Tc-99m 3-phase bone scan lower extremity
e. No ideal imaging exam

Suspected septic arthritis.

a. *X-ray area of interest* is the most appropriate (9).
b. US area of interest is usually appropriate, but there is a better choice here. Exam is most useful for the hip (8).
c. MRI area of interest is usually appropriate, but there is a better choice here. Use as follow-up study as needed (7).
d. Tc-99m 3-phase bone scan lower extremity is usually appropriate, but there is a better choice here. Use as follow-up study as needed (7).

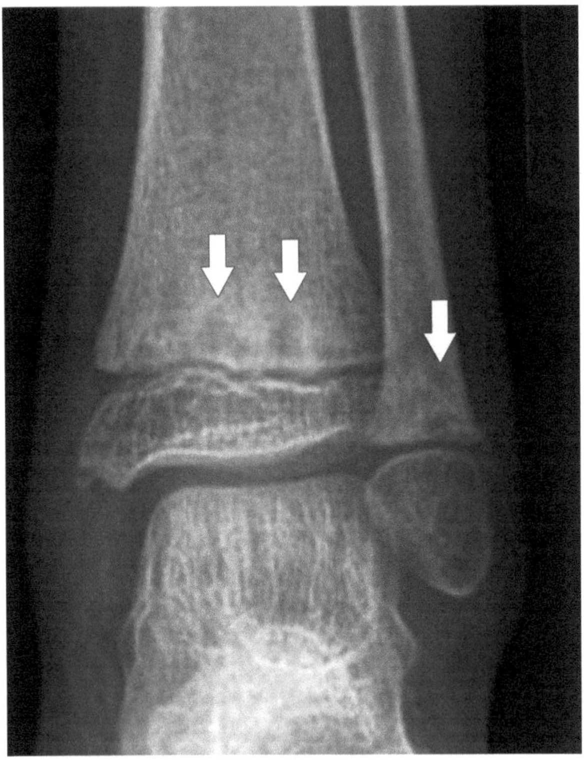

Fig. 7.29 Osteomyelitis. Ankle X-ray AP view shows metaphyseal irregularities (*arrows*) of tibia and fibula

7.12 Suspected Physical Abuse

A 1-year-old girl suspected victim of physical abuse with no focal signs or symptoms.

a. X-ray skeletal survey
b. CT head
c. MRI head
d. Tc-99m bone scan whole body
e. No ideal imaging exam

Child 2 years or less with no focal signs or symptoms.

a. *X-ray skeletal survey* is the most appropriate. Exam includes at least 2 views of the skull (9).
b. CT head is usually not appropriate (2).
c. MRI head may sometimes be appropriate. May be useful for evidentiary purposes (5).
d. Tc-99m bone scan whole body may sometimes be appropriate. May be useful for evidentiary purposes (4).

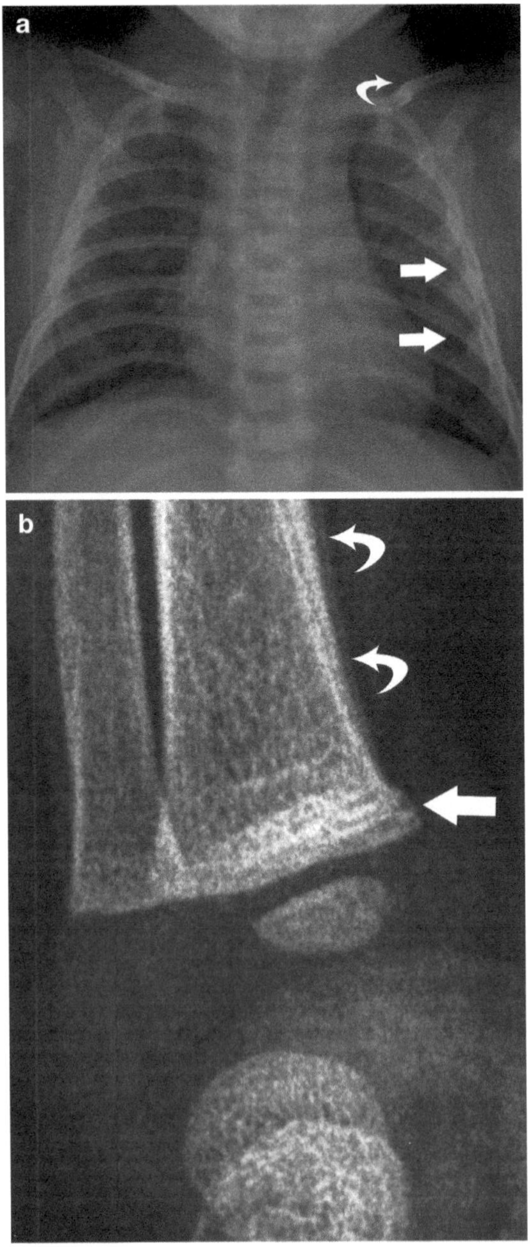

Fig. 7.30 Child abuse. Skeletal survey chest X-ray (**a**) shows healing left rib (*arrow*) and clavicular (*curved arrow*) fractures. Ankle X-ray (**b**) shows a distal tibial metaphyseal corner fracture (*arrow*) with periosteal reaction (*curved arrows*)

A 1-year-old girl suspected victim of physical abuse with history of head trauma and no focal signs or symptoms. Neurologic exam is normal.

a. X-ray skeletal survey
b. CT head
c. MRI head
d. Tc-99m bone scan whole body
e. No ideal imaging exam

Child 2 years or less with head trauma by history but no focal findings or neurologic abnormality on exam.

a. *X-ray skeletal survey* is the most appropriate. Exam includes at least 2 views of the skull (9).
b. CT head may sometimes be appropriate (6).
c. MRI head is usually appropriate, but there is a better choice here (7).
d. Tc-99m bone scan whole body may sometimes be appropriate. May be useful for evidentiary purposes (4).

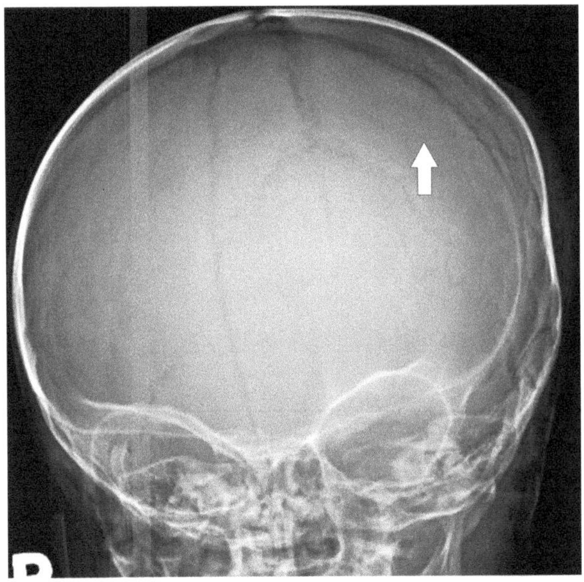

Fig. 7.31 Child abuse. Skull X-ray AP view shows a left parietal skull fracture (*arrow*)

A 1-year-old boy suspected victim of physical abuse with seizures.

a. US head
b. CT head
c. MRI head
d. Tc-99m bone scan whole body
e. No ideal imaging exam

Child up to age 5 years with seizures or neurologic signs and symptoms, with or without physical findings.

a. US head is usually not appropriate (2).
b. *CT head* is the most appropriate (9).
c. MRI head is usually appropriate, but there is a better choice here (8).
d. Tc-99m bone scan whole body may sometimes be appropriate. May be useful for evidentiary purposes (4).

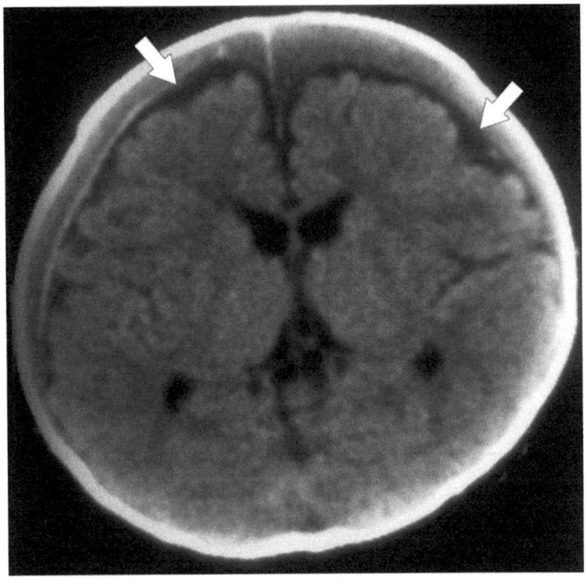

Fig. 7.32 Child abuse. Head CT without contrast demonstrates bilateral subdural hematoma (*arrow*)

A 5-year-old girl suspected victim of child abuse with visceral injuries discrepant with provided history.

a. US head
b. CT head
c. MRI head
d. Tc-99m bone scan whole body
e. No ideal imaging exam

Child of any age with visceral injuries discrepant with history and inconclusive physical and laboratory examinations.

a. US head is usually not appropriate (2).
b. *CT head* is the most appropriate (9).
c. MRI head is usually appropriate, but there is a better choice here (8).
d. Tc-99m bone scan whole body may sometimes be appropriate. May be useful in for evidentiary purposes (4).

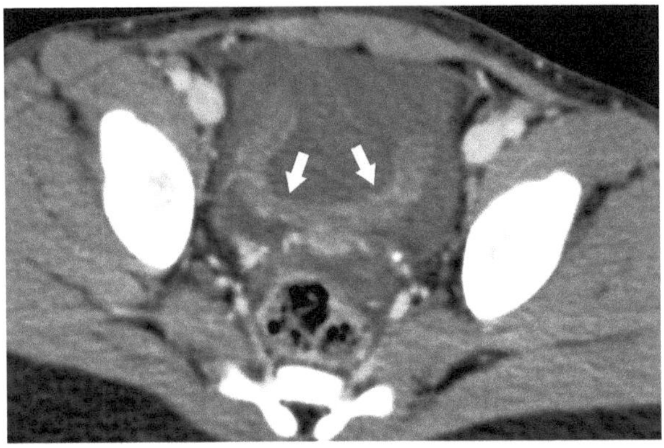

Fig. 7.33 Child abuse. Abdominopelvic CT with contrast shows a large hematoma (*arrows*) in the bladder

Thoracic Imaging

8

8.1 Acute Respiratory Illness[1]

A 51-year-old woman with cough, sputum production, chest pain, or dyspnea.

a. X-ray chest
b. CT chest without contrast
c. Ga-67 scan lung
d. Tc-99m DTPA scan lung
e. No ideal imaging exam

[1] Acute respiratory illness is defined as cough, sputum production, chest pain, or dyspnea.

S.I. Lee, J.H. Thrall, *Choosing the Correct Radiologic Test*,
DOI 10.1007/978-3-642-15772-1_8, © Springer-Verlag Berlin Heidelberg 2013

Older than age 40 years.

a. *X-ray chest* is the most appropriate (8).
b. CT chest without contrast may sometimes be appropriate (4).
c. Ga-67 scan lung is usually not appropriate (NA).
d. Tc-99m DTPA scan lung is usually not appropriate (NA).

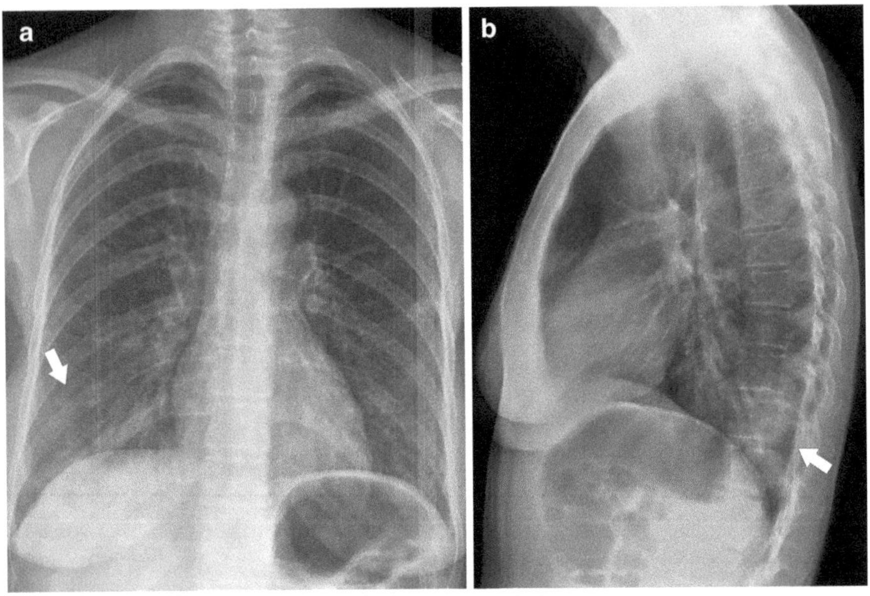

Fig. 8.1 Pneumonia. Chest X-ray posteroanterior (**a**) and lateral (**b**) views show pneumonia (*arrows*) in the right lower lobe

A 74-year-old man with known dementia with cough, sputum production, chest pain, or dyspnea.

a. X-ray chest
b. CT chest without contrast
c. Ga-67 scan lung
d. Tc-99m DTPA scan lung
e. No ideal imaging exam

Dementia, any age.

a. *X-ray chest* is the most appropriate (8).
b. CT chest without contrast may sometimes be appropriate (4).
c. Ga-67 scan lung is usually not appropriate (NA).
d. Tc-99m DTPA scan lung is usually not appropriate (NA).

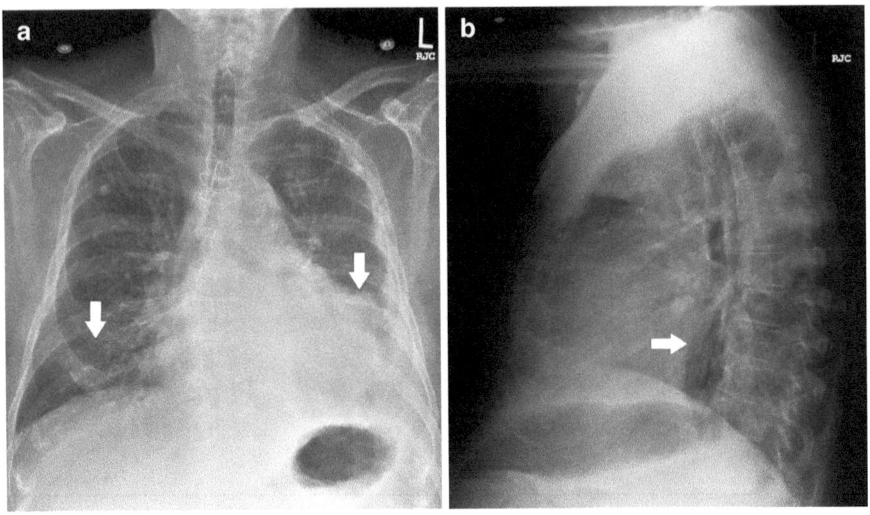

Fig. 8.2 Aspiration pneumonia. Chest X-ray posteroanterior (**a**) and lateral (**b**) views show pneumonia (*arrows*) bilaterally in the lower lobes

A 32-year-old man with cough, sputum production, chest pain, or dyspnea who is otherwise healthy and has no risk factors.

a. X-ray chest
b. CT chest without contrast
c. Ga-67 scan lung
d. Tc-99m DTPA scan lung
e. No ideal imaging exam

Younger than age 40 years, negative physical exam, and no other signs, symptoms, or risk factors.

a. X-ray chest may sometimes be appropriate (4).
b. CT chest without contrast is usually not appropriate (1).
c. Ga-67 scan lung is usually not appropriate (NA).
d. Tc-99m DTPA scan lung is usually not appropriate (NA).
e. *No ideal imaging exam* is the correct answer.

A 25-year-old man with cough, sputum production, chest pain, or dyspnea. Exam reveals unilateral decrease in breath sounds.

a. X-ray chest
b. CT chest without contrast
c. Ga-67 scan lung
d. Tc-99m DTPA scan lung
e. No ideal imaging exam

Less than 40 years old, positive physical exam or other risk factors.

a. *X-ray chest* is the most appropriate (9).
b. CT chest without contrast may sometimes be appropriate (4).
c. Ga-67 scan lung is usually not appropriate (NA).
d. Tc-99m DTPA scan lung is usually not appropriate (NA).

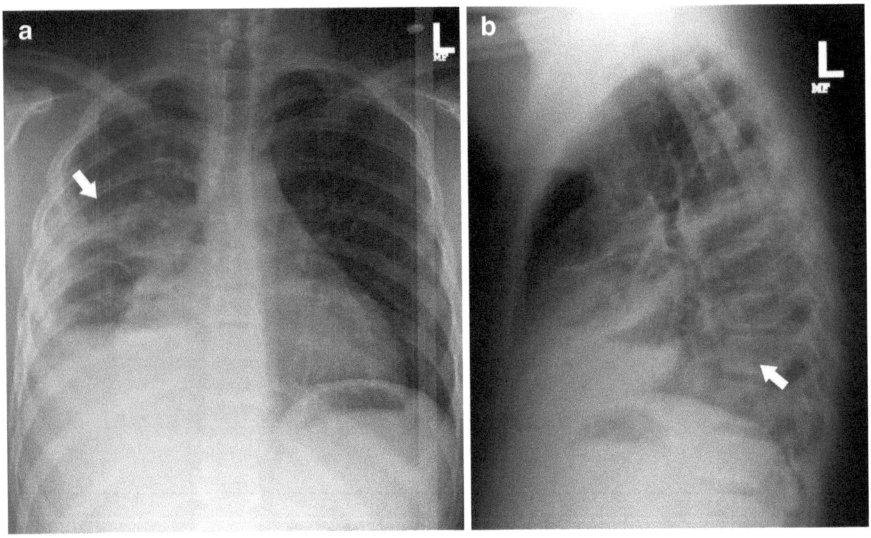

Fig. 8.3 Pneumonia. Chest X-ray posteroanterior (**a**) and lateral (**b**) chest views show pneumonia (*arrows*) in the right lower lobe

A 32-year-old man with cough, sputum production, chest pain, or dyspnea from uncomplicated asthma.

a. X-ray chest
b. CT chest without contrast
c. Ga-67 scan lung
d. Tc-99m DTPA scan lung
e. No ideal imaging exam

Acute asthma, uncomplicated.

a. X-ray chest may sometimes be appropriate (4).
b. CT chest without contrast is usually not appropriate (1).
c. Ga-67 scan lung is usually not appropriate (NA).
d. Tc-99m DTPA scan lung is usually not appropriate (NA).
e. *No ideal imaging exam* is the correct answer.

A 77-year-old woman with cough, sputum production, chest pain, or dyspnea from asthma. Pneumonia is suspected.

a. X-ray chest
b. CT chest without contrast
c. Ga-67 scan lung
d. Tc-99m DTPA scan lung
e. No ideal imaging exam

Acute asthma. Suspect pneumonia or pneumothorax.

a. *X-ray chest* is the most appropriate (9).
b. CT chest without contrast is usually not appropriate (2).
c. Ga-67 scan lung is usually not appropriate (NA).
d. Tc-99m DTPA scan lung is usually not appropriate (NA).

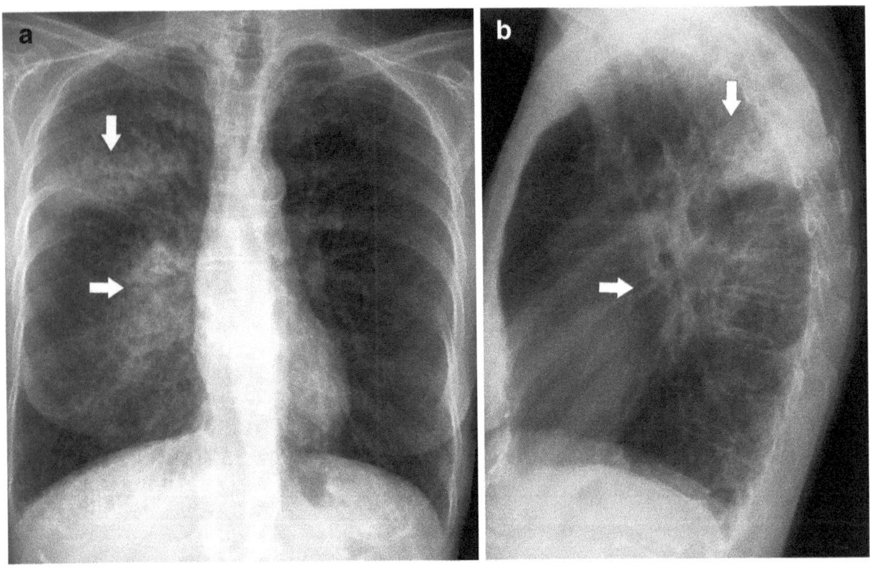

Fig. 8.4 Pneumonia in an asthmatic patient. Chest X-ray posteroanterior (**a**) and lateral (**b**) views show hyperinflated lungs with flattened diaphragms and multifocal pneumonia (*arrows*) in the right lung

A 30-year-old woman with cough, sputum production, chest pain, or dyspnea. She is neutropenic with a fever.

a. X-ray chest
b. CT chest without contrast
c. Ga-67 scan lung
d. Tc-99m DTPA scan lung
e. No ideal imaging exam

Febrile, neutropenic.

a. *X-ray chest* is the most appropriate (9).
b. CT chest without contrast is usually not appropriate (2).
c. Ga-67 scan lung is usually not appropriate (NA).
d. Tc-99m DTPA scan lung is usually not appropriate (NA).

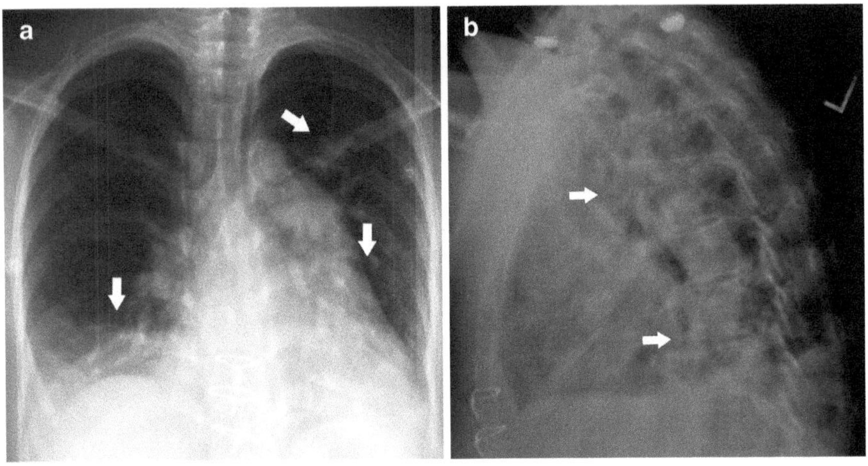

Fig. 8.5 Pneumonia in a neutropenic patient. Chest X-ray posteroanterior (**a**) and lateral (**b**) views show multifocal pneumonia (*arrows*) bilaterally

8.2 Acute Respiratory Illness[1] in HIV-Positive Patient

A 40-year-old man, HIV positive, with cough, sputum production, chest pain, or dyspnea.

a. X-ray chest
b. CT chest without contrast
c. Ga-67 scan lung
d. Tc-99m DTPA scan lung
e. No ideal imaging exam

Cough, dyspnea, chest pain, fever.

a. *X-ray chest* is the most appropriate (9).
b. CT chest without contrast is usually not appropriate (NA).
c. Ga-67 scan lung is usually not appropriate (NA).
d. Tc-99m DTPA scan lung is usually not appropriate (NA).

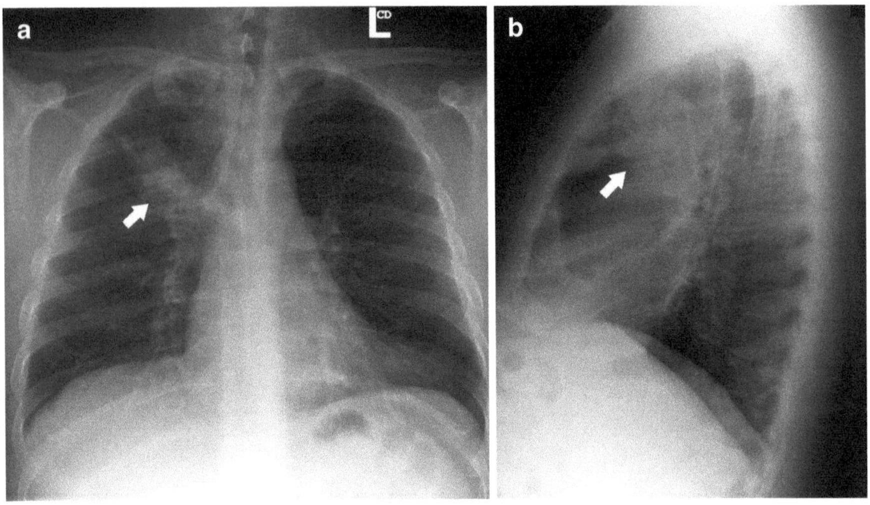

Fig. 8.6 Pneumonia. Chest X-ray posteroanterior (**a**) and lateral (**b**) views show pneumonia (*arrows*) in the right upper lobe

A 48-year-old man, HIV positive, with cough, sputum production, chest pain, or dyspnea. Chest X-ray is nonspecific.

a. CT chest without contrast
b. MRI chest
c. Ga-67 scan lung
d. Tc-99m DTPA scan lung
e. No ideal imaging exam

Negative, equivocal, or nonspecific chest radiograph.

a. *CT chest without contrast* is the most appropriate (8).
b. MRI chest is usually not appropriate (NA).
c. Ga-67 scan lung is usually appropriate, but there is a better choice here (7).
d. Tc-99m DTPA scan lung is usually not appropriate (2).

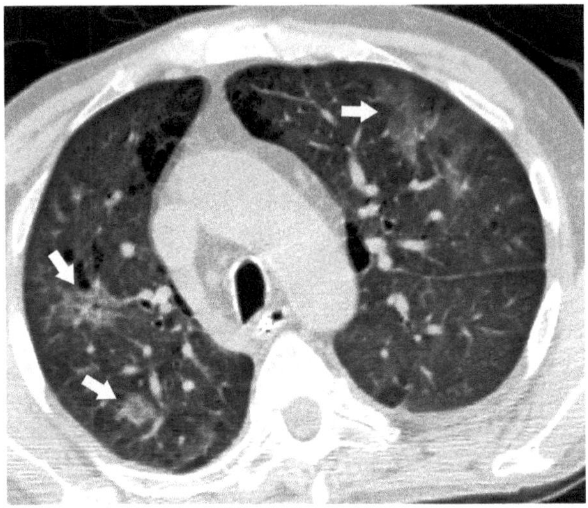

Fig. 8.7 Pneumocystis carinii pneumonia. Chest CT through the upper thorax shows multifocal bilateral air "ground glass" opacities (*arrow*)

A 34-year-old man, HIV positive, with cough, sputum production, chest pain, or dyspnea. Chest X-ray shows diffuse confluent opacities.

a. CT chest without contrast
b. MRI chest
c. Ga-67 scan lung
d. Tc-99 m DTPA scan lung
e. No ideal imaging exam

Positive chest radiograph, diffuse confluent opacities.

a. CT chest without contrast may sometimes be appropriate (6).
b. MRI chest is usually not appropriate (NA).
c. Ga-67 scan lung is usually not appropriate (2).
d. Tc-99 m DTPA scan lung is usually not appropriate (2).
e. *No ideal imaging exam* is the correct answer.

A 46-year-old man, HIV positive, with cough, sputum production, chest pain, or dyspnea. Chest X-ray shows adenopathy suspected of noninfectious origin.

a. CT chest
b. MRI chest
c. Ga-67 scan lung
d. Tc-99 m DTPA scan lung
e. No ideal imaging exam

Positive chest radiograph, noninfectious disease suspected.

a. *CT chest* is the most appropriate, if neoplasm is suspected (8).
b. MRI chest is usually not appropriate (NA).
c. Ga-67 scan lung is usually not appropriate (2).
d. Tc-99 m DTPA scan lung is usually not appropriate (2).

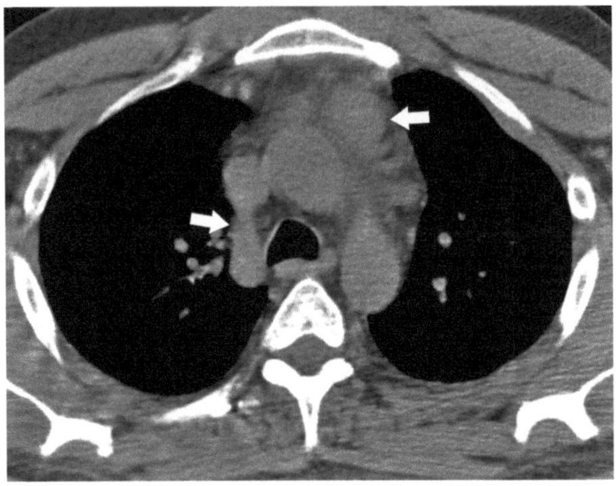

Fig. 8.8 Lymphoma in an HIV-positive patient. Chest CT without contrast through the midthorax shows mediastinal adenopathy (*arrows*)

8.3 Chronic Dyspnea

A 58-year-old woman with chronic dyspnea. Physical exam is positive for pulmonary findings.

a. X-ray chest
b. CT chest
c. CTA chest (noncoronary)
d. Tc-99mV/Q scan lung
e. No ideal imaging exam

Any age, positive physical examination.

a. *X-ray chest* is the most appropriate (9).
b. CT chest is usually not appropriate (NA).
c. CTA chest (noncoronary) is usually not appropriate (NA).
d. Tc-99mV/Q scan lung is usually not appropriate (NA).

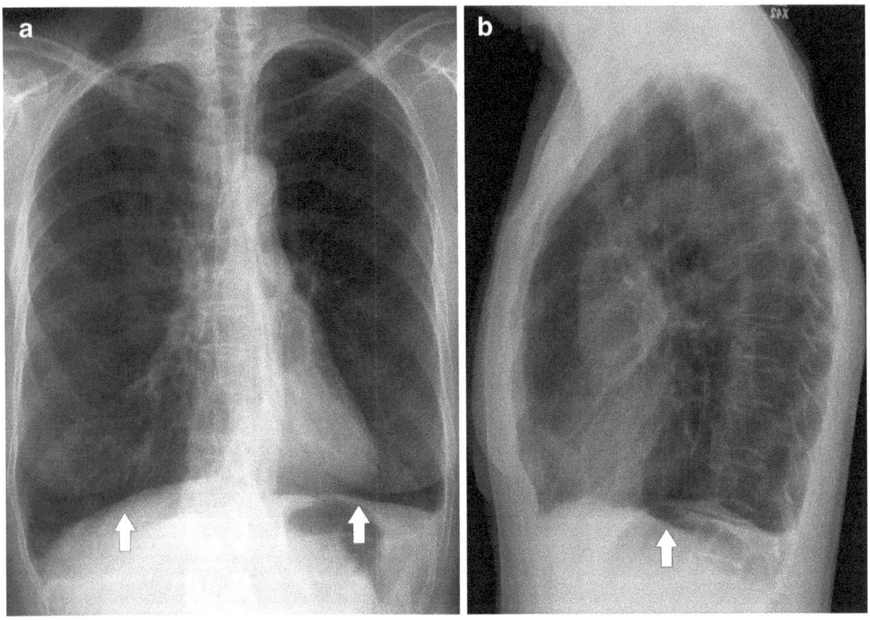

Fig. 8.9 Emphysema. Chest X-ray posteroanterior (**a**) and lateral (**b**) views show hyperinflated lungs and flattened diaphragm (*arrows*)

A 66-year-old man with chronic dyspnea. Physical exam is negative for pulmonary findings.

a. X-ray chest
b. CT chest
c. CTA chest (noncoronary)
d. Tc-99mV/Q scan lung
e. No ideal imaging exam

Any age, negative physical examination.

a. *X-ray chest* is the most appropriate. A negative chest radiograph does not rule out infiltrative lung disease (8).
b. CT chest is usually not appropriate (NA).
c. CTA chest (noncoronary) is usually not appropriate (NA).
d. Tc-99mV/Q scan lung is usually not appropriate (NA).

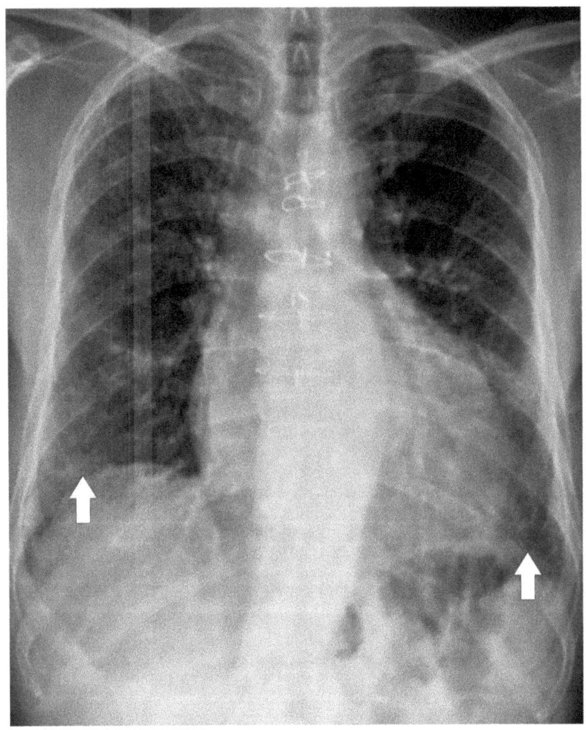

Fig. 8.10 Pulmonary fibrosis. Chest X-ray posteroanterior view shows fine subpleural linear and nodular opacities (*arrows*)

8.4 Hemoptysis

A 78-year-old woman with a 45-pack-year smoking history reports hemoptysis.

a. X-ray chest
b. CTA chest (noncoronary)
c. MRI chest
d. Tc-99m DTPA scan lung
e. No ideal imaging exam

Two risk factors (>40 years old and >40-pack-year history).

a. *X-ray chest* is the most appropriate. Obtain exam as baseline and repeat when clinically indicated (9).
b. CTA chest (noncoronary) may sometimes be appropriate. Use to evaluate source of bleeding (i.e., systemic or pulmonary artery vascular supply) (5).
c. MRI chest is usually not appropriate (NA).
d. Tc-99m DTPA scan lung is usually not appropriate (NA).

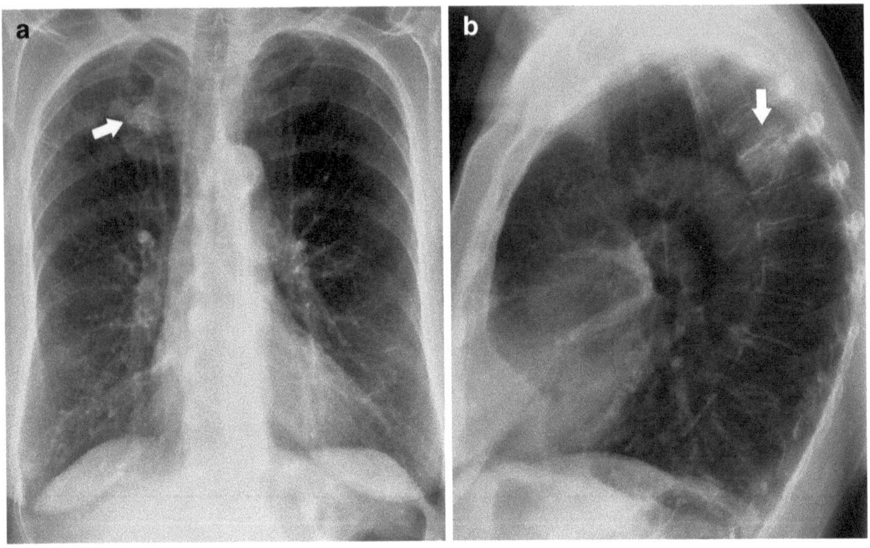

Fig. 8.11 Lung cancer in a patient with emphysema. Chest X-ray posteroanterior (**a**) and lateral (**b**) views show a 3-cm mass in the right upper lobe (*arrows*)

An 82-year-old woman with hemoptysis with no findings of cardiopulmonary compromise.

a. CT chest
b. CTA chest (noncoronary)
c. Tc-99m DTPA scan lung
d. Angiographic embolization bronchial artery
e. No ideal imaging exam

Massive hemoptysis without cardiopulmonary compromise.

a. *CT chest* is the most appropriate. CT with contrast is preferred as it may show source of bleeding (9).
b. CTA chest (noncoronary) may sometimes be appropriate. Use to evaluate source of bleeding (i.e., systemic or pulmonary artery vascular supply), especially before bronchial artery embolization (5).
c. Tc-99m DTPA scan lung is usually not appropriate (NA).
d. Angiographic embolization bronchial artery is usually appropriate, but there is a better choice here (8).

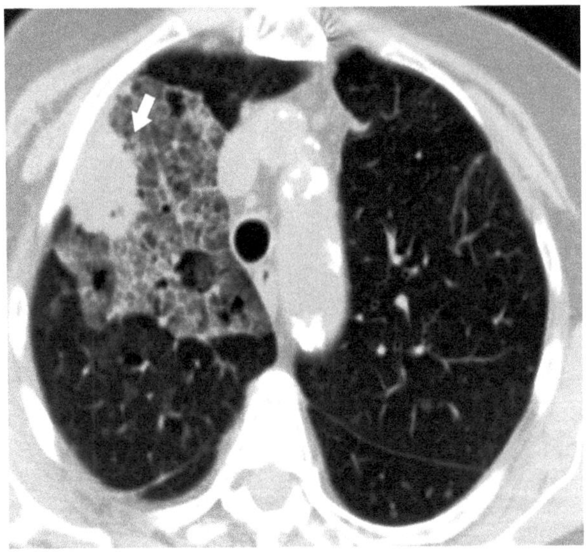

Fig. 8.12 Bleeding lung cancer. Chest CT shows a right upper lobe mass (*arrow*) and surrounding ground glass opacity and interlobar thickening consistent with hemorrhage

8.5 Rib Fractures

A 60-year-old man with suspected rib fractures.

a. X-ray chest
b. X-ray rib views
c. CT chest
d. Tc-99m bone scan ribs
e. No ideal imaging exam

Adult.

a. *X-ray chest* is the most appropriate. Obtain PA view (8).
b. X-ray rib views may sometimes be appropriate (5).
c. CT chest is usually not appropriate (3).
d. Tc-99m bone scan ribs is usually not appropriate (2).

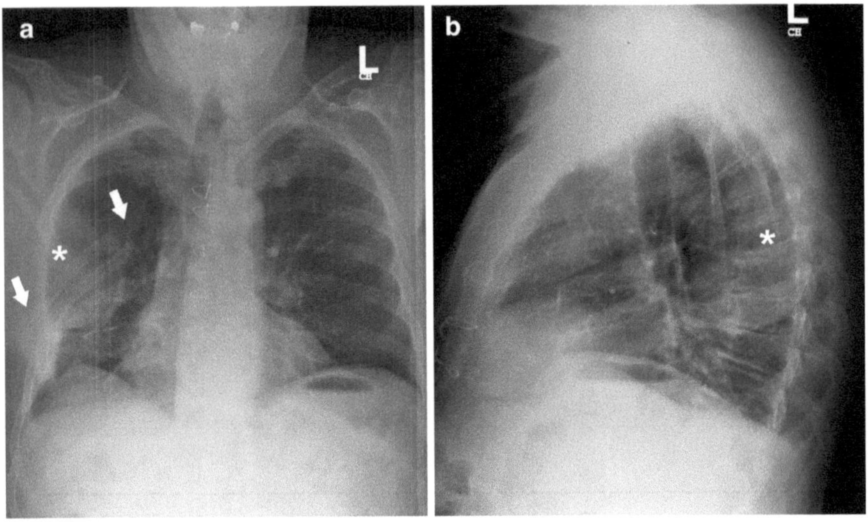

Fig. 8.13 Rib fracture. Chest X-ray posteroanterior (**a**) and lateral (**b**) views show multiple rib fractures (*arrows*) and a lung contusion (*star*)

8.6 Hospital Admission or Preoperative Imaging

A 62-year-old man admitted for elective surgery.

a. X-ray chest
b. CT chest
c. CTA chest (noncoronary)
d. Nuclear medicine myocardial perfusion scan
e. No ideal imaging exam

Asymptomatic; history and physical unremarkable.

a. X-ray chest is usually not appropriate (2).
b. CT chest is usually not appropriate (NA).
c. CTA chest (noncoronary) is usually not appropriate (NA).
d. Nuclear medicine myocardial perfusion scan is usually not appropriate (NA).
e. *No ideal imaging exam* is the correct answer.

A 43-year-old man admitted for elective surgery. Evaluation is positive for acute cardiopulmonary findings.

a. X-ray chest
b. CT chest
c. CTA chest (noncoronary)
d. Nuclear medicine myocardial perfusion scan
e. No ideal imaging exam

Acute cardiopulmonary findings by history or physical.

a. *X-ray chest* is the most appropriate (9).
b. CT chest is usually not appropriate (NA).
c. CTA chest (noncoronary) is usually not appropriate (NA).
d. Nuclear medicine myocardial perfusion scan is usually not appropriate (NA).

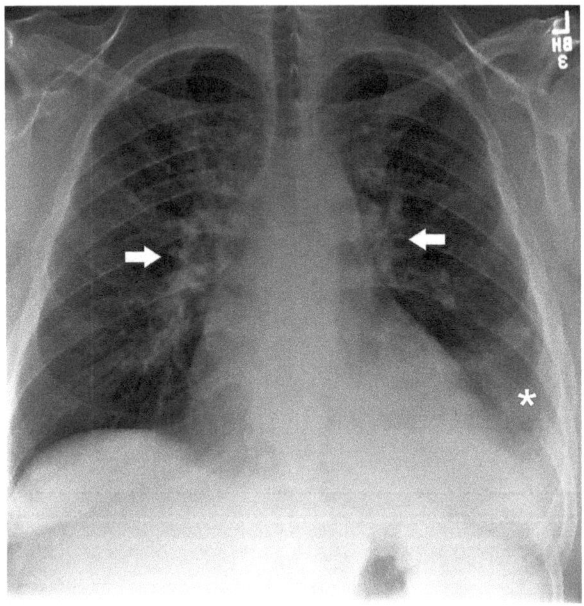

Fig. 8.14 Pulmonary edema. Chest X-ray posteroanterior view shows cardiomegaly, bilateral hilar prominence (*arrows*), and left pleural effusion (*star*)

A 75-year-old man admitted for elective surgery. Patient has a history of chronic cardiopulmonary disease, and a chest X-ray within the past 6 months is available.

a. X-ray chest
b. CT chest
c. CTA chest (noncoronary)
d. Nuclear medicine myocardial perfusion scan
e. No ideal imaging exam

Chronic cardiopulmonary disease in the elderly (>age 70), previous chest radiograph within 6 months available.

a. X-ray chest may sometime be appropriate (6).
b. CT chest is usually not appropriate (NA).
c. CTA chest (noncoronary) is usually not appropriate (NA).
d. Nuclear medicine myocardial perfusion scan is usually not appropriate (NA).
e. *No ideal imaging exam* is the correct answer.

An 88-year-old woman admitted for elective surgery. Patient has a history of chronic cardiopulmonary disease, and no chest X-ray within the past 6 months is available.

a. X-ray chest
b. CT chest
c. CTA chest (noncoronary)
d. Nuclear medicine myocardial perfusion scan
e. No ideal imaging exam

Chronic cardiopulmonary disease in the elderly (>age 70), previous chest radiograph within 6 months not available.

a. *X-ray chest* is the most appropriate (8).
b. CT chest is usually not appropriate (NA).
c. CTA chest (noncoronary) is usually not appropriate (NA).
d. Nuclear medicine myocardial perfusion scan is usually not appropriate (NA).

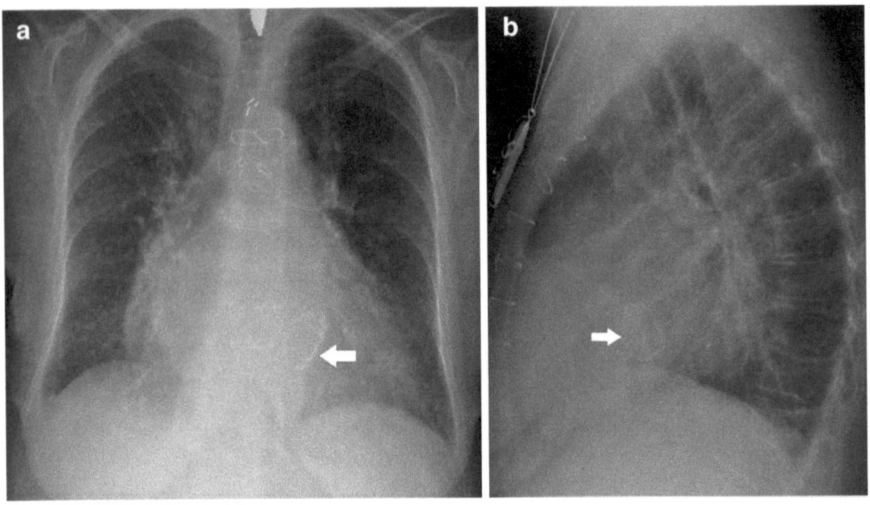

Fig. 8.15 Cardiomegaly. Chest X-ray posteroanterior (**a**) and lateral (**b**) views reveal an enlarged heart and a prosthetic mitral valve (*arrow*)

8.7 Uncomplicated Hypertension

A 64-year-old man with hypertension. He has no complications such as coronary heart disease, congestive heart failure, stroke, atrial fibrillation, or transient ischemia attacks.

a. X-ray chest
b. CT chest
c. CTA chest (noncoronary)
d. Myocardial perfusion scan
e. No ideal imaging exam

a. X-ray chest may sometimes be appropriate (5).
b. CT chest is not rated in appropriateness.
c. CTA chest (noncoronary) is usually not appropriate (NA).
d. Myocardial perfusion scan is usually not appropriate (NA).
e. *No ideal imaging exam* is the correct answer.

8.8 Solitary Pulmonary Nodule

A 62-year-old woman with 1.5-cm nodule seen on chest X-ray. There is low clinical suspicion for cancer.

a. CT chest without contrast
b. CT chest with contrast
c. Watchful waiting with CT chest on follow-up
d. MRI chest with or without contrast
e. No ideal imaging exam

Nodule ≥1 cm, low clinical suspicion for cancer.

a. *CT chest without contrast* is the most appropriate. Use to detect occult calcifications, fat, and bronchus sign (8).
b. CT chest with contrast may sometimes be appropriate. This is probably not indicated if PET has been performed (6).
c. Watchful waiting with CT chest on follow-up may sometimes be appropriate (4).
d. MRI chest with or without contrast is usually not appropriate (2).

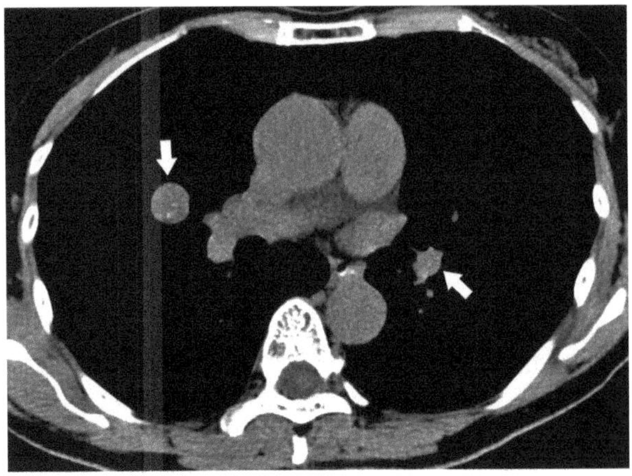

Fig. 8.16 Pulmonary hamartomas. Chest CT without contrast shows soft tissue density nodules (*arrows*), one in each lung. Punctate foci of high-density calcification in each nodule are consistent with hamartomas

A 77-year-old woman with 1.5-cm nodule seen on chest CT without contrast. There is high clinical suspicion for cancer.

a. CT chest with contrast
b. Watchful waiting with CT chest on follow-up
c. MRI chest with or without contrast
d. FDG-PET whole body
e. No ideal imaging exam

Nodule ≥1 cm, moderate to high clinical suspicion for cancer.

a. CT chest with contrast may sometimes be appropriate. This is probably not indicated if PET has been performed (6).
b. Watchful waiting with CT chest on follow-up is usually not appropriate (2).
c. MRI chest with or without contrast is usually not appropriate (2).
d. *FDG-PET whole body* is the most appropriate. Use if nodule is indeterminate on CT (8).

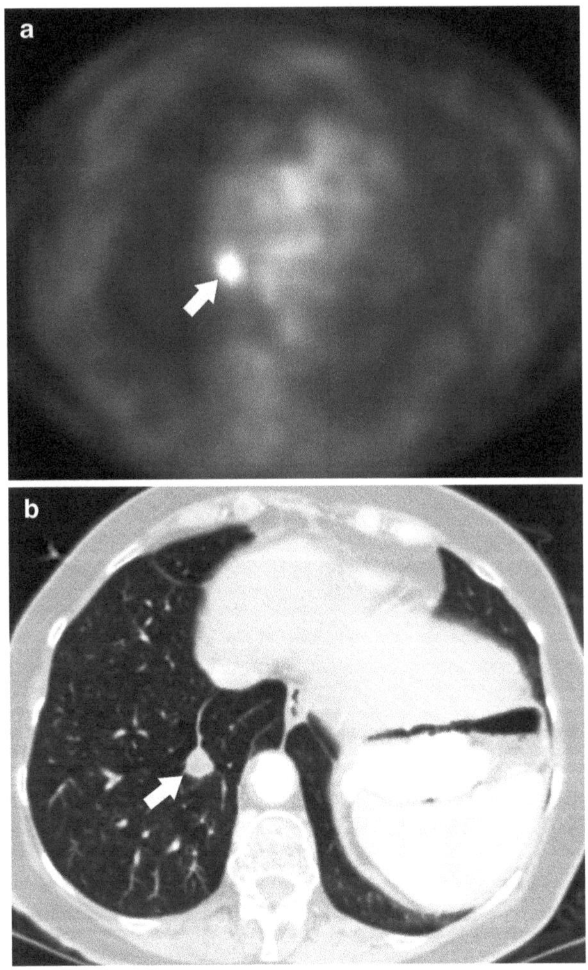

Fig. 8.17 Lung cancer. FDG-PET (**a**) shows a hypermetabolic focus (*arrow*) which on the concurrent chest CT (**b**) corresponds to a 1.5 cm in right lower lobe lung nodule

A 55-year-old woman with 0.8-cm nodule seen on chest X-ray. There is low clinical suspicion for cancer.

a. CT chest
b. Watchful waiting with CT chest on follow-up
c. MRI chest
d. FDG-PET whole body
e. No ideal imaging exam

Nodule ≤1 cm, low clinical suspicion for cancer.

a. CT chest is usually appropriate, but there is a better choice here (7).
b. *Watchful waiting with CT chest on follow-up* is the most appropriate (8).
c. MRI chest is usually not appropriate (1).
d. FDG-PET whole body is usually not appropriate (3).

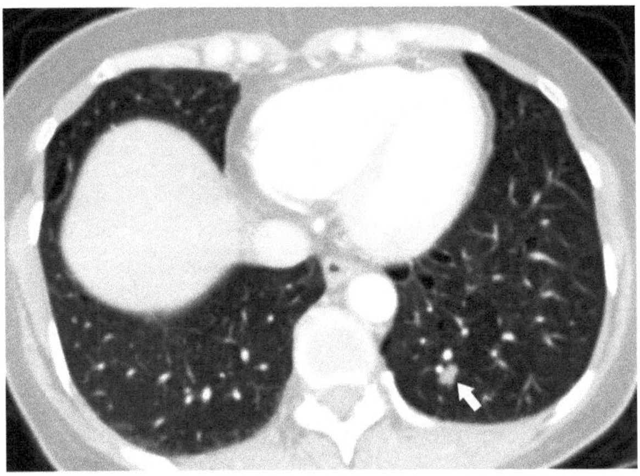

Fig. 8.18 Benign pulmonary nodule. Chest CT shows an 8-mm nodule in the left lower lobe (*arrow*) which has remained stable in size over 2 years and is, therefore, considered benign

A 50-year-old woman with 0.8-cm nodule seen on chest X-ray. There is high clinical suspicion for cancer.

a. CT chest without contrast
b. Watchful waiting with CT chest on follow-up
c. FDG-PET whole body
d. Transthoracic needle biopsy
e. No ideal imaging exam

Nodule ≤1 cm, moderate to high clinical suspicion for cancer.

a. *CT chest* is the most appropriate (8).
b. Watchful waiting with CT chest on follow-up may sometimes be appropriate (5).
c. FDG-PET whole body is usually not appropriate (2).
d. Transthoracic needle biopsy may sometimes be appropriate (6).

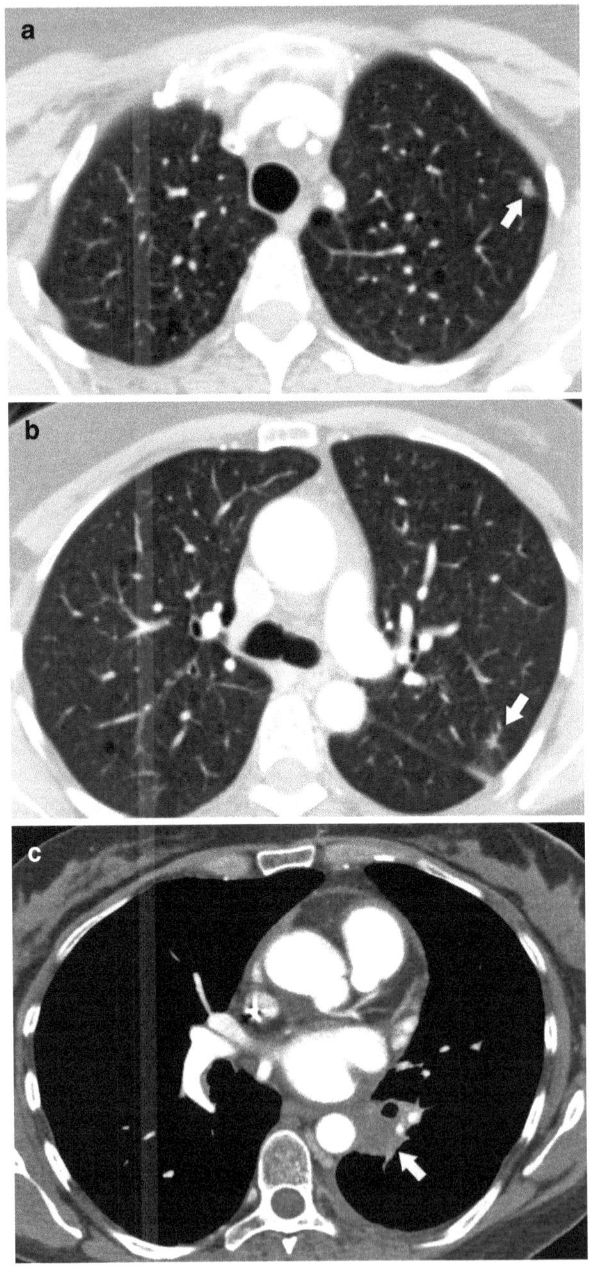

Fig. 8.19 Lung cancer. Chest CT with contrast in lung windows (**a**, **b**) shows multiple spiculated <1-cm left upper lobe pulmonary nodules (*arrows*) and in soft tissue windows (**c**) shows adenopathy (*arrow*)

Urologic Imaging

9

9.1 Renal Trauma

A 30-year-old man with blunt abdominal trauma and microscopic hematuria. Isolated renal trauma is suspected.

a. X-ray abdomen and pelvis
b. US kidneys and bladder
c. US abdomen for free fluid
d. CT abdomen and pelvis with contrast
e. No ideal imaging exam

S.I. Lee, J.H. Thrall, *Choosing the Correct Radiologic Test*,
DOI 10.1007/978-3-642-15772-1_9,

Blunt abdominal trauma with microscopic hematuria and no suspicion of associated abdominal injury.

a. X-ray abdomen and pelvis may sometimes be appropriate (4).
b. US kidneys and bladder is usually not appropriate (2).
c. US abdomen for free fluid may sometimes be appropriate (4).
d. CT abdomen and pelvis with contrast may sometimes be appropriate (4).
e. *No ideal imaging exam* is the correct answer.

A 30-year-old man with blunt abdominal trauma and hematuria. Renal trauma associated with multisystem injury is suspected.

a. X-ray abdomen and pelvis
b. US kidneys and bladder
c. US abdomen for free fluid
d. CT abdomen and pelvis with contrast
e. No ideal imaging exam

Blunt abdominal trauma and suspicion of multisystem trauma, with hematuria.

a. X-ray abdomen and pelvis is usually appropriate, but there is a better choice here. It detects associated fractures (7).
b. US kidneys and bladder may sometimes be appropriate (4).
c. US abdomen for free fluid may sometimes be appropriate (4).
d. *CT abdomen and pelvis* with contrast is the most appropriate. It detects associated injuries (9).

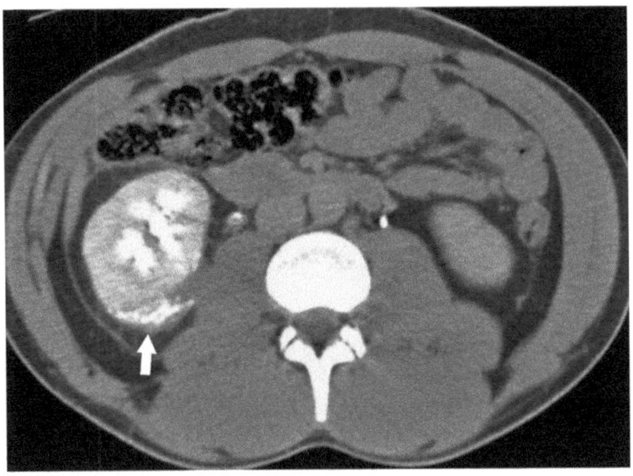

Fig. 9.1 Renal fracture with urine leak from blunt trauma. Abdominal CT with contrast in the delayed phase reveals extrarenal leakage (*arrow*)

A 30-year-old man with penetrating abdominal injury. Renal trauma is suspected.

a. X-ray abdomen and pelvis
b. US kidneys and bladder
c. US abdomen for free fluid
d. CT abdomen and pelvis with contrast
e. No ideal imaging exam

Penetrating abdominal injury and suspicion of multisystem trauma, with or without hematuria.

a. X-ray abdomen and pelvis may sometimes be appropriate (4).
b. US kidneys and bladder is usually not appropriate (2).
c. US abdomen for free fluid may sometimes be appropriate (4).
d. *CT abdomen and pelvis* with contrast is the most appropriate (9).

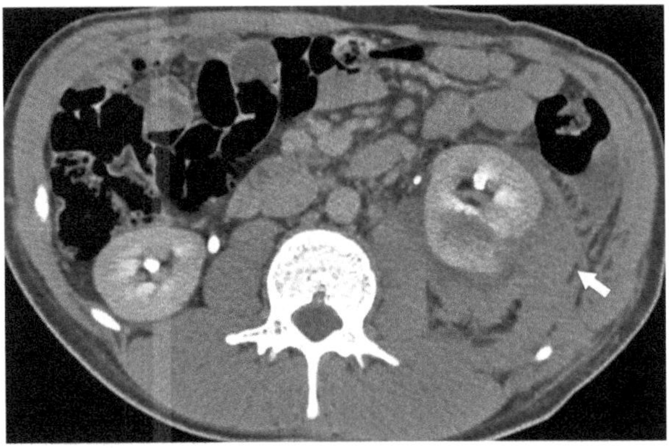

Fig. 9.2 Renal injury from penetrating trauma. Abdominal CT with contrast shows perinephric hematoma and renal injury from a stab wound (*arrow*)

9.2 Suspected Lower Urinary Tract Trauma

A 24-year-old man with penetrating trauma to the lower abdomen and pelvis. Bladder injury is suspected.

a. X-ray abdomen
b. X-ray retrograde urethrogram
c. Transabdominal US pelvis (bladder and urethra)
d. CT pelvis with bladder contrast (CT cystography)
e. No ideal imaging exam

Penetrating trauma, lower abdomen/pelvis.

a. X-ray abdomen may sometimes be appropriate. It is used for any question of foreign body (e.g. bullet) (5).
b. X-ray retrograde urethrogram is usually not appropriate. Do not use if urethral injury from foreign body (e.g. knife, bullet) is suspected (2).
c. Transabdominal US pelvis (bladder and urethra) is usually not appropriate. Ultrasound is usually not definitive (2).
d. *CT pelvis with bladder contrast* (*CT cystography*) is the most appropriate. CT cystogram and X-ray retrograde cystogram are equivalent (8).

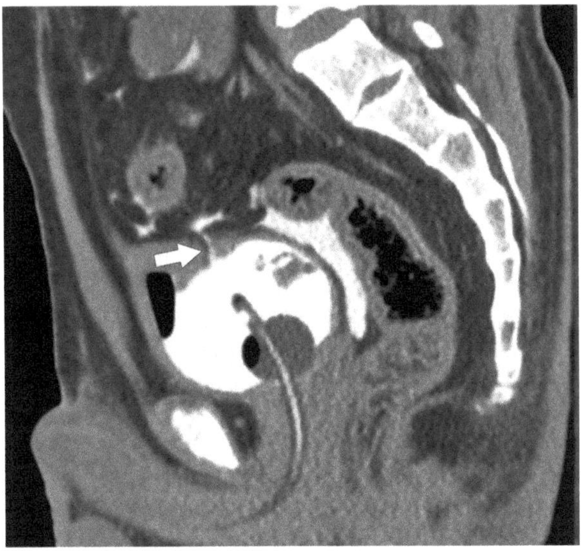

Fig. 9.3 Intraperitoneal bladder rupture. Pelvic CT cystogram sagittal reconstruction image shows a contrast-filled bladder containing a Foley balloon and extravasation of contrast through a defect in the bladder dome (*arrow*) into the intraperitoneal space

A 34-year-old man with blunt trauma to the lower abdomen and pelvis. Bladder injury is suspected.

a. X-ray retrograde urethrogram
b. Transabdominal US pelvis (bladder and urethra)
c. CT pelvis with bladder contrast (CT cystography)
d. Angiography of pelvis (bladder)
e. No ideal imaging exam

Blunt trauma, lower abdomen/pelvis.

a. X-ray retrograde urethrogram may sometimes be appropriate. It is necessary if pelvic fracture is present (5).
b. Transabdominal US pelvis (bladder and urethra) is usually not appropriate. Ultrasound is usually not definitive (2).
c. *CT pelvis with bladder contrast* (*CT cystography*) is the most appropriate (8).
d. Angiography of pelvis (bladder) is usually not appropriate. It is used for persistent bleeding prior to embolotherapy (3).

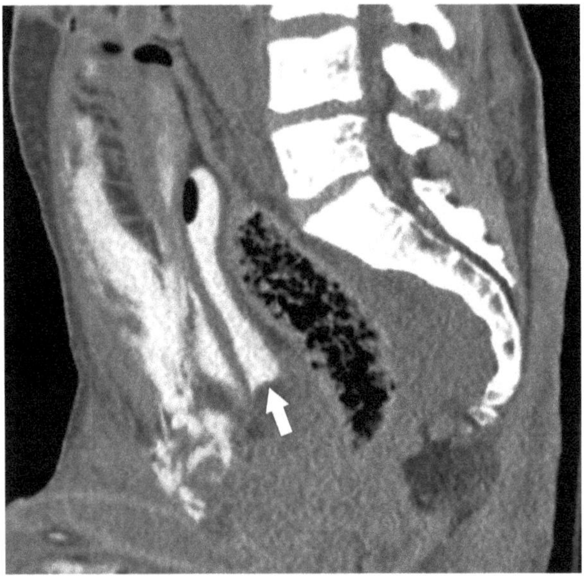

Fig. 9.4 Extraperitoneal bladder rupture. Pelvic CT cystogram sagittal reconstruction image shows a contrast-filled bladder (*arrow*) and extravasation of contrast into the prevesicular space

A 19-year-old man with blunt trauma to the perineum. Urethral injury is suspected.

a. X-ray retrograde urethrogram
b. Transabdominal US pelvis (bladder and urethra)
c. CT pelvis (CT cystography)
d. Angiogram pelvis (bladder)
e. No ideal imaging exam

Blunt perineal trauma in the male (straddle injury).

a. *X-ray retrograde urethrogram* is the most appropriate (9).
b. Transabdominal US pelvis (bladder and urethra) is usually not appropriate. Transabdominal ultrasound is not definitive (1).
c. CT pelvis (CT cystography) is usually not appropriate (1).
d. Angiogram pelvis (bladder) is usually not appropriate. It is used for persistent bleeding prior to embolotherapy (1).

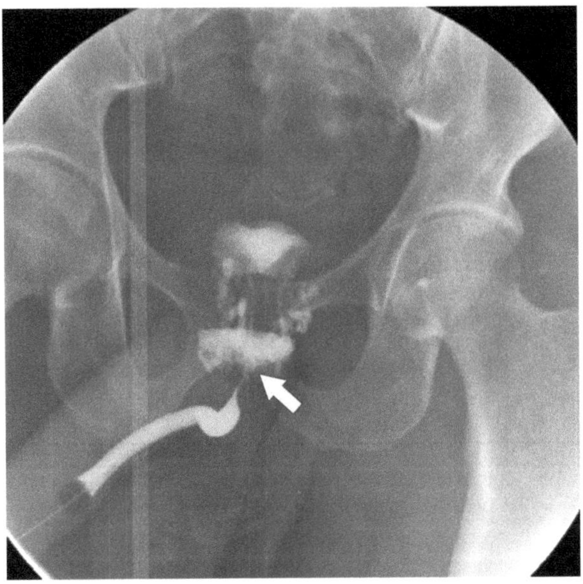

Fig. 9.5 Urethral tear. X-ray retrograde urethrogram oblique anteroposterior view shows contrast extravasation (*arrow*) from a tear at the membranous urethra

9.3 Acute Onset Flank Pain with Suspicion of Stone Disease

A 32-year-old man presents with acute onset of left flank pain suspicious for kidney stones. He reports no such prior episodes.

a. X-ray abdomen
b. X-ray intravenous urography
c. US kidneys and bladder with Doppler and X-ray abdomen
d. CT abdomen and pelvis without contrast
e. No ideal imaging exam

Suspicion of stone disease.

a. X-ray abdomen is usually not appropriate. It is most useful in patients with known stone disease (1).
b. X-ray intravenous urography is usually appropriate, but there is a better choice here (7).
c. US kidneys and bladder with Doppler and X-ray abdomen may sometimes be appropriate. It is the preferred exam in pregnancy, in patients who are allergic to iodinated contrast, and if CT is not available (6).
d. *CT abdomen and pelvis without contrast* is the most appropriate. A reduced-dose technique is preferred (8).

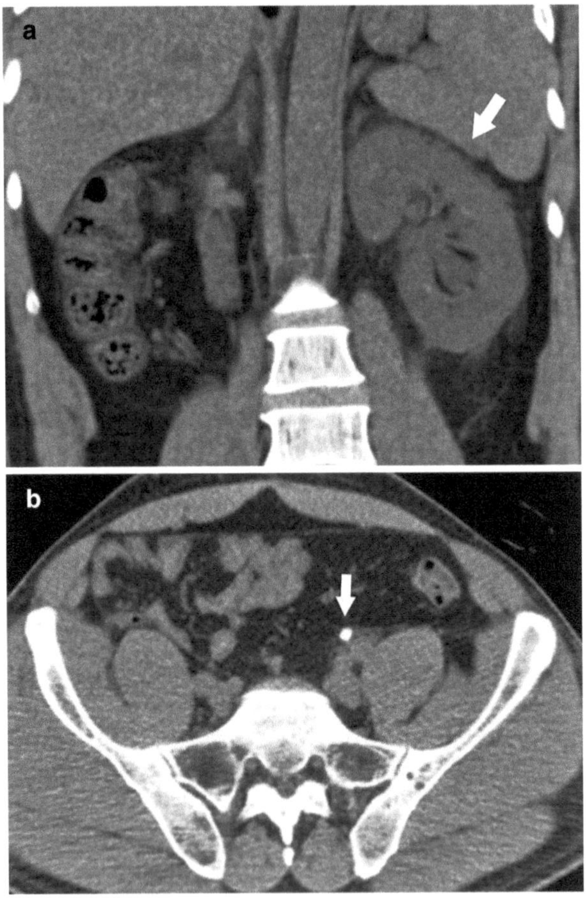

Fig. 9.6 Obstructive urolithiasis. Abdomen and pelvic CT without contrast coronal reconstruction image (**a**) shows moderate left hydronephrosis (*arrow*). An axial image through the midpelvis (**b**) reveals a left ureteral stone (*arrow*)

A 32-year-old man presents with acute onset of left flank pain suspicious for kidney stones. He reports previous episodes of symptomatic kidney stones.

a. X-ray abdomen
b. X-ray intravenous urography
c. US kidneys and bladder with Doppler and X-ray abdomen
d. MRI abdomen and pelvis
e. No ideal imaging exam

Recurrent symptoms of stone disease.

a. X-ray abdomen may sometimes be appropriate. It is good for baseline and follow-up post treatment (6).
b. X-ray intravenous urography is usually not appropriate (2).
c. *US kidneys and bladder with Doppler and X-ray abdomen* is the most appropriate. Low-dose CT of the abdomen and pelvis without contrast is also acceptable here (7).
d. MRI abdomen and pelvis is usually not appropriate (2).

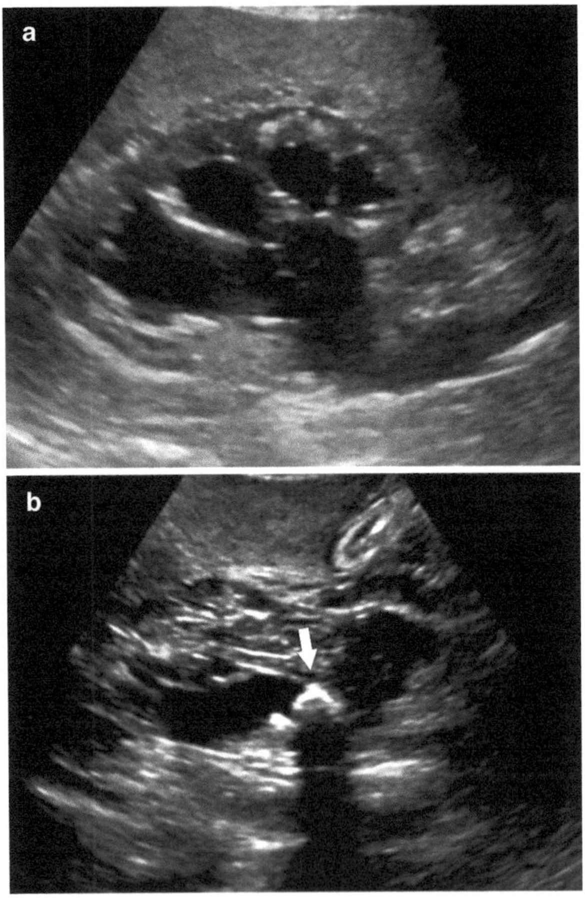

Fig. 9.7 Obstructive urolithiasis. Renal ultrasound sagittal view of the right kidney (**a**) and ureter (**b**) shows right hydronephrosis and obstructing stone (*arrow*) in the midureter

9.4 Acute Pyelonephritis

A 22-year-old previously healthy woman with acute pyelonephritis.

a. X-ray intravenous urography
b. US kidneys and bladder
c. CT abdomen and pelvis without and with contrast
d. Tc-99m DMSA scan kidney
e. No ideal imaging exam

Uncomplicated patient.

a. X-ray intravenous urography is usually not appropriate. Studies show that imaging adds little to management if the patient responds to therapy within 72 h (1).
b. US kidneys and bladder is usually not appropriate. Studies show that imaging adds little to management if the patient responds to therapy within 72 h (1).
c. CT abdomen and pelvis without and with contrast is usually not appropriate. Studies show that imaging adds little to management if the patient responds to therapy within 72 h (1).
d. Tc-99m DMSA scan kidney is usually not appropriate. Studies show that imaging adds little to management if the patient responds to therapy within 72 h (1).
e. *No ideal imaging exam* is the correct answer.

A 24-year-old diabetic woman with acute pyelonephritis. She re-presents with worsening symptoms while being treated.

a. X-ray intravenous urography
b. US kidneys and bladder and X-ray abdomen
c. CT abdomen and pelvis without and with contrast
d. Tc-99m DMSA scan kidney
e. No ideal imaging exam

Complicated patient (e.g., diabetes, immunocompromised, history of stones, prior renal surgery, not responding to therapy).

a. X-ray intravenous urography is usually not appropriate (2).
b. US kidneys and bladder and X-ray abdomen may sometimes be appropriate (6).
c. *CT abdomen and pelvis without and with contrast* is the most appropriate (8).
d. Tc-99m DMSA scan kidney is usually not appropriate. It cannot differentiate renal parenchymal disease from a perinephric process (3).

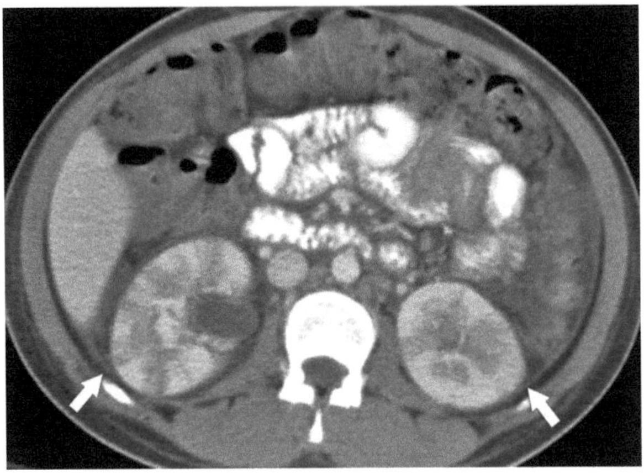

Fig. 9.8 Pyelonephritis. Abdomen and pelvic CT with contrast in a patient shows enlarged kidneys with a striated nephrogram (*arrows*) consistent with uncomplicated but persistent pyelonephritis

9.5 Hematuria

A 50-year-old presents with new-onset hematuria. He has no history of renal disease.

a. X-ray abdomen
b. US kidneys and bladder
c. CT abdomen and pelvis without and with contrast (CT urography)
d. MRI abdomen and pelvis without and with contrast (MR urography)
e. No ideal imaging exam

All patients except those with generalized renal parenchymal disease or young females with hemorrhagic cystitis.

a. X-ray abdomen is usually not appropriate. It is assumed that an abdomen film will be part of the indicated intravenous urogram. If an intravenous urogram is not performed, X-ray abdomen may be performed along with US (2).
b. US kidneys and bladder may sometimes be appropriate. This may miss ureteral and urothelial lesions. Abdominal X-ray, retrograde pyelography, and cystoscopy are useful adjuncts (5).
c. *CT abdomen and pelvis without and with contrast* (*CT urography*) is the most appropriate (9).
d. MRI abdomen and pelvis without and with contrast (MR urography) may sometimes be appropriate (5).

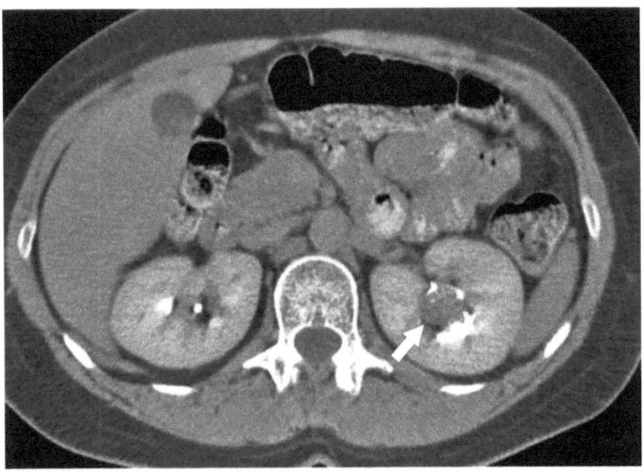

Fig. 9.9 Transitional cell carcinoma. Abdominal CT with contrast shows a soft tissue mass (*arrow*) in the left renal pelvis

A 22-year-old man with history of glomerulonephropathy, now with hematuria.

a. X-ray intravenous urography
b. US kidneys and bladder
c. CT abdomen and pelvis without and with contrast (CT urography)
d. MRI abdomen and pelvis without and with contrast (MR urography)
e. No ideal imaging exam

Due to generalized renal parenchymal disease.

a. X-ray intravenous urography is usually not appropriate (1).
b. *US kidneys and bladder* is the most appropriate. Use for renal volume and morphology and as a localizer for biopsy (8).
c. CT abdomen and pelvis without and with contrast (CT urography) is usually not appropriate (2).
d. MRI abdomen and pelvis without and with contrast (MR urography) is usually not appropriate (1).

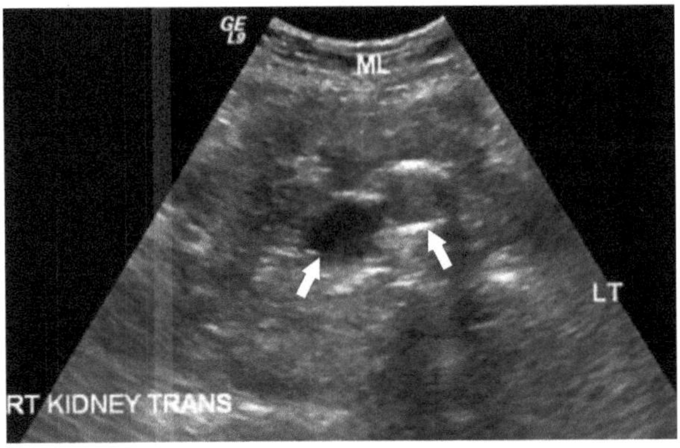

Fig. 9.10 Horseshoe kidney. Renal US transverse image of the midline abdomen shows a fused right and left kidney (ML) anterior to the aorta and inferior vena cava (*arrows*)

9.6 Renovascular Hypertension

A 52-year-old man with hypertension suspected of renovascular origin. His renal function is normal.

a. US kidney with Doppler
b. CTA abdomen
c. Angiotensin-converting-enzyme inhibitor renal scan
d. Angiogram renal arteries (arteriogram kidneys)
e. No ideal imaging exam

High index of suspicion of renovascular hypertension and normal renal function.

a. US kidney with Doppler may sometimes be appropriate. It is useful if there is a dedicated team of physicians and technologists who are skilled in the examination (6).
b. *CTA abdomen* is the most appropriate. It is similar to MRA in accuracy but requires intravenous iodinated contrast (8).
c. Angiotensin-converting-enzyme inhibitor renal scan may sometimes be appropriate. Although the technique has not been standardized, it appears to have a relatively high sensitivity and specificity in patients with normal renal function (6).
d. Angiogram renal arteries (arteriogram kidneys) may sometimes be appropriate. It is considered the gold standard for diagnosing renal artery stenosis but is invasive. It probably is not indicated as primary diagnostic method but reserved for confirmation and for angioplasty or stent placement (4).

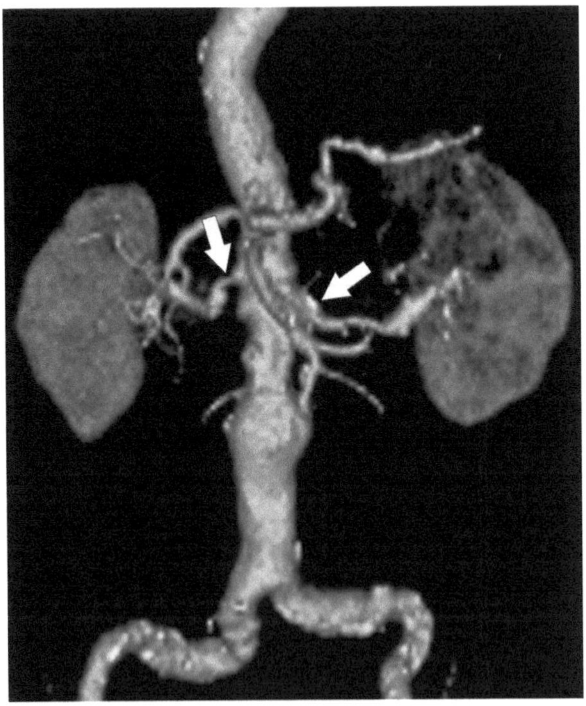

Fig. 9.11 Bilateral renal artery stenoses. Abdominal CTA volume-rendered 3-D reconstruction image shows narrowing (*arrows*) at the origins of the renal arteries bilaterally

A 51-year-old man with hypertension suspected of renovascular origin. He has diminished renal function.

a. X-ray intravenous urography
b. MRA abdomen with contrast
c. Angiotensin-converting-enzyme inhibitor renal scan
d. Angiogram of renal arteries (arteriogram kidneys)
e. No ideal imaging exam

High index of suspicion of renovascular hypertension and diminished renal function.

a. X-ray intravenous urography is usually not appropriate. It is significantly less sensitive than other exams and uses contrast (2).
b. *MRA abdomen with contrast* is the most appropriate. It is useful in older patients with atherosclerotic vascular disease with diminished renal function who are the most likely to have proximal renal artery stenosis (8).
c. Angiotensin-converting-enzyme inhibitor renal scan may sometimes be appropriate. Although diminished renal function can affect the sensitivity and specificity of the exam, it is still reliable as a screening tool (4).
d. Angiogram of renal arteries (arteriogram kidneys) may sometimes be appropriate. It is often used to guide angioplasty or stent placement (4).

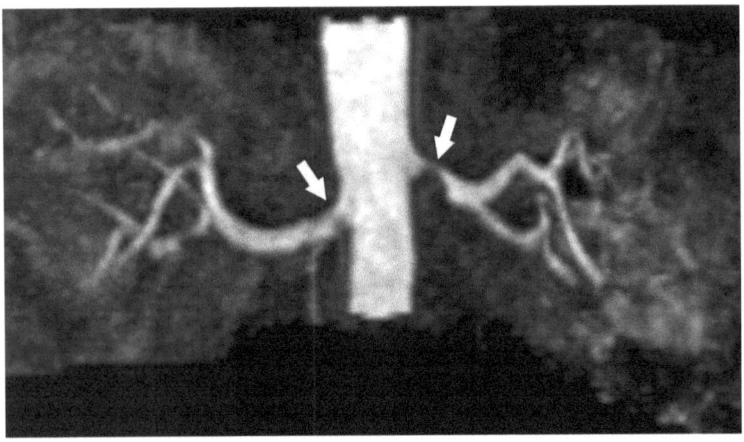

Fig. 9.12 Bilateral renal artery stenoses. Abdominal MRA with contrast maximal intensity projection image shows narrowing (*arrows*) at the origins of the renal arteries bilaterally

A 50-year-old man with "essential" hypertension. Renovascular etiology is considered unlikely.

a. US kidney with Doppler
b. CTA abdomen
c. MRA abdomen with contrast
d. Angiotensin-converting-enzyme inhibitor renal scan
e. No ideal imaging exam

Low index of suspicion of renovascular hypertension ("essential" hypertension).

a. US kidney with Doppler is usually not appropriate (1).
b. CTA abdomen is usually not appropriate (1).
c. MRA abdomen with contrast is usually not appropriate (1).
d. Angiotensin-converting-enzyme inhibitor renal scan is usually not appropriate (1).
e. *No ideal imaging exam* is the correct answer.

9.7 Renal Failure

A 43-year-old woman with acute renal failure.

a. US kidneys and bladder
b. CT abdomen
c. MRA abdomen
d. Tc-99m MAG3 scan kidneys
e. No ideal imaging exam

Acute renal failure, unspecified.

a. *US kidneys and bladder* is the most appropriate. Perform preferably with Doppler (9).
b. CT abdomen is usually not appropriate. Use to evaluate for ureteral obstruction due to retroperitoneal diseases, masses, and tumors. Noncontrast helical CT is more sensitive than abdominal X-ray for calculi (3).
c. MRA abdomen may sometimes be appropriate. Newer techniques with gadolinium are very effective for renal artery evaluation. It evaluates for renal vein or inferior vena caval thrombosis (4).
d. Tc-99m MAG3 scan kidneys may sometimes be appropriate. It assesses global and differential renal function and prognosis for recovery (5).

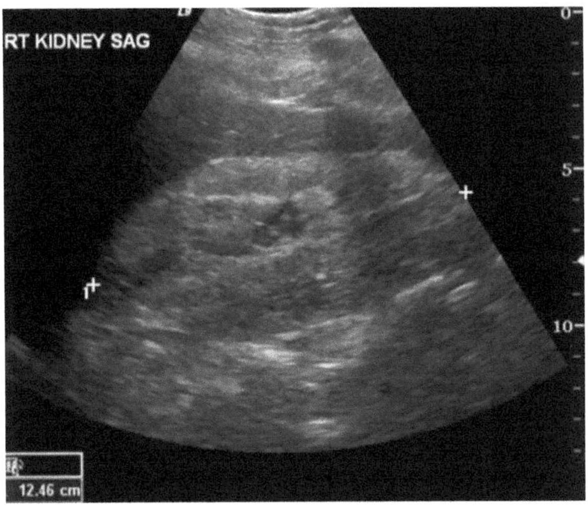

Fig. 9.13 Acute tubular necrosis. Renal ultrasound shows a normal-sized right kidney (*calipers*) with an echogenic cortex. The left kidney looked similar

A 75-year-old man with chronic renal failure.

a. US kidneys and bladder
b. CT abdomen
c. MRA abdomen (kidneys)
d. Tc-99m MAG3 scan kidneys
e. No ideal imaging exam

Chronic renal failure.

a. *US kidneys and bladder* is the most appropriate. Perform preferably with Doppler (9).
b. CT abdomen is usually not appropriate. Use to evaluate for ureteral obstruction due to retroperitoneal diseases, masses, and tumors. Noncontrast helical CT is more sensitive than abdominal X-ray for calculi (3).
c. MRA abdomen may sometimes be appropriate. It allows noninvasive evaluation of renal arteries. Perform preferably with contrast (6).
d. Tc-99m MAG3 scan kidneys is usually not appropriate. It assesses global and differential renal function and prognosis for recovery (3).

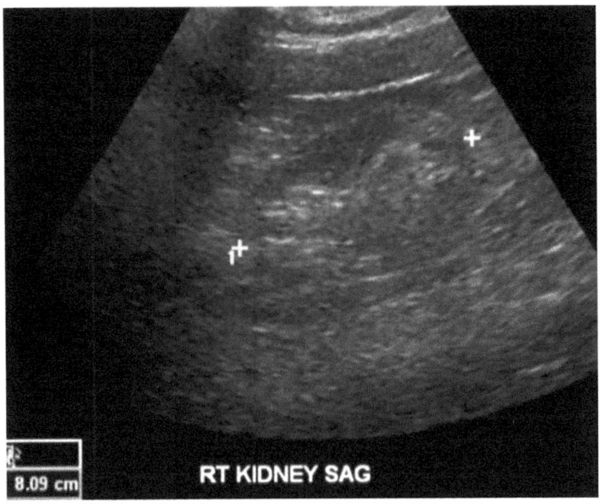

Fig. 9.14 Renal atrophy. Renal ultrasound demonstrates small right kidney (*calipers*) with an echogenic cortex that is consistent. The left kidney looked similar

9.8 Recurrent Lower Urinary Tract Infections in Women

A 25-year-old woman presents with recurrent bladder infections. She is otherwise healthy.

a. X-ray intravenous urography
b. X-ray voiding cystourethrography
c. US kidneys and bladder
d. CT abdomen and pelvis without and with contrast
e. No ideal imaging exam

With no underlying risk factors.

a. X-ray intravenous urography is usually not appropriate. It is not cost effective in this group (2).
b. X-ray voiding cystourethrography is usually not appropriate (2).
c. US kidneys and bladder is usually not appropriate (2).
d. CT abdomen and pelvis without and with contrast is usually not appropriate (2).
e. *No ideal imaging exam* is the correct answer.

A 50-year-old woman presents with recurrent bladder infections which has been increasing in frequency and unresponsive to conventional therapy.

a. X-ray intravenous urography
b. X-ray voiding cystourethrography
c. US kidneys and bladder
d. CT abdomen and pelvis without and with contrast
e. No ideal imaging exam

Patients who are nonresponders to conventional therapy, get frequent reinfections, and have known underlying risk factors.

a. X-ray intravenous urography may sometimes be appropriate. It may be used in young women but will not detect abscesses or small stones (4).
b. X-ray voiding cystourethrography may sometimes be appropriate. It assesses for reflux, bladder or urethral fistula, or prolapse (6).
c. US kidneys and bladder is usually not appropriate (3).
d. *CT abdomen and pelvis without and with contrast* is the most appropriate (7).

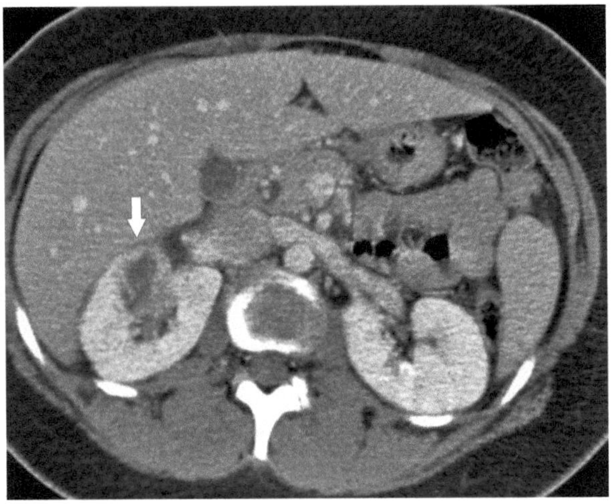

Fig. 9.15 Renal abscess. Abdominal CT with contrast shows an abscess (*arrow*) in the right kidney

9.9 Obstructive Voiding Symptoms Secondary to Prostate Disease

A 60-year-old man with symptoms of bladder outlet obstruction from prostatic hypertrophy. His renal function is normal.

a. X-ray intravenous urography
b. X-ray voiding cystourethrography
c. US kidneys
d. US pelvis (bladder and prostate)
e. No ideal imaging exam

Normal renal function.

a. X-ray intravenous urography is usually not appropriate. Appropriateness rating would be higher if significant residual urine is present. In patients with stones, hematuria, or atypical history, the study may be warranted (3).
b. X-ray voiding cystourethrography is usually not appropriate. Consider this in men younger than age 50 with symptoms (2).
c. US kidneys may sometimes be appropriate. Appropriateness rating would be higher if significant residual urine was present. It evaluates for hydronephrosis (5).
d. *US pelvis (bladder and prostate)* is the most appropriate. If there is significant residual postvoid residual urine volume in the bladder, evaluation of upper tracts is indicated. Gives estimate of prostate size and bladder wall thickness (7).

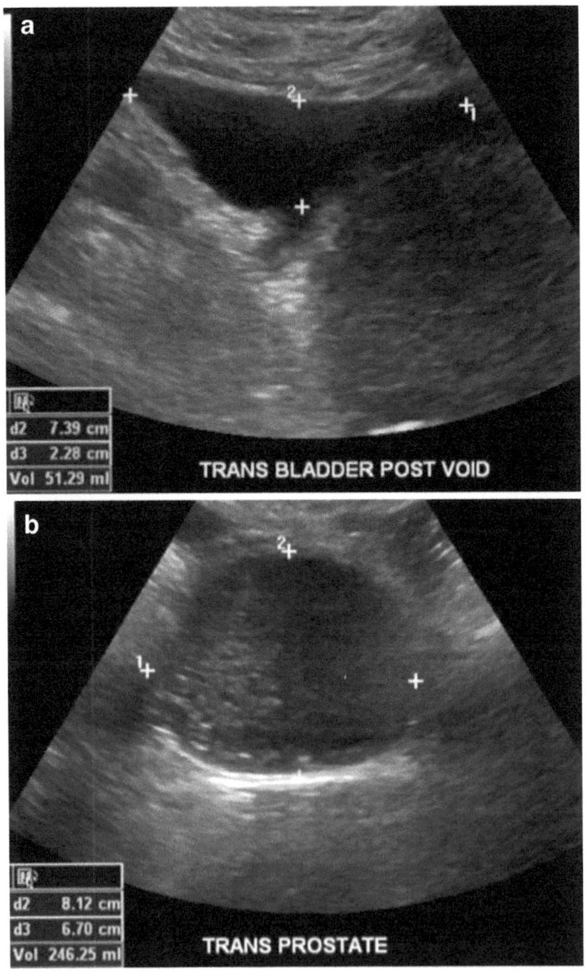

Fig. 9.16 Bladder outlet obstruction and prostatic hypertrophy. Pelvic US transverse views of the bladder (**a**) and prostate (**b**) after urinary voiding show a moderate-sized bladder residual and a markedly enlarged prostate gland

A 60-year-old man with symptoms of bladder outlet obstruction from prostatic hypertrophy. He has abnormal serum renal function tests.

a. X-ray abdomen
b. X-ray intravenous urography
c. X-ray voiding cystourethrography
d. US kidneys
e. No ideal imaging exam

Increased blood urea nitrogen and/or creatinine.

a. X-ray abdomen is usually not appropriate. Use to exclude calculi. It can be used in association with US (3).
b. X-ray intravenous urography is usually not appropriate. Other studies are better for evaluating the same structures (2).
c. X-ray voiding cystourethrography is usually not appropriate. Consider this in men younger than age 50 with symptoms (2).
d. *US kidneys* is the most appropriate. Use to evaluate for hydronephrosis (8).

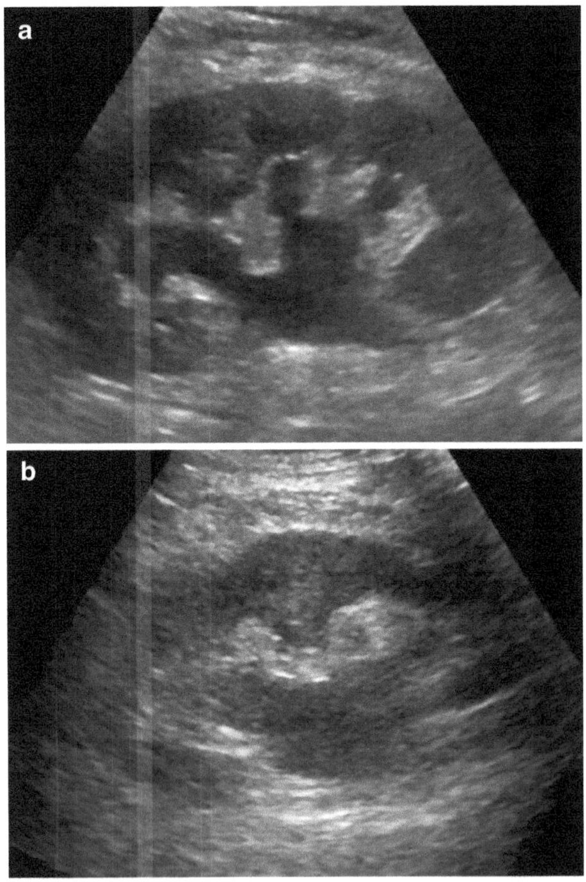

Fig. 9.17 Bilateral hydronephrosis. Renal ultrasound shows moderate hydronephrosis of the right (**a**) and left (**b**) kidneys

9.10 Acute Onset Scrotal Pain

A 28-year-old male patient with acute onset left scrotal pain. He reports no history of scrotal trauma or mass.

a. US scrotum without Doppler
b. US scrotum with Doppler
c. MRI scrotum
d. Ga-67 or In-111 white blood cell scan scrotum
e. No ideal imaging exam

Without trauma, without antecedent mass.

a. US scrotum without Doppler is usually not appropriate. Gray-scale US alone is relatively insensitive to earliest changes of decreased or absent perfusion (1).
b. *US scrotum with Doppler* is the most appropriate. It is an excellent study that is generally available and has high sensitivity and specificity but is operator and equipment dependent. It must be performed in a timely manner (9).
c. MRI scrotum is usually not appropriate. It may be helpful if other tests are inconclusive but must be performed in short time frame (3).
d. Ga-67 or In-111 white blood cell scan scrotum is usually not appropriate. Diagnosis or infection is not obtainable in a reasonable time frame (1).

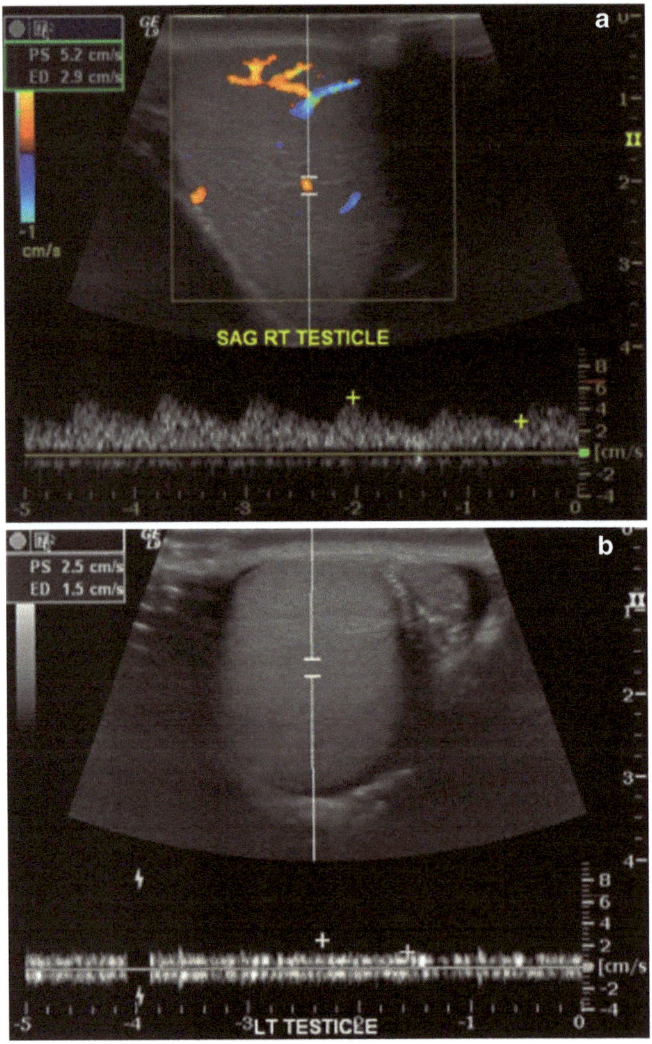

Fig. 9.18 Left testicular torsion. Scrotal ultrasound with Doppler demonstrates pulsatile arterial waveforms in the right (**a**) but not in the left (**b**) testicle

Vascular Imaging 10

10.1 Blunt Chest Trauma

A 70-year-old man with blunt chest trauma. Aortic injury is suspected.

a. CT chest without contrast
b. CTA chest (noncoronary)
c. MRA chest (noncoronary)
d. Angiogram thoracic aorta
e. No ideal imaging exam

S.I. Lee, J.H. Thrall, *Choosing the Correct Radiologic Test*,
DOI 10.1007/978-3-642-15772-1_10, © Springer-Verlag Berlin Heidelberg 2013

Suspected aortic injury.

a. CT chest without contrast may sometimes be appropriate. It is useful to detect mediastinal hematoma when contrast is contraindicated (6).
b. *CTA chest* (*noncoronary*) is the most appropriate (9).
c. MRA chest (noncoronary) may sometimes be appropriate. It is of limited practicality but can be an alternative when iodinated contrast is contraindicated (5).
d. Angiogram thoracic aorta is usually appropriate, but there is a better choice here (8).

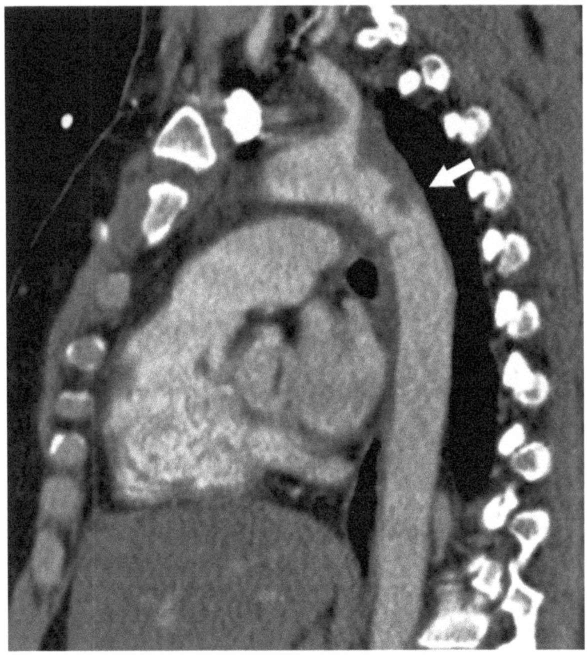

Fig. 10.1 Aortic arch injury. Chest CTA sagittal reconstruction image shows an aortic arch tear (*arrow*)

10.2 Blunt Abdominal Trauma

A 22-year-old man with blunt abdominal trauma. He is hemodynamically unstable.

a. US chest, abdomen, and pelvis to screen for free fluid (FAST scan)
b. US abdomen and pelvis to evaluate organs
c. CT chest, abdomen, and pelvis with contrast
d. Arteriogram with possible embolization abdomen and pelvis
e. No ideal imaging exam

Unstable patient.

a. *US chest, abdomen, and pelvis to screen for free fluid* (*FAST scan*) is the most appropriate. It allows for rapid assessment and is patient condition permitting (8).
b. US abdomen and pelvis to evaluate organs is usually not appropriate (3).
c. CT chest, abdomen, and pelvis with contrast is usually appropriate, but there is a better choice here. Clinical judgment is needed on stability of patient versus need for diagnostic information (7).
d. Arteriogram with possible embolization abdomen and pelvis may sometimes be appropriate (5).

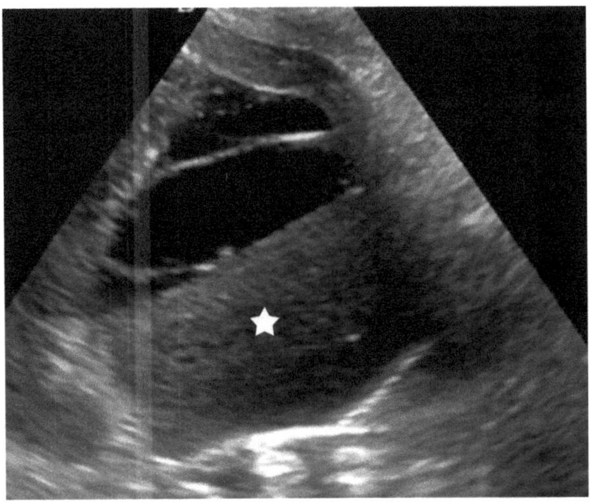

Fig. 10.2 Hemoperitoneum. Abdomen ultrasound shows complex fluid with dependent layering debris (*star*) consistent with blood

A 47-year-old woman with blunt abdominal trauma. She is hemodynamically stable.

a. US chest, abdomen, and pelvis to screen for free fluid (FAST scan)
b. US abdomen and pelvis to evaluate organs
c. CT chest, abdomen, and pelvis with contrast
d. Angiogram abdomen and pelvis with possible embolization
e. No ideal imaging exam

Stable patient.

a. US chest, abdomen, and pelvis to screen for free fluid (FAST scan) may sometimes be appropriate (5).
b. US abdomen and pelvis to evaluate organs is usually not appropriate (3).
c. *CT chest, abdomen, and pelvis with contrast* is the most appropriate (9).
d. Arteriogram abdomen and pelvis with possible embolization abdomen and pelvis may sometimes be appropriate (5).

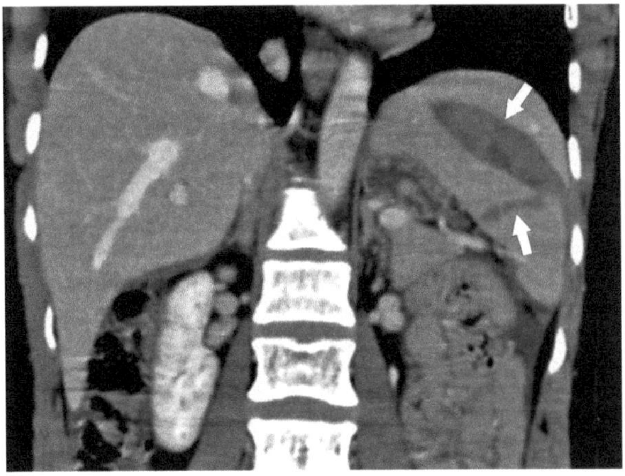

Fig. 10.3 Splenic laceration. Abdomen CT with intravenous contrast coronal reformation image shows splenic lacerations (*arrows*) containing hematoma

10.3 Hematemesis

A 24-year-old man with a history of alcoholism now with hematemesis.

a. X-ray chest
b. US liver with Doppler
c. Tc-99m-labeled red blood cell scan
d. Visceral angiogram
e. No ideal imaging exam

History of alcoholism or liver disease.

a. *X-ray chest* is the most appropriate (8).
b. US liver with Doppler may sometimes be appropriate (6).
c. Tc-99m-labeled red blood cell scan may sometimes be appropriate (6).
d. Visceral angiogram may sometimes be appropriate (6).

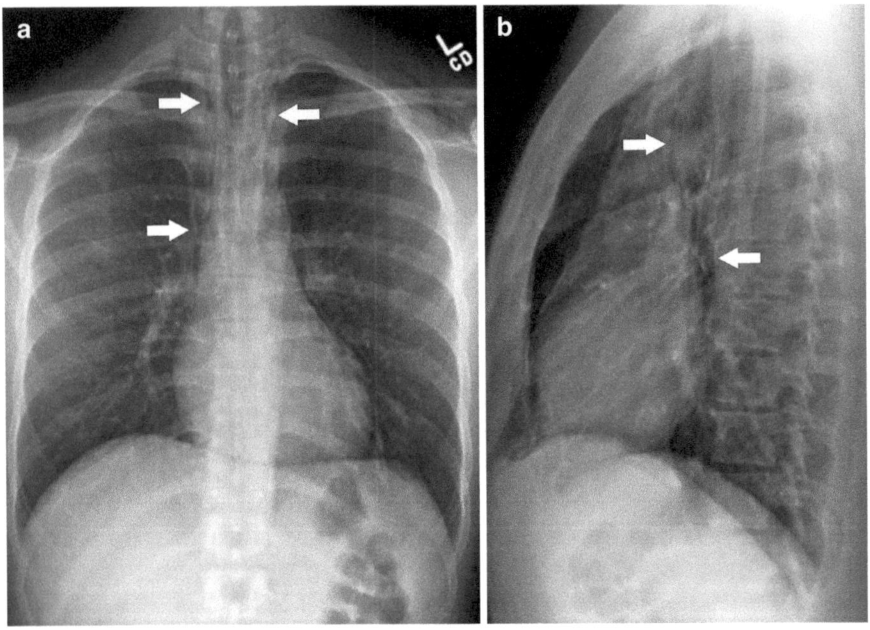

Fig. 10.4 Pneumomediastinum. Chest X-ray posteroanterior (**a**) and lateral (**b**) views reveal mediastinal air (*arrows*) from an esophageal tear

A 74-year-old woman with no history of alcoholism or liver disease now with hematemesis.

a. US liver with Doppler
b. CT abdomen
c. Tc-99m-labeled red blood cell scan
d. Visceral angiogram
e. No ideal imaging exam

No history of alcoholism or liver disease.

a. US liver with Doppler may sometimes be appropriate (4).
b. CT abdomen may sometimes be appropriate (4).
c. Tc-99m-labeled red blood cell scan may sometimes be appropriate (6).
d. *Visceral angiogram* is the most appropriate (8).

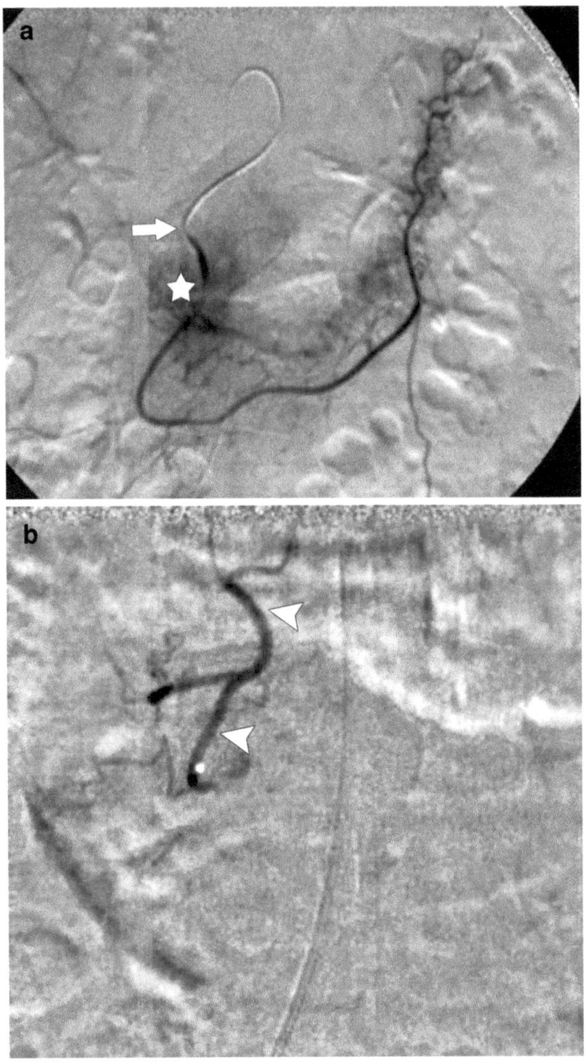

Fig. 10.5 Duodenal angiodysplasia. Visceral angiogram with catheter (*arrow*) in the gastroduodenal artery origin in the arterial phase (**a**) shows a blush of contrast in the proximal third portion of the duodenum (*star*). The venous phase (**b**) reveals an early draining vein (*arrowheads*)

10.4 Pulsatile Abdominal Mass

A 79-year-old man with a pulsatile abdominal mass on physical exam.

a. US abdominal aorta
b. CT abdomen without contrast
c. CTA abdomen
d. MRA abdomen
e. No ideal imaging exam

a. *US abdominal aorta* is the most appropriate. It serves as an initial examination but may be limited by body habitus or acoustic window (9).
b. CT abdomen without contrast is usually appropriate, but there is a better choice here. It is preferred for symptomatic patients and is suitable for patients in whom US is not useful (8).
c. CTA abdomen is usually appropriate, but there is a better choice here. It enables preinterventional planning (7).
d. MRA abdomen may sometimes be appropriate. It is an alternative to CTA but cannot detect calcium. Site-specific expertise is important (6).

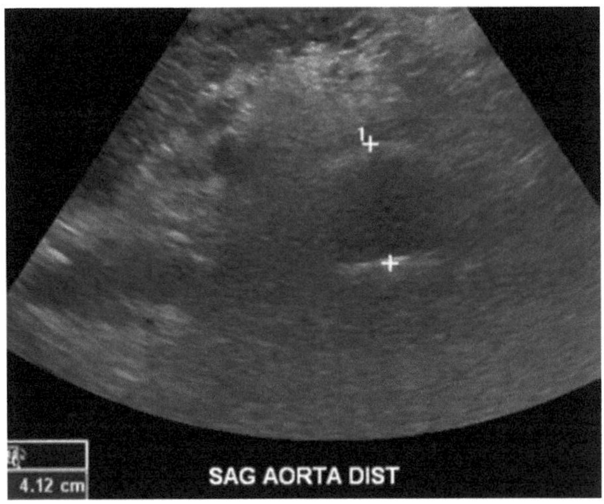

Fig. 10.6 Abdominal aortic aneurysm. Abdomen ultrasound sagittal view of aorta shows a 4.1-cm infrarenal aortic aneurysm (*calipers*)

10.5 Suspected Upper Extremity Deep Vein Thrombosis

A 48-year-old man with suspected upper extremity deep venous thrombosis.

a. US upper extremity with Doppler
b. CTA chest (noncoronary)
c. MRA chest (noncoronary) without and with contrast
d. Venography upper extremity and superior vena cava
e. No ideal imaging exam

a. *US upper extremity with Doppler* is the most appropriate. It is standard for arm veins. Other modalities are required for evaluating central veins (8).
b. CTA chest (noncoronary) is usually appropriate, but there is a better choice here. Contrast injection on asymptomatic side is preferred. It serves as an alternative to MRA for evaluating central veins (7).
c. MRA chest (noncoronary) without and with contrast is usually appropriate, but there is a better choice here. Contrast injection on asymptomatic side is preferred. It is used to evaluate central veins (7).
d. Venography upper extremity and superior vena cava is usually appropriate, but there is a better choice here. Although the gold standard, it is generally reserved for inconclusive noninvasive studies (7).

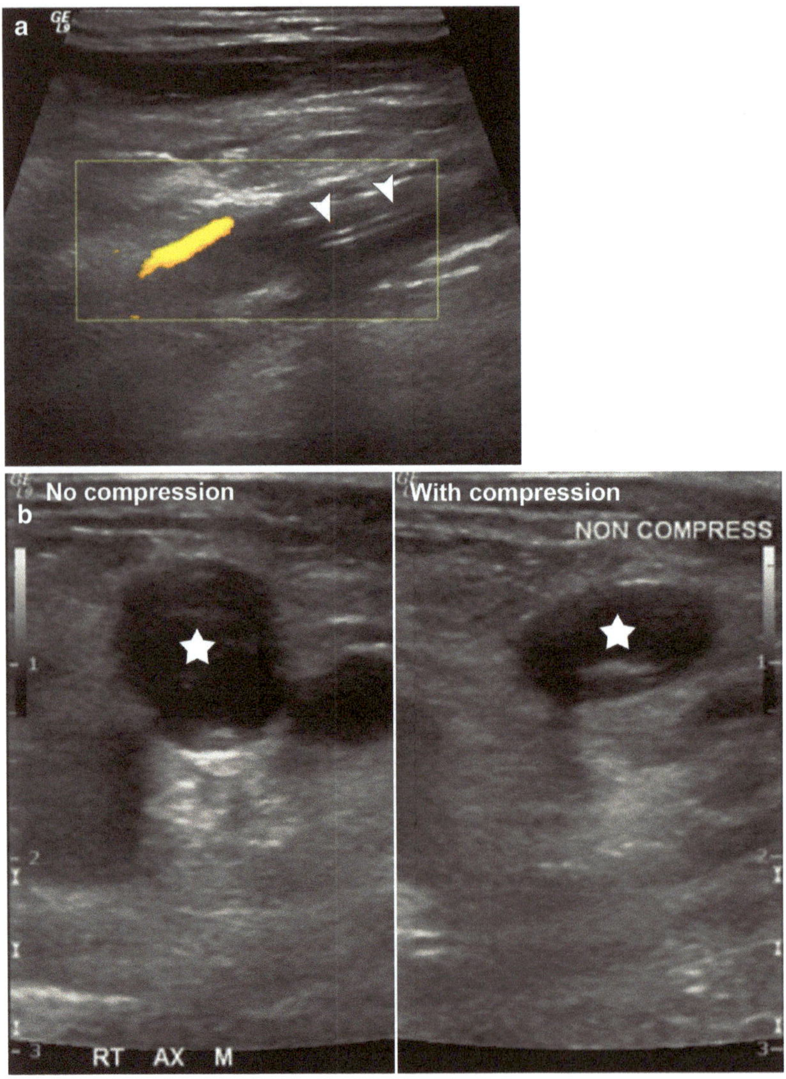

10.6 Suspected Lower Extremity Deep Vein Thrombosis

A 72-year-old man with suspected lower extremity deep venous thrombosis.

a. US lower extremity with Doppler
b. CT pelvis with contrast
c. MRI venography lower extremity
d. Venography pelvis
e. No ideal imaging exam

Fig. 10.7 Right arm deep venous thrombosis. Right upper extremity ultrasound Doppler image of the subclavian vein (**a**) demonstrates no blood flow and a catheter (*arrowheads*) in place. Gray-scale images (**b**) show a noncompressible right axillary vein (*stars*) indicating intraluminal thrombus

a. *US lower extremity with Doppler* is the most appropriate. Perform with venous compression (9).
b. CT pelvis with contrast may sometimes be appropriate. It is used as an adjunct to CT pulmonary arteriogram done for suspected pulmonary embolus (6).
c. MRI venography lower extremity may sometimes be appropriate (6).
d. Venography pelvis may sometimes be appropriate. Use when other studies are equivocal or an intervention is planned (6).

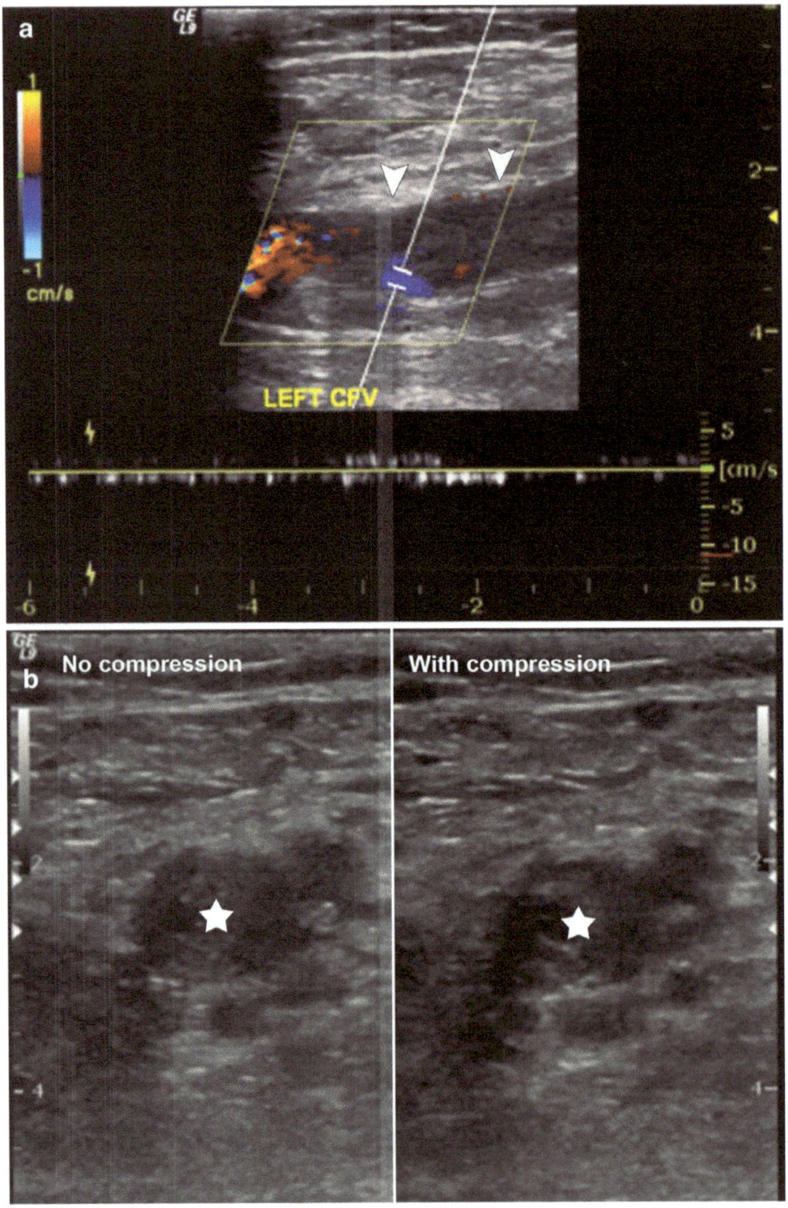

10.7 Sudden Onset of Cold, Painful Leg

An 83-year-old woman with history of left femoral artery stent now presents with sudden onset of a cold painful leg.

a. US lower extremity with Doppler
b. CTA lower extremity
c. MRA lower extremity
d. Arteriogram of aorta and bilateral lower extremity
e. No ideal imaging exam

Fig. 10.8 Left leg deep venous thrombosis. Left lower extremity ultrasound Doppler image (**a**) demonstrates no blood flow (*arrowheads*) in the common femoral vein which on gray-scale images (**b**) is noncompressible (*stars*) indicating intraluminal thrombus

a. US lower extremity with Doppler may sometimes be appropriate. Limitations include heavily calcified vessels and operator dependency (5).
b. CTA lower extremity is usually appropriate, but there is a better choice here. Distal abdominal aorta should be included (7).
c. MRA lower extremity is usually appropriate, but there is a better choice here. Distal abdominal aorta should be included (7).
d. *Arteriogram of aorta and bilateral lower extremity* is the most appropriate (8).

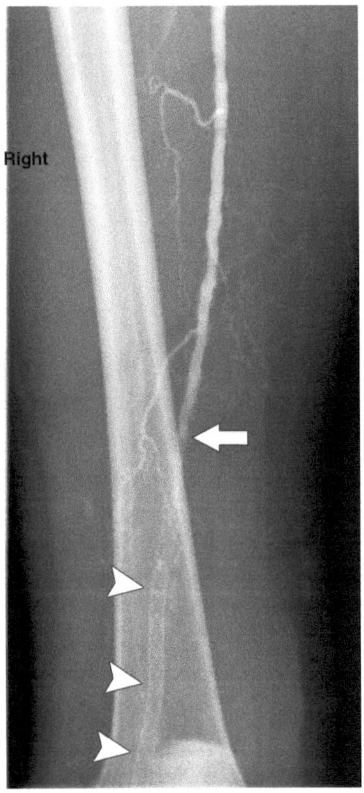

Fig. 10.9 Occluded left superficial femoral artery stent. Right leg angiogram with contrast injection proximal to the stent reveals lack of contrast flow (*arrow*) into the stent (*arrowheads*)

10.8 Claudication

A 73-year-old man with claudication and an abnormal noninvasive hemodynamic exam.

a. Noninvasive hemodynamic exam short-interval follow-up
b. US lower extremity with Doppler
c. MRA lower extremity with contrast
d. Arteriogram lower extremity
e. No ideal imaging exam

Suspected Vascular Etiology.

a. Noninvasive hemodynamic exam short-interval follow-up is not rated in appropriateness.
b. US lower extremity with Doppler may sometimes be appropriate (6).
c. *MRA lower extremity with contrast* is the most appropriate (8).
d. Arteriogram lower extremity is usually appropriate, but there is a better choice here. It is indicated to guide intervention once vascular diagnosis is established by noninvasive hemodynamic studies and/or physical exam (7).

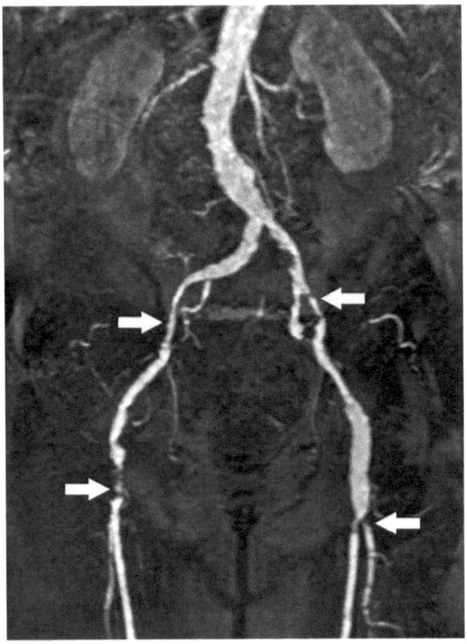

Fig. 10.10 Bilateral leg atherosclerosis. Lower extremity MRA maximal intensity projection image shows irregular caliber of the iliac and superficial femoral arteries with segments of severe stenosis (*arrows*)

Women's Imaging

11

11.1 Abnormal Vaginal Bleeding

A 54-year-old postmenopausal woman with vaginal bleeding.

a. US pelvis transabdominal
b. US pelvis transvaginal
c. US hysterosonogram
d. MRI pelvis with contrast
e. No ideal imaging exam

S.I. Lee, J.H. Thrall, *Choosing the Correct Radiologic Test*,
DOI 10.1007/978-3-642-15772-1_11, © Springer-Verlag Berlin Heidelberg 2013

Postmenopausal vaginal bleeding. First study.

a. US pelvis transabdominal is usually appropriate, but there is a better choice here (8).
b. *US pelvis transvaginal* is the most appropriate (9).
c. US hysterosonogram may sometimes be appropriate (6).
d. MRI pelvis with contrast is usually not appropriate (2).

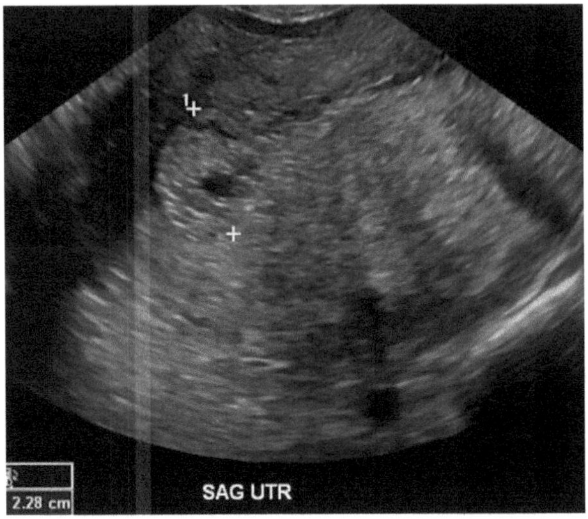

Fig. 11.1 Endometrial cancer. Pelvic ultrasound transvaginal sagittal view of the uterus reveals an abnormally thick endometrium (*calipers*)

A 58-year-old postmenopausal woman with vaginal bleeding. Transvaginal ultrasound shows endometrial thickness of <5 mm.

a. US pelvis transabdominal
b. US hysterosonogram
c. CT pelvis with contrast
d. MRI pelvis with contrast
e. No ideal imaging exam

Postmenopausal vaginal bleeding, endometrium <5 mm by transvaginal ultrasound.

a. US pelvis transabdominal may sometimes be appropriate (4).
b. US hysterosonogram is usually not appropriate (2).
c. CT pelvis with contrast is usually not appropriate (2).
d. MRI pelvis with contrast is usually not appropriate (2).
e. *No ideal imaging exam* is the correct answer.

A 52-year-old postmenopausal woman with vaginal bleeding. Transvaginal ultrasound shows endometrial thickness of ≥5 mm.

a. US pelvis transabdominal
b. US pelvis with Doppler
c. US hysterosonogram
d. MRI pelvis with contrast
e. No ideal imaging exam

Postmenopausal vaginal bleeding, endometrium ≥5 mm by transvaginal ultrasound.

a. US pelvis transabdominal may sometimes be appropriate (4).
b. US pelvis with Doppler may sometimes be appropriate (4).
c. *US hysterosonogram* is the most appropriate (8).
d. MRI pelvis with contrast is usually not appropriate (2).

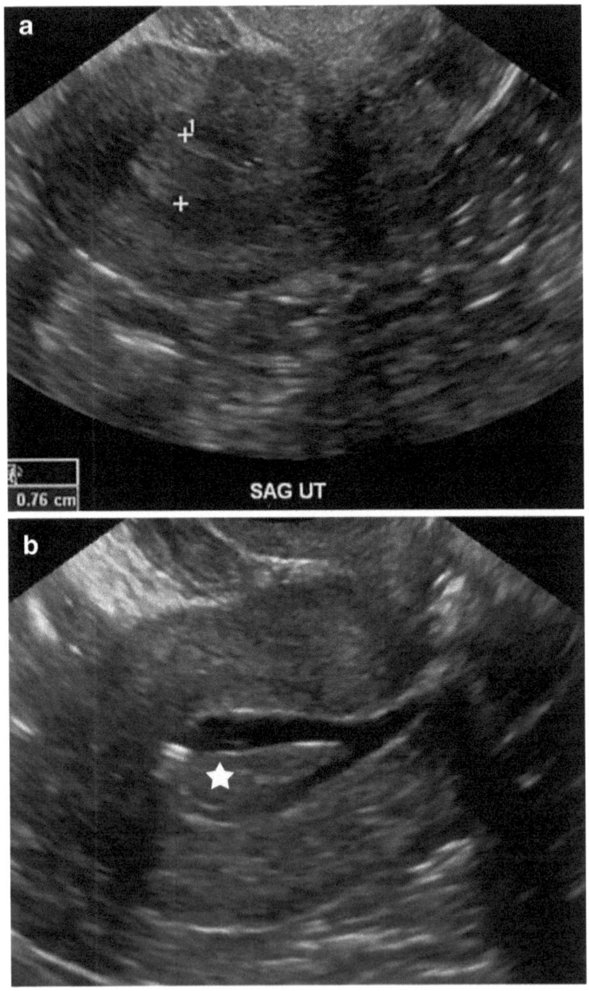

Fig. 11.2 Endometrial polyp. Sagittal view of the uterus on transvaginal ultrasound (**a**) shows an abnormally thick endometrium (*calipers*). The concurrent hysterosonogram (**b**) reveals an underlying endometrial polyp (*star*) originating from the fundal endometrium

A 36-year-old premenopausal woman with abnormal vaginal bleeding.

a. US pelvis transabdominal
b. US pelvis transvaginal
c. US hysterosonogram
d. MRI pelvis with contrast
e. No ideal imaging exam

Premenopausal vaginal bleeding. First study.

a. US pelvis transabdominal is usually appropriate, but there is a better choice here (8).
b. *US pelvis transvaginal* is the most appropriate (9).
c. US hysterosonogram may sometimes be appropriate (4).
d. MRI pelvis with contrast is usually not appropriate (2).

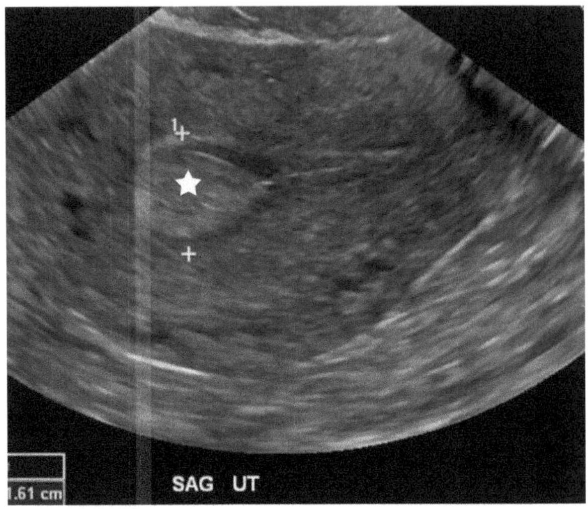

Fig. 11.3 Endometrial polyp. Sagittal view of the uterus on transvaginal ultrasound shows endometrium which is of normal thickness (*calipers*) but contains a focal lesion (*star*) corresponding to a polyp

A 34-year-old premenopausal woman with abnormal vaginal bleeding. Transvaginal ultrasound shows endometrial thickness <16 mm.

a. US pelvis transabdominal
b. US pelvis with Doppler
c. US hysterosonogram
d. MRI pelvis with contrast
e. No ideal imaging exam

Premenopausal vaginal bleeding, endometrium <16 mm by transvaginal ultrasound.

a. US pelvis transabdominal may sometimes be appropriate (4).
b. US pelvis with Doppler may sometimes be appropriate (5).
c. US hysterosonogram may sometimes be appropriate (6).
d. MRI pelvis with contrast is usually not appropriate (2).
e. *No ideal imaging exam* is the correct answer.

A 47-year-old premenopausal woman with abnormal vaginal bleeding. Transvaginal ultrasound shows endometrial thickness ≥16 mm.

a. US pelvis with Doppler
b. US hysterosonogram
c. CT pelvis with contrast
d. MRI pelvis with contrast
e. No ideal imaging exam

Premenopausal vaginal bleeding, endometrium ≥16 mm by transvaginal ultrasound.

a. US pelvis with Doppler may sometimes be appropriate (5).
b. *US hysterosonogram* is the most appropriate (7).
c. CT pelvis with contrast is usually not appropriate (2).
d. MRI pelvis with contrast may sometimes be appropriate (4).

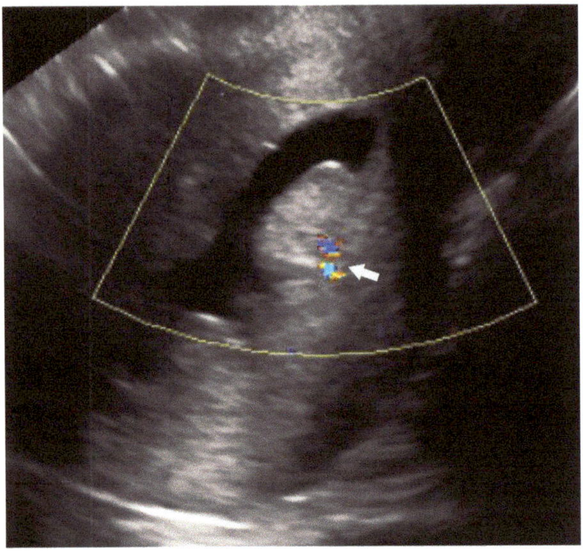

Fig. 11.4 Endometrial polyp. Sagittal view of the uterus on a hysterosonogram with color Doppler reveals a polyp originating from the posterior endometrium with a characteristic feeding vessel (*arrow*)

11.2 First Trimester Bleeding

A 28-year-old woman with vaginal bleeding and a positive serum pregnancy test and in the first trimester of pregnancy.

a. US pelvis transvaginal
b. US pelvis Doppler
c. US hysterosonogram
d. MRI pelvis
e. No ideal imaging exam

Positive urine or serum pregnancy test.

a. *US pelvis transvaginal* is the most appropriate (9).
b. US pelvis Doppler may sometimes be appropriate (4).
c. US hysterosonogram is not rated in appropriateness.
d. MRI pelvis may sometimes be appropriate (4).

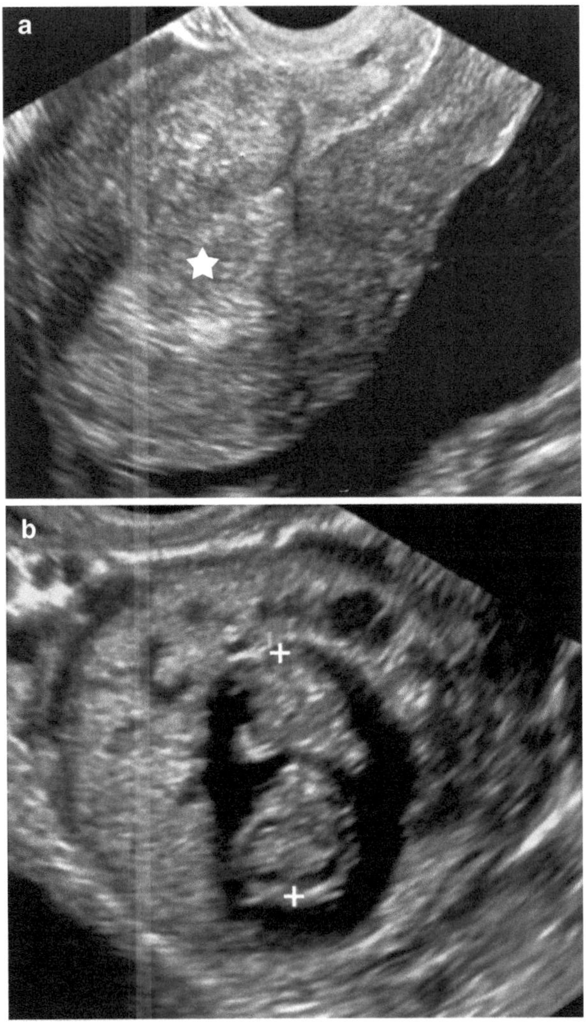

Fig. 11.5 Ectopic pregnancy. Transvaginal pelvic ultrasound sagittal view of uterus (**a**) shows no gestation in the endometrial cavity (*star*). Coronal view of the left adnexa (**b**) reveals the gestation with a fetus (*calipers*)

11.3 Acute Pelvic Pain in the Reproductive Age Group

A 32-year-old woman with acute pelvic pain suspected of gynecologic origin. Serum β-hCG is positive.

a. X-ray abdomen
b. US pelvis transvaginal
c. CT pelvis with or without abdomen
d. MRI pelvis with or without abdomen
e. No ideal imaging exam

Gynecological etiology suspected, serum β-hCG positive.

a. X-ray abdomen is not rated in appropriateness.
b. *US pelvis transvaginal* is the most appropriate. Both transvaginal and transabdominal US should be performed if possible (9).
c. CT pelvis with or without abdomen is usually not appropriate. Add abdominal CT as indicated (2).
d. MRI pelvis may sometimes be appropriate if US is inconclusive or nondiagnostic. Add abdominal MRI as indicated (6).

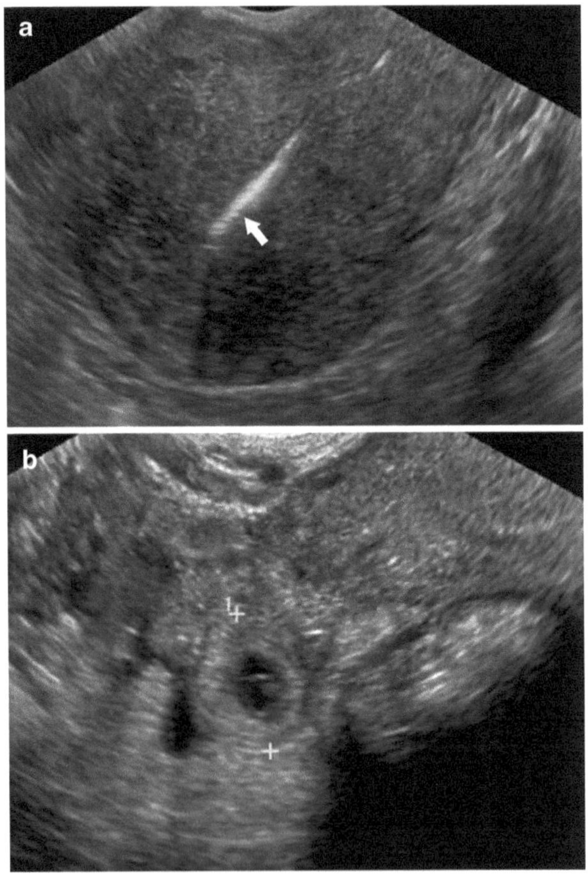

Fig. 11.6 Ectopic pregnancy. Transvaginal pelvic ultrasound at midline (**a**) shows no pregnancy and an intrauterine device (*arrow*) in the endometrial cavity. Image of the right adnexa (**b**) show a gestational sac with a yolk sac (*calipers*)

A 32-year-old woman with acute pelvic pain suspected of gynecologic origin. Serum β-hCG is negative.

a. X-ray abdomen
b. US pelvis transvaginal
c. CT pelvis with or without abdomen
d. MRI pelvis with or without abdomen
e. No ideal imaging exam

Gynecological etiology suspected, serum β-hCG negative.

a. X-ray abdomen is usually not appropriate (NA).
b. *US pelvis transvaginal* is the most appropriate. Both transvaginal and transabdominal US should be performed if possible (9).
c. CT pelvis may sometimes be appropriate if ultrasound is inconclusive or nondiagnostic and MRI is not available. In young women undergoing repeat imaging, cumulative radiation dose should be considered. Add abdominal CT as indicated (5).
d. MRI pelvis with or without abdomen may sometimes be appropriate if US is inconclusive or nondiagnostic. Add abdominal MRI as indicated (6).

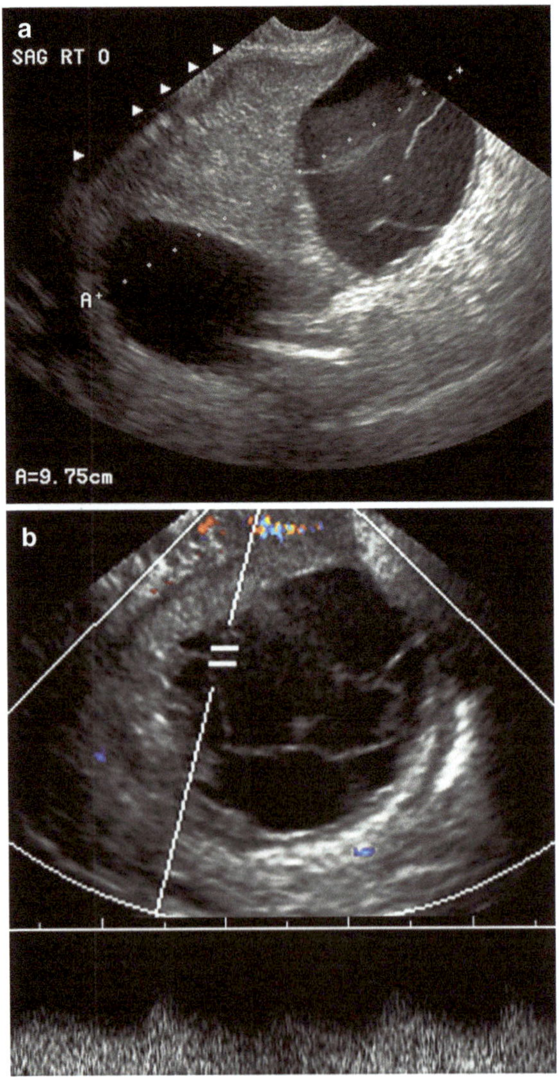

Fig. 11.7 Ovarian torsion. Transvaginal pelvic ultrasound on gray-scale imaging (**a**) shows an enlarged right ovary (*calipers*). Despite torsion, Doppler imaging (**b**) in torsed ovaries usually demonstrates arterial blood flow (spectral scale below) and is therefore not helpful in making this diagnosis

A 32-year-old woman with acute pelvic pain suspected of nongynecologic origin. Serum β-hCG is positive.

a. X-ray abdomen
b. US abdomen and pelvis transabdominal
c. CT abdomen and pelvis
d. MRI abdomen and pelvis
e. No ideal imaging exam

Nongynecological etiology suspected, serum β-hCG positive.

a. X-ray abdomen is usually not appropriate (NA).
b. *US abdomen and pelvis transabdominal* is the most appropriate. Add transvaginal US as indicated (9).
c. CT abdomen and pelvis is usually not appropriate (3).
d. MRI abdomen and pelvis is usually appropriate, but there is a better choice here (8).

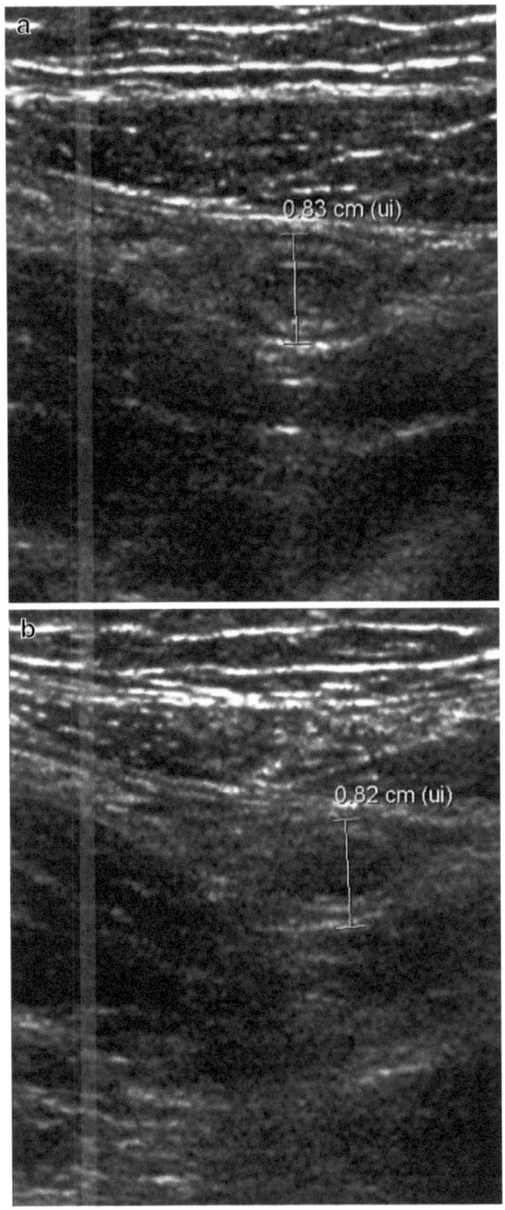

Fig. 11.8 Appendicitis. Transabdominal pelvic ultrasound of the right lower quadrant without (**a**) and with (**b**) compression reveals a blind-ending noncompressible loop of bowel (*calipers*) that measures >6 mm in thickness

A 32-year-old woman with acute pelvic pain suspected of nongynecologic origin. Serum β-hCG is negative.

a. X-ray abdomen
b. US pelvis transvaginal
c. CT abdomen and pelvis
d. MRI abdomen and pelvis
e. No ideal imaging exam

Nongynecologic etiology suspected, serum β-hCG negative.

a. X-ray abdomen is usually not appropriate (NA).
b. US pelvis transvaginal may sometimes be appropriate (4).
c. *CT abdomen and pelvis* is the most appropriate (9).
d. MRI abdomen and pelvis is usually not appropriate. It is used to avoid radiation exposure of CT in a young patient (3).

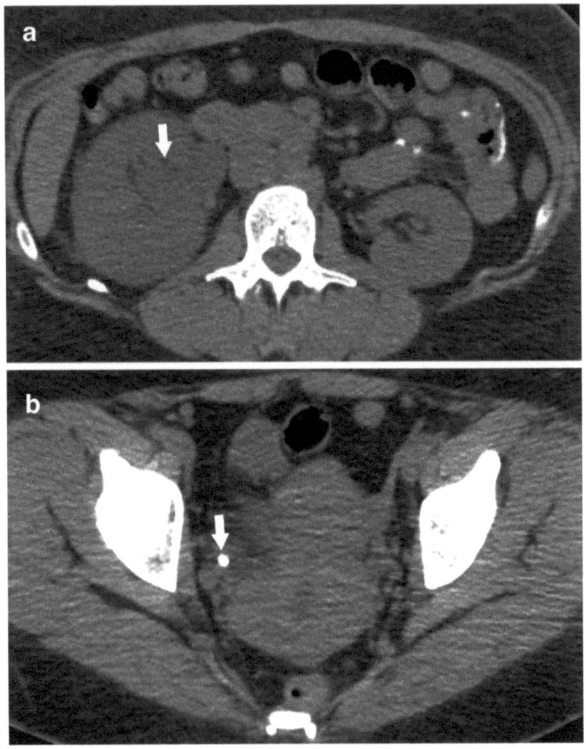

Fig. 11.9 Obstructive urolithiasis. Abdominopelvic CT without contrast at the level of the kidneys (**a**) shows right hydronephrosis (*arrow*). Image at the pelvis (**b**) reveals a stone (*arrow*) at the right ureteropelvic junction

11.4 Clinically Suspected Adnexal Mass

A 32-year-old premenopausal woman with a clinically suspected adnexal mass. She is not pregnant.

a. US pelvis transvaginal
b. CT pelvis with contrast
c. MRI pelvis with contrast
d. FDG-PET whole body
e. No ideal imaging exam

Reproductive age female (not pregnant). Initial evaluation.

a. *US pelvis transvaginal* is the most appropriate. Transabdominal and Doppler ultrasound may be added depending on the clinical circumstances (9).
b. CT pelvis with contrast is usually not appropriate (3).
c. MRI pelvis with contrast may sometimes be appropriate. It is used if US inconclusive or technically limited (5).
d. FDG-PET whole body is usually not appropriate (1).

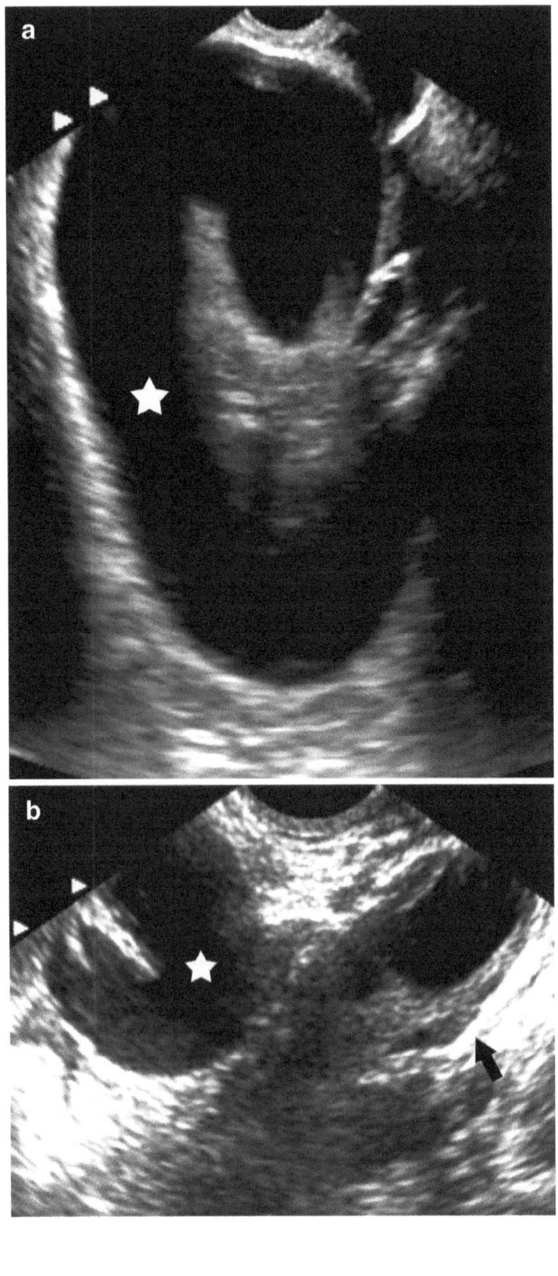

Fig. 11.10 Hydrosalpinx. Transvaginal pelvic ultrasound (**a**, **b**) shows a tubular cystic structure (*star*) in the left adnexa and a normal separate left ovary (*arrow*)

A 32-year-old premenopausal woman with a mixed solid and cystic or completely solid adnexal mass that is persistent on follow-up. She is not pregnant.

a. CT pelvis with contrast
b. MRI pelvis with contrast
c. FDG-PET whole body
d. Image-guided aspiration or biopsy
e. No ideal imaging exam

Reproductive age female (not pregnant) with complex or solid mass that is persistent or enlarging on pelvic sonography at short-term follow-up.

a. CT pelvis with contrast is usually appropriate, but there is a better choice here. Use to stage suspected ovarian cancer or to evaluate for primary malignancy in suspected metastases (7).
b. *MRI pelvis with contrast* is the most appropriate. Use if nonsurgical management is elected and malignancy cannot be excluded (8).
c. FDG-PET whole body is usually not appropriate. Not appropriate for tissue characterization of adnexal lesions (2).
d. Image-guided aspiration or biopsy is usually not appropriate (NA).

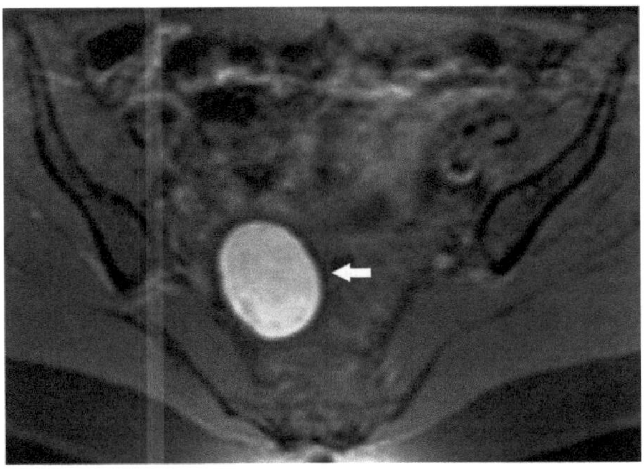

Fig. 11.11 Endometrioma. Pelvic MRI axial T1-weighted image with fat saturation shows a homogeneous intensely bright cyst (*arrow*) in the right ovary

A 62-year-old postmenopausal woman with clinically suspected adnexal mass.

a. US pelvis transvaginal
b. CT pelvis with contrast
c. MRI pelvis with contrast
d. FDG-PET whole body
e. No ideal imaging exam

Postmenopausal female (>12 months amenorrhea). Initial evaluation.

a. *US pelvis transvaginal* is the most appropriate. Transabdominal and Doppler ultrasound may be added depending on the clinical circumstances (9).
b. CT pelvis with contrast is usually not appropriate (2).
c. MRI pelvis with contrast may sometimes be appropriate. Use for further evaluation of the mass if ultrasound is inconclusive (5).
d. FDG-PET whole body is usually not appropriate (2).

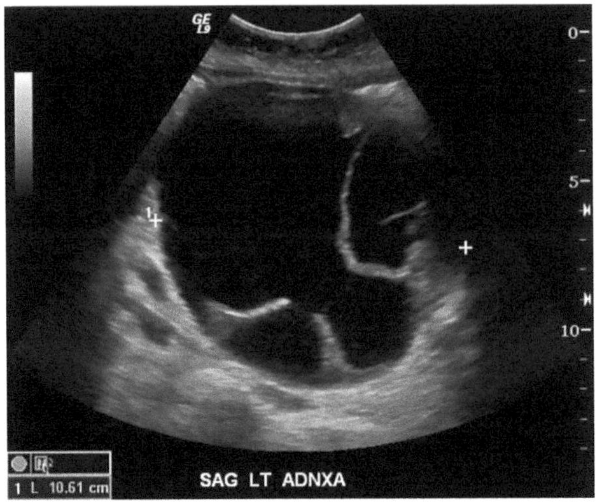

Fig. 11.12 Ovarian cystadenoma. Transvaginal pelvic ultrasound shows a mixed solid and cystic mass (*calipers*) in the left adnexa. A normal left ovary was not seen

11.5 Ovarian Cancer Screening

A 55-year-old woman with low risk for ovarian cancer presents for screening.

a. US pelvis transabdominal
b. US pelvis transvaginal
c. CT pelvis
d. MRI pelvis
e. No ideal imaging exam

Premenopausal or postmenopausal female, low risk.

a. US pelvis transabdominal is usually not appropriate (2).
b. US pelvis transvaginal is usually not appropriate (2).
c. CT pelvis is usually not appropriate (2).
d. MRI pelvis is usually not appropriate (2).
e. *No ideal imaging exam* is the correct answer.

A 28-year-old premenopausal woman with family history of ovarian cancer presents for screening.

a. US pelvis transabdominal
b. US pelvis transvaginal
c. CT pelvis
d. MRI pelvis
e. No ideal imaging exam

Premenopausal female: high risk (personal history or family history).

a. US pelvis transabdominal may sometimes be appropriate (4).
b. *US pelvis transvaginal* is the most appropriate (7).
c. CT pelvis is usually not appropriate (2).
d. MRI pelvis is usually not appropriate (2).

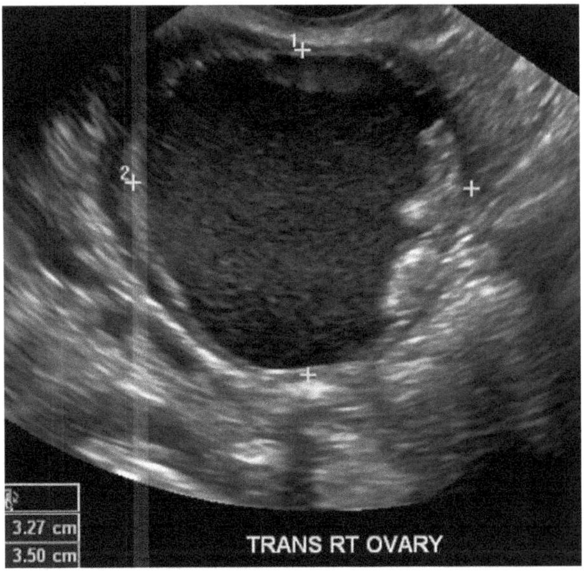

Fig. 11.13 Borderline ovarian tumor. Transvaginal pelvic ultrasound transverse of the right ovary reveals a small mixed solid and cystic mass (*calipers*)

A 59-year-old woman with elevated serum CA125 presents for ovarian cancer screening.

a. US pelvis transabdominal
b. US pelvis transvaginal
c. CT pelvis
d. MRI pelvis
e. No ideal imaging exam

Postmenopausal female: high risk (personal history or family history or elevated CA 125).

a. US pelvis transabdominal may sometimes be appropriate (4).
b. *US pelvis transvaginal* is the most appropriate (8).
c. CT pelvis is usually not appropriate (2).
d. MRI pelvis is usually not appropriate (2).

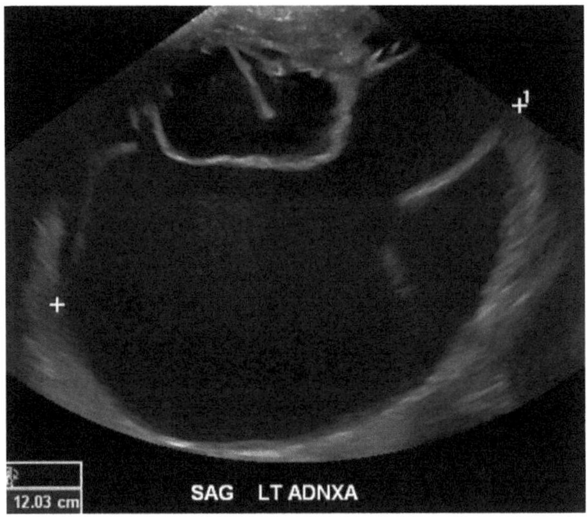

Fig. 11.14 Ovarian cancer. Transvaginal pelvic ultrasound sagittal view of the left adnexa reveals a large mixed solid and cystic mass (*calipers*)

Index

S.I. Lee, J.H. Thrall, *Choosing the Correct Radiologic Test*,
DOI 10.1007/978-3-642-15772-1, © Springer-Verlag Berlin Heidelberg 2013

FSC
www.fsc.org
MIX
Papier | Fördert
gute Waldnutzung
FSC® C083411

Kolibri 360 GmbH
Ferdinand-Jühlke-Straße 7
99095 Erfurt, Deutschland
produktsicherheit@kolibri360.de